Epilepsies of Childhood

POSTGRADUATE PAEDIATRICS SERIES

Under the General Editorship of

JOHN APLEY
CBE, MD, BS, FRCP

Emeritus Consultant Paediatrician,
United Bristol Hospitals

Epilepsies of Childhood

NIALL V. O'DONOHOE
MD, FRCP(I), DCH

Lecturer in Paediatric Neurology, Trinity College, Dublin.
Consultant Paediatric Neurologist, Our Lady's Hospital for Sick Children,
The Children's Hospital, Temple Street, and The National Children's
Hospital, Dublin. Paediatrician, Mater Misericordiae Hospital, Dublin.

BUTTERWORTHS
London - Boston
Sydney - Wellington - Durban - Toronto

United Kingdom London	Butterworth & Co (Publishers) Ltd 88 Kingsway, WC2B 6AB
Australia Sydney	Butterworth Pty Ltd 586 Pacific Highway, Chatswood, NSW 2067 Also at Melbourne, Brisbane, Adelaide and Perth
Canada Toronto	Butterworth & Co (Canada) Ltd 2265 Midland Avenue, Scarborough, Ontario, M1P 4S1
New Zealand Wellington	Butterworths of New Zealand Ltd T & W Young Building, 77–85 Customhouse Quay, 1, CPO Box 472
South Africa Durban	Butterworth & Co (South Africa) Ltd 152–154 Gale Street
USA Boston	Butterworth (Publishers) Inc 10 Tower Office Park, Woburn, Mass. 01801

First published 1979

© Butterworth & Co (Publishers) Ltd, 1979

ISBN 0 407 00138 7

```
British Library Cataloguing in Publication Data

O'Donohoe, Niall V
    Epilepsies of childhood. – (Postgraduate
    paediatrics series).
    1. Epilepsy in children
    I. Title   II. Series
    618.9'28'53        RJ496.E6        79–40722

    ISBN 0-407-00138-7
```

Typeset by Butterworths Litho Preparation Department
Printed and bound by Camelot Press Ltd, Southampton, Hants.

Dedicated to Barbara

Editor's Foreword

'Age influences disease' and a chronological approach has clarified our understanding of many childhood disturbances. In the epilepsies it is surely essential, for maturation (that goes with age) provides the critical variable in all seizure disorders, as Ounsted pointed out. Why do fits occur rarely in the premature infant, most commonly in the few years following later infancy, and then decline in frequency in the years afterwards ? We have learned a great deal from many disciplines about how the contributory causes vary with the patient's age. No less important, we are learning how and why the clinical presentations take the different forms we may see in the panorama of growth. Based on the newer understanding, therapy – both preventive and remedial – can be applied more effectively to the fits themselves and to the patient who suffers them.

This book is the more logical and persuasive because of Dr O'Donohoe's chronological presentation, and he makes it glow with his rich and extensive clinical experience. At the same time experimental and research contributions, culled from many sources, are woven into the texture of his argument and inform the intensely practical advice he offers about both diagnosis and treatment.

Dr O'Donohoe has the gift of conveying the sense of complex scientific concepts in lucid words that clinicians will appreciate. With his delightfully personal writing, what could have been a dull collection of dry facts, and details of drugs, comes to life. The result is a book combining down-to-earth experience and perspective with literary charm. When clinicians refer to it, both for up-to-date ideas and for details of treatment, many will surely go on reading for the sheer enjoyment which he shares with them.

John Apley

Preface

Convulsive disorders have their highest incidence in childhood and seizures are among the most frequent symptoms presenting to the paediatrician and the paediatric neurologist. They cause parents great anxiety and doctors are often perplexed and confused by the problems they create. Public attitudes about epilepsy are still, unfortunately, rooted in prejudice and superstition.

There have been remarkable advances in the understanding and treatment of epilepsy in recent times, although the communication of new knowledge of the subject has been made difficult by an abundance of classifications and by misleading and outdated terminology. However, the *International Classification of the Epilepsies,* first introduced in 1969, is being accepted gradually and is providing an international language of epilepsy for the first time.

I have attempted in this book to describe the epilepsies of childhood in a more or less chronological sequence, while using the terminology of the *International Classification* and emphasizing the important influences of age, growth and developmental status on the type of epilepsy which develops.

Although the book is written primarily for general paediatricians at all stages of their careers, I hope that others, including specialist and community paediatricians, specialists in mental handicap, child psychiatrists and family doctors may find it useful and interesting.

My own interest in epilepsy derives from the fortunate experience of working with the late Dr Paul Sandifer at the Hospital for Sick Children, Great Ormond Street, in the late 1950s. I owe a special debt to the late Dr Ronald MacKeith, one of the greatest international paediatricians of his generation, who ensured that I joined the mainstream of British and European paediatric neurology. Dr Christopher Ounsted and Dr David Taylor of the Park Hospital for Children, Oxford, have influenced my thinking about childhood epilepsy profoundly and their work is referred to frequently in this book.

I am greatly indebted to my excellent EEG technician, Miss Geraldine Monaghan, who has taught me much about the EEG and epilepsy, and to Miss Catherine Condron who typed my manuscript. The Research Centre at Our Lady's Hospital for Sick Children, Dublin, helped with a generous grant.

Above all, I must thank Dr John Apley for suggesting the book and for his constant advice and encouragement during the writing of it.

Niall V. O'Donohoe

Contents

ix

CHAPTER 1

Epilepsy: History and Statistics

Epilepsy is not easily defined. The words 'epilepsy' and 'epileptic' are of Greek origin and have the same root as the verb meaning 'to seize' or 'to attack'. The word epilepsy means simply 'to be seized' in a passive sense. The idea of a disease seizing a man goes back to the old magic concept that all diseases were 'attacks' or seizures by gods or demons. Since epilepsy was the demoniac disease par excellence, the term gradually acquired a more particular meaning and came to signify an epileptic seizure. Epilepsy acquired its name because it attacked or seized both the senses and the mind. This concept of epilepsy is of ancient origin and was already in use, as were the terms 'epilepsy' and 'epileptic', in Hippocratic times (Temkin, 1971).

However, although 'epilepsy' and 'epileptic' were used in the earliest times as designations of both epileptic attacks and epileptic persons, the term epilepsy did not mean the underlying disease which the physicians preferred to refer to as 'the sacred disease' (morbus divinus). This name arose from the belief, common from antiquity to the relatively recent past, that diseases were phenomena more or less dependent on the supernatural and were considered to be a divine retribution for wickedness or a consequence of possession by spirits. Epilepsy, more than any other condition, was susceptible to explanation in these terms. Temkin (1971) has written: 'In the struggle between the magic and the scientific conception, the latter has gradually emerged victorious in the western world. But the fight has been long and eventful, and in it epilepsy held one of the key positions.'

The battle was first joined around 400 BC when Hippocrates attacked the supernatural explanation of epilepsy in the book on 'The Sacred Disease' (Chadwick and Mann, 1950). The alleged divine character, the author or authors argued, was merely a shelter for ignorance and fraudulent malpractice. Epilepsy, it was claimed, was not more divine than any other disease, but, like all diseases, it was hereditary with its cause residing in the brain — a brain overflowing with a superfluity of phelgm, one of the four humours. Epilepsy, therefore, should be treated not by magic but by diet and drugs. Unfortunately the mythology surrounding epilepsy persisted, including a supposed link between epilepsy and lunacy and the idea that epilepsy could be caused by the influence of the cycle of the moon. The various ideas connecting epilepsy, madness, possession and similar states with the moon and other stars spawned a rich astrological literature through the centuries and even up to present day.

Having the sacred disease did not do the unfortunate sufferer much good. The epileptic was regarded as unclean; whoever touched him might become prey to the demon. It was thought that spitting would keep the demon away and throw back contagion, and thus one could escape infection. The magic concept, according to which epilepsy was a contagious disease, was one of the factors that made the epileptic's life a misery and gave him a social stigma. It was a disgraceful disease and the unfortunate person who felt an attack coming on rushed home or to a deserted place where he covered his head. To the ancients the epileptic was an object of horror and disgust, and throughout almost all of history those afflicted have been viewed with anxiety and fear. No other illness has set individuals apart so far, so often and so long, and these attitudes persist to the present day despite the quite frequent association of greatness and genius with the condition (Socrates, Julius Caesar, Napoleon, Dostoevski, Dante and Handel, to name a few).

From the time of hippocrates physicians wrote about 'convulsions', particularly with reference to children, without clearly defining the meaning of the term and its relationship to epilepsy. There was an awareness in medical writing about children that convulsions in early childhood might have a different prognostic significance from epileptic seizures in older persons, but for a long time terminology remained confused. Attitudes to children with epilepsy were unenlightened and often cruel until well into the nineteenth century, and they frequently suffered the general fate of epileptics in being confined with insane persons.

The enlightenment of the eighteenth century and advances in neurology in the nineteenth century led to improved knowledge and understanding of epilepsy and to the final abandonment of the idea of demoniacal possession as a cause. The National Hospital for the Paralysed and Epileptic in London was opened in 1860 and during the early years of that decade the work of the great John Hughlings Jackson began in that hospital. In 1873 this produced a broad definition of epilepsy which is still perfectly valid: 'Epilepsy is the name for occasional, sudden, excessive, rapid and local discharges of grey matter.' According to his definition there was not just one form of the disease, but many epilepsies: one of these was a type of unilateral epilepsy with a characteristic march of clinical events which bears his name. Hughlings Jackson's former assistant W. R. Gowers published his important book *Epilepsy and Other Chronic Convulsive Diseases* in 1881, which incorporated many of Hughlings Jackson's ideas and attempted to differentiate epilepsy from conditions such as hysteria and migraine.

The epoch-making discovery of the human electroencephalogram (EEG) and the first publication of his observations on it by Hans Berger in 1929 (Gloor, 1974) provided the tool which facilitated the separation of epilepsy from other conditions and offered visual proof of Hughlings Jackson's theories. The subsequent explosion of knowledge about the EEG in epilepsy over the next two decades culminated in the publication of the classic *Atlas of Electroencephalography* by F. A. and E. L. Gibbs (1952). Other important milestones in the scientific understanding of epilepsy were Penfield and Jasper's (1954) *Epilepsy and the Functional Anatomy of the Human Brain* which dealt in detail with the neuroanatomy and neurosurgery of epilepsy, and William Lennox's great book *Epilepsy and Related Disorders*, which was published in 1960 at the end of his long life devoted to the study of epilepsy and the care of its victims.

Lennox (1960) wrote that epilepsy was a disturbance of the normal rhythms of the brain. 'The rhythm of the body when orderly spells health. Dysrhythmia is a disease. Of all the systems of the body, the central nervous system is most nearly cyclic in function, and recurrent irregularity of its rhythm most profoundly disturbs the functions of both body and mind.' Lennox regarded epilepsy as an anarchy of cell function just as cancer is an anarchy of cell growth.

The manifestations of epilepsy are legion and no single symptom is essential. Lennox (1960) quoted Boerhaave (1974) as follows: 'For there is no one gesture, inflexion, or posture of the body known, which it has not shewn at some time, and it emulates all the motions of running, walking, turning, bending forwards, lying down, standing upright, or keeping the body in a very stiff and almost insuperable action.' The manifestations of epilepsy may appear as disturbances of consciousness or be evinced by sensory, visceral or motor signs, or present as perversions of ideation, emotion or mood. Some patients may experience all of these symptoms, others only one or two, and the symptomatology and intensity of the disturbances may vary from time to time. They may also experience what Lennox called the horror of epilepsy, quoting Margiad Evans (1953) as follows: 'Ever since a second convulsion I have been incredulous of all things firm and material. The light has held patches of invisible darkness. Time has become as rotten as worm-eaten wood, the earth under me is full of trap-doors and the sense of being, which is life and all that surrounds and creates it, a thing taken and given irresponsibly and without warning as children snatch at a toy.'

It is important to realize that all forms of epilepsy, as Hughlings Jackson wrote, arise from recurring excessive neuronal discharges occurring somewhere in the brain. Sometimes the site of origin can be easily identified while at other times no epileptic focus can be found. However, whatever their source the discharges frequently spread to other parts of the brain and even to the central nervous system as a whole. It must also be remembered that, as a rule, epilepsy is a chronic recurring disorder, and that many upsets in homeostasis originating outside the central nervous system may provoke disturbances of the brain culminating in epileptic phenomena identical with those caused by epilepsy itself. Anyone may have a fit given the right circumstances. These sporadic disturbances must be distinguished from epilepsy which is a recurring condition. Furthermore, the diagnosis must be made positively, based on careful history and clinical observations, and not just by exclusion. The label of epilepsy is, unfortunately, still too pejorative for mistakes to be made. In making a diagnosis, it is better to err on the side of 'not epilepsy' and subsequently to correct one's mistake than to apply a mistaken diagnosis of epilepsy which may be difficult to rectify later.

EPIDEMIOLOGY: PREVALENCE AND INCIDENCE

The study of the epidemiology of epilepsy is beset with problems since epilepsy is often a hidden disease. This makes the accumulation of accurate statistics on the prevalence and incidence of seizures difficult and unreliable. Prevalence refers to the ratio of those people affected by a particular disorder to those not affected at a given time. Incidence refers to the number of new cases of a disorder within a given population in a given time period and may also be expressed as a percentage.

The survey of Pond, Bidwell and Stein (1960) was comprehensive and gave an overall prevalence rate of 6.2/1000 population with an inception rate of new cases of 0.7/1000/year. These authors included every type of epileptic fit. Kurtzke et al. (1973) stated that the best evidence available indicated the prevalence of convulsive disorders as about 4–6/1000 population at the time of publishing their book. They further emphasized that all prevalence rates must be considered as minimal estimates. Taking a reasonable estimate of prevalence as 5/1000 would mean that there were about one million people with epilepsy in the USA. The Epilepsy Foundation of America and the National

Institute of Neurological Diseases and Stroke in the USA have produced higher estimates of up to four million people with some form of epilepsy living in the USA (*Basic Statistics on the Epilepsies*, 1975). Epileptic patients outnumber those with any other serious neurological disease, with the probable exception of cerebrovascular disease. Roger (1970) has written a comprehensive review of the literature on the epidemiology of epilepsy in Europe and North America.

Prevalence in childhood

Convulsions are the commonest problem encountered in paediatric neurology. It has been estimated that 90 per cent of those who develop symptoms of epilepsy do so before the age of 20 years. The inception rates of new cases per year are highest in the youngest age groups, they fall off during childhood, rise again in the age range 10–20 years, and then fall off rapidly among adults (*Epilepsy in Society*, 1971). According to Miller *et al.* (1960) in Newcastle upon Tyne, 7.2 per cent of the children in the 'Thousand Family Survey' had had one convulsion or more by the age of five years, and 20 per cent of these children had died. All but one of the deaths occurred under the age of one year and were ascribed mainly to birth trauma and infections. Millichap (1968) estimated that approximately 3 per cent of the population of the USA under five years of age were affected by febrile convulsions. Various studies have indicated that in Great Britain the prevalence of epilepsy in schoolchildren is in the order of 8/1000 (*People with Epilepsy*, 1969). This means that there must be almost 60 000 schoolchildren in that country who are subject to epilepsy, and the inception rate of new cases is between 2 and 4/1000/year. However, it is generally believed that only about half of the schoolchildren with epilepsy are known to the school health authorities in Great Britain.

Cooper (1965), in a survey of epilepsy seen in general practice, found that among eight-year-old children with epilepsy there was an excess in the group classified as average or below average in performance at school, and others have commented on reading retardation in children with epilepsy. Learning difficulties in children with epilepsy are probably due to several different causes including underlying brain damage, the effects of long-term medication and also to the fragmentation of attention by subclinical discharges. These various aspects of the problem are discussed in detail elsewhere.

It is clear, therefore, that epilepsy is common in childhood and that affected children are vulnerable medically and educationally, in addition to facing considerable social difficulties as a result of their seizures. Epilepsy in childhood, just as in adults, is a family problem which will have an impact on and modify the lives of all the family members. Looked at from the medical standpoint, the complexity of the problems facing the child with epilepsy and his parents is such as to make it impossible for any one discipline to deal adequately with all of them, and a team approach is essential. The many facets of epilepsy make it difficult to define concisely. David Taylor (1969) has attempted it as follows: 'Epilepsy is a phenomenon, it scarcely warrants being called a symptom and it is not a disease.' However, we need not take too much time trying to define epilepsy, but rather try to understand it; to a considerable extent this is now possible.

REFERENCES

Basic Statistics on the Epilepsies (1975) Washington, DC: Epilepsy Foundation of America

Boerhaave, H. (1724) *Boerhaave's Aphorisms: Concerning the Knowledge and Cure of Diseases*. London: William and John Innys

Cooper, J. E. (1965). 'Epilepsy in a longitudinal survey of 5000 children'. *Br. med. J.* **1**, 1020–1022

Chadwick, J., Mann, W. (1950). Translators. 'The Sacred Disease'. In *The Medical Works of Hippocrates*. Oxford: Blackwell Scientific

Epilepsy in Society (1971) London: Office of Health Economics

Evans, M. (1953). *A Ray of Darkness*, p. 191. New York: Roy Publishers

Gibbs, F. A. and Gibbs, E. L. (1952) *Atlas of Electroencephalography, Vol. 2: Epilepsy*. Cambridge, Mass: Addison Wesley

Gloor, P. (1974). 'Hans Berger – psychophysiology and the discovery of the human electroencephalogram.' In *Epilepsy. Proceedings of the Hans Berger Centenary Symposium*, pp. 353–373. Eds. P. Harris and C. Mawdsley. Edinburgh, London, New York: Churchill Livingstone

Gowers, W. R. (1881). *Epilepsy and Other Chronic Convulsive Diseases: Their Causes, Symptoms and Treatment*. London: Churchill

Jackson, J. Hughlings (1931–32). *Selected Writings of John Hughlings Jackson*, p. 100. Ed. J. Taylor, London: Hodder and Stoughton

Kurtzke, J. F., Kurland, L. T., Goldberg, I. D., Choi, N. W. and Reeder, F. A. (1973). 'Convulsive disorders.' In *Epidemiology of Neurologic and Sense Organ Disorders*, pp. 15–40. APHA Monograph Series on Vital and Health Statistics Ed. L. T. Kurland, J. F. Hurtzke and I. D. Goldberg. Cambridge, Mass: Harvard Press

Lennox, W. G. (1960). *Epilepsy and Related Disorders*. 2 Vols. London: J and A. Churchill

Miller, F. J. W., Court, S. D. M., Walton, W. S. and Knox, E. G. (1960). *Growing up in Newcastle-upon-Tyne*, pp. 164–173. London: Nuffield Foundation, Oxford University Press

Millichap, J. G. (1968). *Febrile Convulsions*. New York: Macmillan

Penfield, W. and Jasper, H. (1954). *Epilepsy and the Functional Anatomy of the Human Brain*. Boston: Little, Brown and Company and London: J. and A. Churchill

People with Epilepsy (1969). London: HMSO

Pond, D. A., Bidwell, B. H. and Stein, L. (1960). 'A survey of epilepsy in fourteen general practices. I: Demographic and medical data.' *Psychiatria, neurol. neurochir.* **63**, 217–236

Roger, J. (1970). 'Epidemiology of epilepsy in European and North American populations.' *Afr. J. med. Sci.* **1**, 237–245

Taylor, D. C. (1969). 'Some psychiatric aspects of epilepsy.' In *Current Problems in Neuropsychiatry*, pp. 106–109. Ed. R. N. Herrington. Ashford, Kent: Headley Brothers

Temkin, O. (1971). *The Falling Sickness*, 2nd edn. Baltimore and London: Johns Hopkins

CHAPTER 2

Problems of Classification and Aetiology, Including Genetic Aspects

Classification in general is a method of conveying information. The important components of any classification are accurate nomenclature, arrangement and grouping. The terminology and classification of epilepsy have evolved over many years creating a profusion of interchangeable and confusing descriptive terms. Denis Williams (1976) said that there are as many classifications as there are needs to classify. Marsden (1976) defined the problem of classification as a need to evolve a single code to cover three basically incompatible systems of classification, namely, that of clinical signs and symptoms of the fit, that relating to the anatomical and electrophysiological evidence of the source of the fit and that defining the aetiology of the fit. Any classification employed must be useful and should reflect the needs of the user.

To the paediatrician and paediatric neurologist the chronological aspects of epilepsy through infancy, childhood and adolescence are particularly interesting, and a chronological approach will, to a large extent, be adopted in this book (see *Figures 3.1* and *4.1*). It is often difficult to convince doctors dealing exclusively or predominantly with adults that paediatrics is not just medicine (or neurology) in small people. The factors of age, growth and development exert their influences constantly and certainly not least in the problems of childhood epilepsy. Ounsted (1971) wrote that: 'for all seizure disorders, maturation is the critical variable', and Lennox (1960) said that: 'the type of epilepsy which occurs in a child represents a confluence of age, heredity, and structural brain abnormality'.

The simplest, time-honoured classification of epilepsy is to divide it into idiopathic and symptomatic epilepsy, and this is still in wide clinical use. Another popular and practical classification has been pithily stated by Williams (1968) in a discussion on the management of epilepsy. 'For our present purpose there are two kinds of epilepsy, general and focal. The general epilepsies fall into two groups, petit mal and grand mal. There are only two kinds of petit mal, absences and myoclonic fits without disorders of consciousness, and they both have as their electrical accompaniment a generalised three-a-second spike-wave discharge of characteristic kind. There is only one kind of grand mal, and it in effect constitutes a unit of disturbed consciousness and behaviour. All other forms of epilepsy are focal, whatever their behavioural or experimental accompaniments, and however elaborate or unitary may be their nature.'

An international committee was convened by the *International League Against Epilepsy* to consider the formulation of a comprehensive classification of epilepsy which would include the type of clinical seizure, the type of EEG seizure, the EEG interictal expression, the anatomical substrate and aetiology and the age of the patient. The product of this committee was published in 1969 and is now generally known as the *International Classification* (Gastaut, 1969, 1970). Epileptic seizures were classified as follows:

1. Partial seizures or those beginning locally. These fits were further subdivided into those with elementary symptomatology, generally without impairment of consciousness; those with complex symptomatology, generally with impairment of consciousness; and partial seizures becoming secondarily generalized.
2. Generalized seizures or those which were bilaterally symmetrical and without local onset. These included petit mal absences, bilateral massive myoclonus, infantile spasms, clonic and/or tonic seizures, tonic-clonic seizures (grand mal) and atonic and akinetic seizures.
3. Unilateral seizures.
4. Unclassifiable seizures.

Merlis (1970) modified the classification as follows:

1. Generalized epilepsies
   (*a*) Primary generalized epilepsies including petit mal and grand mal
   (*b*) Secondary generalized epilepsies
   (*c*) Undetermined generalized epilepsies
2. Partial (focal, local) epilepsies which include Jacksonian and temporal lobe seizures
3. Unclassifiable epilepsies.

The *International Classification* has its critics and various modifications have been suggested, but its great virtue is that it is being used internationally and enables individuals from different countries to speak a common language of epilepsy. For example, the much misused term 'petit mal' can now be used to mean just one type of primary generalized epilepsy and not a variety of minor attacks of many different types and aetiologies. As far as is possible and applicable the *International Classification* will be used as a framework in this book.

However, we must not be misled into thinking that this more elaborate categorization of epileptic phenomena necessarily deepens our knowledge and understanding of epilepsy. Hughlings Jackson's (1931) concept of a seizure as being due to 'an occasional, an excessive and a disorderly discharge of nerve tissue' has not been bettered as an explanation of the chronic recurrent paroxysmal disorder which constitutes epilepsy. It must be remembered, however, as Marsden (1976) has emphasized, that epilepsy consists of more than just having fits. The person with epilepsy has a predisposition to recurrent fits determined by a variety of causes, some identifiable and many unknown. The individual attack may be triggered by a precipitating cause and the actual symptoms of the attack are determined by the electrical and biochemical events which occur in the brain during the seizure. Physical, behavioural, intellectual and social consequences derive from epilepsy and may be as important or more significant for the patient than the actual seizures.

AGE AND EPILEPSY

In children, as already emphasized, the factors of *age, growth and development* exert constant influences in determining whether or not epilepsy develops. Fits are rare in the premature baby because of the undeveloped state of his nervous system; however, they are more common in the full-term baby, rare in the early months of life, very common between six months and four years and decline in frequency until puberty. The varying *convulsive threshold* or inherent susceptibility to convulse at different ages is only partly determined by the state of anatomical maturation of the brain at the time and by the degree of cerebral damage, if any, which is present.

There is now evidence that epilepsy involves variations of the normal *physicochemical mechanisms* of cells. Epileptogenesis concerns masses of cells in which both the threshold of stimulation is lower than normal and the increased susceptibility to discharge can occur spontaneously when the necessary conditioning and precipitating mechanisms develop. The resting membrane potential of the neuronal cell has been shown to depend on the selective permeability of the cell membrane to sodium and potassium ions. It is highly permeable to potassium and poorly permeable to sodium. This results in a high intracellular potassium level and a low intracellular sodium level under normal circumstances. However, the delicate balance of the resting potentials of cell membranes may be altered in a number of ways, for example, by changes in the concentration of extracellular ions, by sudden mechanical or chemical stimulation and by pathophysiological alteration of the membrane as a result of genetic fault, disease processes or damage from whatever cause. When this balance is upset the semipermeable characteristics alter permitting sodium and potassium to diffuse across the membrane resulting in the ionic gradients and their associated potentials changing. An action potential is created briefly on the surface of the cell, and this is an effective stimulus to neighbouring portions of the cell membrane from which the electrical potential spreads along the axons, always away from the point of impulse generation. Synaptic transmission involves impulse transmission in one direction from the end branches of the axons of one neurone to the dendrites or body of another neurone. Neurotransmitter agents are required for the passage of the impulse in this way and the multiple functions of the central nervous system require a highly integrated system of excitatory and inhibitory neurotransmitter substances. These include acetylcholine, norepinephrine, serotonin, dopamine and γ-aminobutyric acid (GABA). Enzyme mechanisms, acting on these neurotransmitters, also have an important role.

The concept that increased permeability to ions is involved in epileptogenicity is now accepted and it appears that all convulsions, no matter how they are induced, result in a depletion of potassium and an increase in sodium concentrations in neuronal cells. A defect in the active transport of sodium and potassium appears to be closely associated with the mechanisms involved in the generation of seizures. Derangements of the excitatory neurotransmitter mechanisms in the central nervous system, such as acetylcholine, are probably also involved in epileptogenesis. Derangements in the synthesis of the powerful inhibitory substance GABA are also considered important because they produce an alteration in the normal excitatory/inhibitory balance of the brain towards the excitatory side. For example, there is evidence that pyridoxal phosphate is essential for the synthesis of GABA, and that metabolic or dietary pyridoxine deficiency may result in convulsions in infancy. The new anticonvulsant, sodium valproate, appears to act by preventing the breakdown of GABA. Those interested in obtaining further information about these important neurochemical matters are referred to the books by Schmidt and Wilder (1968) and Aird and Woodbury (1974).

It may be postulated, therefore, in the case of infants and children, that not only does the anatomical maturation of the developing nervous system play an important part in deciding when seizures will occur and what form they will take but also that variations in the balance between inhibitory and excitatory brain systems during maturation play a significant role in determining the convulsive threshold or the individual's susceptibility to convulsions at any particular age. Furthermore, nervous tissue can be rendered hyperexcitable by changes in the body's homeostasis acting diffusely. These include fever, hypoxia, hypocalcaemia, hypoglycaemia, over-hydration and alterations in acid-base balance. Extraneous factors such as the administration of convulsant drugs; the too rapid withdrawal of anticonvulsant drugs, especially barbiturates; overdosage with various drugs producing drug toxicity and various toxins act in a similar way on the nervous system. Emotional disturbance, particularly when acute, and over-fatigue may also act as precipitants of seizures in those with a lowered convulsive threshold or with established epilepsy.

GENETIC FACTORS AND COUNSELLING

It is appropriate at this stage to consider the part that genetic influences play in the causation of epilepsy. One of the commonest questions asked by parents and others about epilepsy is 'Is it inherited ?'. The fear of inheriting epilepsy has been present from earliest times and in all cultures. It is closely linked with the prejudice which many people have about individuals suffering from epilepsy. It has led to repressive legislation forbidding people with epilepsy to marry and, in certain countries, the prohibition of immigration of those with epilepsy. The great William Lennox (1960), in his classic work on epilepsy wrote that the subject of heredity was perhaps the most controversial of all queries about epilepsy. He went on to make the following important points:

1. The transmission of a predisposition is a fact and denying this does a disservice to the cause of epilepsy
2. Inheritance is less important in epilepsy than in many other common diseases
3. One argument against people with epilepsy marrying is the supposed incurability of the condition whereas the chances of arrest or complete control are at least as good as in many other chronic disorders such as diabetes mellitus
4. The transmitted traits of the patient and his spouse may be so favourable as to outweigh the undesirable trait of a tendency to seizures
5. A reduction of epilepsy through eugenics has been advocated in a world in which causes of brain injury such as war, violence and crippling accidents are on the increase.

The technical committee of the *French League Against Epilepsy*, with many distinguished specialists participating, investigated the problem for some years and published their findings (Aicardi *et al.*, 1969). All were agreed that epilepsy could not be regarded as a well-defined hereditary trait. With reference to generalized epilepsy, they considered that what is transmitted appears to be a certain 'convulsive predisposition' which is variously expressed as:

1. Simple EEG changes, i.e. paroxysmal discharges without clinical epilepsy
2. Marked photosensitivity
3. Childhood convulsions such as attacks with fever
4. Real clinical and EEG manifestations of primary generalized epilepsy of the petit mal type in children and the grand mal type in children, adolescents and adults.

Another conclusion reached by the technical committee of the *French League Against Epilepsy* was that 'idiopathic epilepsy is inherited as an autosomal dominant trait with variable penetrance; however, it is not the clinical fit which is inherited but the proclivity to convulse' (Aicardi *et al.*, 1969).

Genetic factors play a much less significant role in partial epilepsy although they are important in the type called 'benign focal epilepsy of childhood', to be discussed later. A genetically-determined predisposition to febrile convulsions may result in a child sustaining temporal lobe damage during a prolonged febrile seizure and later going on to develop temporal lobe epilepsy (Ounsted, Lindsay and Norman, 1966).

Genetic factors may act by increasing *the convulsive susceptibility* or lowering *the convulsive threshold* to epilepsy and by causing the transmission of diseases of which fits may be a symptom. Tuberose sclerosis is an obvious example of the latter situation. Genetic factors play only a small part in some of the serious epileptic syndromes of infancy and early childhood such as infantile spasms, and Jeavons and Bower (1964) reported a 5 per cent family history of convulsions in the latter. In febrile convulsions and primary generalized epilepsy of the petit mal type genetic factors are of paramount importance. Primary generalized epilepsy of the grand mal type, still commonly called idiopathic grand mal, is a disorder mainly of the first 20 years of life with a peak age of onset at about seven years. It is certainly solely of genetic origin in a proportion of cases while in others minimal brain injury, either at birth or subsequently, is responsible for the appearance of the epileptogenic lesion after many years of 'ripening'.

Because there are no clear guidelines to the genetics of epilepsy, it is not easy to give *genetic counselling* to prospective parents. Furthermore, as the French Committee emphasized, the inherited condition may be no more than a predisposition to convulse in circumstances which may never arise in an individual child. The overall risk to a child of developing epilepsy, when one parent is epileptic, is between 2 and 3 per cent and where both parents are epileptic it rises steeply to approximately 25 per cent (Brown, 1976). However, one should qualify these figures by saying that the genetic risks are obviously greater when one or both parents suffer or have suffered from a primary generalized epilepsy (or 'idiopathic' epilepsy), in which genetic factors are very important, than when one or both have had a symptomatic generalized or partial epilepsy with a clearly defined acquired cause.

Counselling may also be sought by parents who have one child with epilepsy and who fear that other children they may have will be similarly affected. The answer to this question will depend on the type of epilepsy the affected child suffers from and, if a family history exists, on the nature of the epilepsy in either or both parents. If the child has symptomatic generalized or partial epilepsy due, for example, to birth trauma, and if there is no family history of epilepsy, the risk of subsequent children having epilepsy is that of the incidence of the condition in the general population. If, on the other hand, the child's epileptic state is primary in type and one in which hereditary factors are known to be significant, then the risks of epilepsy for any future siblings of the proband will need to be explained to the parents. Further information concerning these risks will be given in the chapters on the different varieties of epilepsy in childhood and in the chapter on the prevention of epilepsy.

REFERENCES

Aicardi *et al*. (1969). 'General conclusions concerning familial factors in epilepsy.' Technical Committee of the French League Against Epilepsy. *Epilepsia*, **10**, 65–68
Aird, R. B. and Woodbury, D. M. (1974). *The management of Epilepsy*. Illinois: Charles C. Thomas, Springfield
Brown, J. K. (1976). 'Fits in childhood.' In *A Textbook of Epilepsy*, p. 71. Eds J. Laidlaw and A. Richens. Edinburgh, London and New York: Churchill Livingstone
Gastaut, H. (1969). 'Clinical and electroencephalographical classification of epileptic seizures.' *Epilepsia*, **10**, Suppl. pp. 2–21
Gastaut, H. (1970). 'Clinical and electroencephalographical classification of epileptic seizures.' *Epilepsia*, **11**, 102–113
Jackson, J. Hughlings (1931). *Selected Writings of John Hughlings Jackson*, Vol. 1, p. 8. Eds J. Taylor, G. Holmes and F. M. R. Walshe. London: Hodder and Stoughton
Jeavons, P. M. and Bower, B. D. (1964). *Clinics in Developmental Medicine, No. 15: Infantile Spasms*. London: Spastics Society and Heinemann

Lennox, W. G. (1960). *Epilepsy and Related Disorders*. London: J. and A. Churchill

Marsden, C. D. (1976). 'Neurology.' In *A Textbook of Epilepsy*. Eds J. Laidlaw and A. Richens. Edinburgh, London and New York: Churchill Livingstone

Merlis, J. K. (1970). 'Proposal for an International Classification of the Epilepsies.' *Epilepsia*, 11, 114–119

Ounsted, C. (1971). 'Some aspects of seizure disorders.' In *Recent Advances in Paediatrics*, p. 365. Eds D. Gairdner and D. Hull. London: J. and A. Churchill

Ounsted, C., Lindsay, J. M. and Norman, R. M. (1966). *Clinics in Developmental Medicine*, No. 22: *Biological factors in Temporal Lobe Epilepsy*. London: Spastics Society and Heinemann

Schmidt, R. P. and Wilder, B. J. (1968). *Contemporary Neurology Series: Epilepsy*. Oxford: Blackwell Scientific

Williams, D. (1968). 'The management of epilepsy.' *Br. J. hosp. Med.* 2, 702–707

Williams, D. (1976). 'Foreword', *A Textbook of Epilepsy*. Eds J. Laidlaw and A. Richens. Edinburgh, London and New York: Churchill Livingstone

CHAPTER 3

Neonatal Seizures

Seizures occur in just over one per cent of neonates. Like so much else in the newborn, they present special problems in recognition, in determining their cause and in treatment. It is often extremely difficult to distinguish between normal and abnormal behaviour in newborns, and this particularly applies to disorders of movement.

Neonatal seizures are usually partial and always symptomatic. Although there is a very long list (see *Table 3.1*) of possible causes of convulsions at this age, in practice over 90 per cent are due to birth complications, to hypocalcaemia, to hypomagnesaemia or hypoglycaemia or to meningitis. Of the birth complications brain anoxia and ischaemia are the most important factors and usually cause seizures in the first 24–72 hours of life (see *Figure 3.1*). Hypoxic–ischaemic brain injury is the single most important neurological problem occurring in the neonatal period and produces damage by depriving the central nervous system of oxygen. Hypoxaemia diminishes the amount of oxygen available for the brain and ischaemia diminishes the amount of cerebral blood perfusion. The combination of both can lead to death or to the production of one of the serious chronic brain syndromes, namely, mental handicap, cerebral palsy and epilepsy. Hypoxaemia leads to profound biochemical changes in the brain and ischaemia may lead to infarction of the brain. Brain swelling can occur with both and this may further reduce cerebral perfusion. Cerebral necrosis may be another consequence of anoxaemia and ischaemia.

The causes of hypoxia in the newborn are many and may operate before delivery in about half the cases, during delivery in the majority of the remainder and postpartum in about 10 per cent of the infants. Seizures may begin within 6–12 hours of birth in asphyxiated babies.

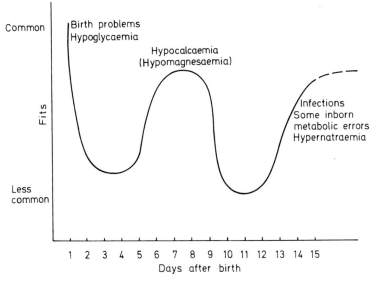

Figure 3.1. Neonatal convulsions. Timing in relation to cause. (From N. V. O'Donohoe, Growing Points in Childhood Epilepsy, 1: The First Six Months, by courtesy of Geigy Pharmaceuticals, Publishers, Macclesfield, Cheshire)

SEIZURE PATTERNS IN NEONATES

Seizure patterns in the neonate are different from those in older infants and children. Generalized tonic-clonic convulsions, so often seen later, are rarely encountered. Usually, the seizure patterns are fragmentary, resembling parts of a generalized seizure. There may be shifting clonic convulsive movements migrating rapidly and in a non-Jacksonian disorderly fashion from one part of the body to other ipsilateral or contralateral areas. Focal clonic convulsions may occur and remain localized to one area or spread to involve one half of the body. Alternating hemiconvulsive seizures, involving first one and then the other half of the body, can occur. Generalized tonic seizures, sometimes resembling episodes of decerebrate rigidity, are not uncommon and may be the presenting clinical feature of intracranial haemorrhage, especially when they occur in premature infants.

Finally, there is a group of seizure phenomena sometimes called *'subtle'* because the clinical correlates are so slight. Indeed, these may be the commonest seizure manifestations in the neonate (Volpe, 1977a). There may be momentary changes in the respiratory rate or even brief periods of apnoea. Nevertheless, it should be emphasized that apnoeic spells, particularly in the premature infant, are more likely to be related to mechanisms other than seizures. When apnoea is a manifestation of a seizure, the spell is almost always accompanied or preceded by one or more of the other subtle manifestations of a seizure. Other subtle phenomena include one or more of the following: tonic horizontal deviation of eyes with or without jerking of the eyes; repetitive blinking or fluttering of the eyelids; drooling, sucking, or other oral buccal lingual movements; 'rowing' or 'swimming' movements of the upper limbs or, less commonly, 'pedalling' movements of the lower limbs; less frequently, vertical deviation of the eyes (usually down) with or without jerking; hyperpnoea and vasomotor phenomena or tonic posturing of a limb or portion of a limb may occur. It is important to realize that, although slight, these clinical changes may signify serious underlying brain injury and that there may, in fact, be dramatic accompanying EEG abnormalities to indicate this.

Jitteriness

It is important to distinguish the movement disorder usually called jitteriness from a convulsion. Jitteriness is a disorder of the newborn and is seen rarely, if ever, in a similar form at a later age. It is characterized by movements with qualities primarily of tremulousness but occasionally of clonus. Volpe (1977a) lists the following four points for distinguishing jitteriness from a seizure:

1. Jitteriness is not accompanied by abnormalities of gaze or extra-ocular movements, unlike seizures
2. Jitteriness is exquisitely stimulus sensitive while seizures are not
3. The dominant movement in jitteriness is tremor, i.e. the alternating movements are rhythmic and of equal rate and amplitude
4. The dominant movement in a seizure is clonic jerking, i.e. the movements have a fast and slow component.

The rhythmic movements of jitteriness can usually be stopped by flexion of the affected limb; however, such a manoeuvre will not affect clonic seizure movements. Conditions commonly involved in the aetiology of jitteriness include hypoxic-ischaemic encephalopathy, hypocalcaemia and drug withdrawal.

Developmental explanation

The reasons for the difference in seizure types in the neonate compared with later infancy and childhood must relate to the developmental state of the nervous system. For a generalized seizure to be possible there must be a certain degree of cortical organization existing to propagate and sustain the electrical discharge, and this is not present in the newborn. Neonatal EEG studies have shown that convulsions are usually of focal cerebral origin, that discharges are frequently limited to one region of the hemisphere and diffuse slowly in the ipsilateral hemisphere or to the contralateral hemisphere and that bilateral synchrony is rare. The reasons for these characteristics are related to the immaturity of the forebrain. The intercellular connections of cortical ganglion cells are incomplete and myelination is deficient in the hemispheres and in the corpus callosum reducing the chances of contralateral spread. Surrounding any epileptic focus there is a population of neurones which develops inhibitory potentials during paroxysmal discharges produced by a mass of cells in the focus. This 'inhibitory surround' limits the local cortical spread of epileptic activity. It has been demonstrated, using intracellular recordings, that these inhibitory postsynaptic potentials are common in immature neocortical neurones and this physiological situation has an influence in creating the high convulsive threshold which exists in the neonate and in early infancy (Purpura, Shofer and Scarff, 1967).

Timing and causes of neonatal seizures

Seizures may occur early in the neonatal period, i.e. in the first 24–72 hours or later at the end of the first week of life. The timing of seizures is closely related to their cause. Volpe (1973, 1977a) has consistently emphasised that the *hypoxic–ischaemic brain insult* is the single most common cause of neonatal convulsions in both premature and full–term infants and, in his series, it accounted for just over 60 per cent of the cases. Characteristically, the attacks begin in the first 24 hours and indeed, in the majority of cases, in the first 12 hours of life. The attacks are usually frequent and severe and may be continuous. Overt seizures are also nearly always associated with subtle attacks. In the premature infant generalized tonic seizures may occur and in the full-term baby multifocal clonic attacks take place. The vast majority of these infants will have shown clinical evidence indicating the occurrence of fetal distress due to intrauterine asphyxia. The common manifestations of this situation are slowing of the fetal heart and/or meconium-stained liquor and a very low Apgar score at birth. Failure to breathe spontaneously at birth adds a postnatal hypoxic–ischaemic insult to the intrauterine insult.

As already emphasized, seizures due to hypoxic-ischaemic insult develop early and are usually severe. Seizures resulting from *cerebral contusion*, which are usually secondary to a traumatic labour (precipitate or prolonged labour, transverse arrest, high forceps extraction, difficult breech delivery, etc.), commonly occur on the second post-natal day and are often truly partial or focal in type. *Primary subarachnoid haemorrhage*, occurring predominantly in premature infants, usually presents with seizures which take place on the second day of life and, between attacks, the baby may seem well giving rise to the description of the 'well baby with seizures'. Periventricular intra-cerebral haemorrhage with intraventricular spread, arising from the subependymal veins in the germinal matrix, is almost exclusively a lesion of the premature infant which may occur from one to three days after severe hypoxia and present with generalized tonic seizures, coma, rapid deterioration and respiratory arrest follows within a few hours. *Subdural haemorrhage*, due to a tear of falx, tentorium or superficial cortical veins, is a traumatic lesion of large babies is now uncommon. Seizures are secondary to associated cerebral contusion and are usually partial or focal in type. They occur in about half the cases and present usually in the first 48 hours of life.

The other important cause of seizures arising in the early neonatal period is *hypoglycaemia*. This is usually considered to be present when the blood glucose level falls below 1.1 mmol/ℓ (20 mg/100ml) in the premature baby and below 1.7 mmol/ℓ (30 mg/100ml) in the full-term infant. However, it should be realized that the actual level of glucose which is required to prevent neurological damage in the neonate is un-known and may be higher than these levels. Hypoglycaemia is most common in small babies (especially those small for gestational age), in the smaller of twins where there is a marked discrepancy in birth weights and in the infants of diabetic or prediabetic mothers. Late feeding of small infants was a contributory cause of hypoglycaemia in the past. The most important factor in the occurrence of neurological damage due to hypoglycaemia is the duration of the hypoglycaemia, therefore early diagnosis and treatment are vital. The neurological symptoms of hypo-glycaemia consist of irritability, drowsiness, hypotonia and, occasionally, apnoea, and these symptoms commonly develop in the second postnatal day. Approximately half the small babies who become hypoglycaemic develop neurological symptoms and about one-quarter of these go on to develop actual seizures. In the larger babies of diabetic mothers neuro-logical symptoms, including seizures, are much less common, possibly because the duration of hypoglycaemia may be only one aetiological factor in causing convulsions in a small infant: hypoxic damage, hypo-calcaemia and even infection may all be associated causes in the same infant. Symptomatic hypoglycaemia should be preventable by moni-toring glucose levels with Dextrostix, by the early feeding of small infants (particularly prematures) or by the administration of intravenous dextrose where early feeding is impossible. As already emphasized, early and vigorous treatment of symptomatic hypoglycaemia, if and when it occurs, is essential to prevent the occurrence of brain damage although this is one instance where prevention is certainly better than cure because symptomatic hypoglycaemia is followed by neurological sequelae, even despite vigorous therapy at the time, in perhaps half of those affected. *Hypocalcaemia,* i.e. serum calcium below 1.7 μmol/ℓ (7 mg/100 ml), may occur in the first 2–3 days of life either in low-birth-weight infants (premature or dysmature) or in association with the complications of birth asphyxia. It may then contribute to the production of seizures but is rarely the primary cause. On the other hand, hypocalcaemia occurring later, i.e. at the age of 6–8 days, is usually the primary cause of the

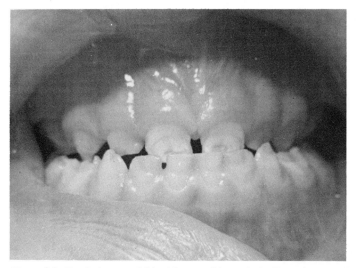

Figure 3.2. Teeth from a child with enamel hypoplasia. Note the typical 'shelf' on the lower incisors and canines. (Courtesy of Dr R. J. Purvis)

clinical features of neonatal tetany which include jitteriness, jaw, knee, and ankle clonus and partial or focal seizures. There may be associated *hypomagnesaemia* or even hypomagnesaemia without hypocalcaemia causing tetany. The incidence of *neonatal tetany* due to hypocalcaemia and/or hypomagnesaemia has shown wide variations in different countries reaching 55 per cent in one Scottish survey (Cockburn *et al.,* 1973). In Volpe's (1977a) series, only a 13 per cent incidence of hypocalcaemia was found to occur which was always complicated by other factors and no single case of typical neonatal tetany of later onset was found. He ascribed these differences to the fact that his unit was receiving selected referrals and to the recent widespread changes in cow's milk preparations with emphasis on their formulas being comparable with human milk. Classic neonatal tetany tended to develop in large full-term infants who fed avidly on a cow's milk mixture in which the ratios of phosphorus to calcium and phosphorus to magnesium were four times higher than in human milk. Hypocalcaemia is rare in breast-fed infants and in infants fed with the modern 'humanized' milks. Infants who have had neonatal tetany may later show enamel hypoplasia of the teeth, the timing of which suggests an antenatal insult during the last trimester (*Figure 3.2*) (Purvis *et al.*, 1973). Maternal vitamin D deficiency may also be the cause of the seasonal variations in the incidence of tetany which is more common in babies born in spring after the relatively sunless months of winter, and may also explain geographical variations in incidence.

There are many other causes of neonatal seizures. An exhaustive list can be found in Brown's (1973) review of convulsions in the newborn period (see *Table 3.1*). The possibility of *infections* being a cause of fits, particularly septicaemia and bacterial or viral meningitis, should never be forgotten. *Structural abnormalities* of the brain may occasionally be responsible but account for less than 5 per cent of the cases. *Barbiturate addiction in the mother* may result in withdrawal fits in the infant (Desmond *et al.*, 1972). *Pyridoxine dependency* is a well known but very rare cause and can be ruled out by injecting pyridoxine 50 mg intravenously, preferably during EEG monitoring, following which the seizures stop in a few minutes. Alternatively, pyridoxine may be given orally (100 mg daily) for a few days.

Disorders of amino-acid metabolism may occasionally present with neonatal seizures and maple syrup urine disease is the one most likely to do so. *Hypernatraemia* associated with dehydration in the salt-losing syndrome of congenital hyperplasia may also lead to seizures. Hypernatraemia may also follow the accidental administration of salt for sugar in a milk feed or the administration of an unsuitable saline intravenous fluid to the newborn. Dehydration in the salt-losing syndrome of congenital adrenal hyperplasia can occur with hyponatraemia and may also lead to seizures. Hyponatraemia may also occur in association with overhydration in infants with meningitis who develop water retention as a result of increased secretion of antidiuretic hormone, and a similar situation may complicate neonatal asphyxia. Water intoxication may occur in the treatment of hypoglycaemia with intravenous glucose infusions resulting in hyponatraemia and a low serum osmolality. Oedema, both peripheral and cerebral, may follow and jitteriness, extensor tonic seizures and even a decerebrate state can be seen. If the correct diagnosis is not made further glucose and water solutions may mistakenly be given with disastrous results.

There are many other rare causes of neonatal seizures. Some, like *hyperbilirubinaemia causing kernicterus*, were once quite common but

TABLE 3.1

The Causes of Convulsions in the First Month of Life (Brown, 1973)

Metabolic

Asphyxia	Hyperbilirubinaemia
Alkalosis	Pyridoxine deficiency
Hypocalcaemia	Pyridoxine dependency
Hypomagnesaemia	Neurolipidosis
Hypoglycaemia	Organic acidurias
Hyponatraemia	Galactosaemia
Water intoxication	Hyperammonaemia
Hypernatraemia	Aminoacidopathies

Intracranial haemorrhage

Traumatic asphyxia
Birth trauma (subdural and subarachnoid)
Intraventricular haemorrhage, low birth weight, asphyxia
Asphyxia, consumption coagulopathy, secondary haemorrhagic disease
Haemorrhagic disease of the newborn (vitamin K deficiency)
Arteriovenous malformations
Berry aneurysms (with coactation of aorta)
Battered baby syndrome (subdural and subarachnoid)
Hypernatraemic dehydration
Thrombocytopenia (drugs to mother, ITP mother, consumption coagulopathy and
  DIC, rhesus haemolytic disease and intrauterine infection)
Idiopathic subarachnoid haemorrhage
Dissecting subependymal haemorrhage and low birth weight

Infections

Meningitis	Congenital taxoplasmosis
Encephalitis	Cytomegalic inclusion disease
Abscess or subdural empyema	Septicaemia with DIC
Rubella encephalitis	Gastroenteritis (biochemical)

Genetic

Familial neonatal convulsions
Neurodermatoses, neurofibromatosis, incontinentia pigmentii and tuberose sclerosis
13/15 trisomy
Congenital cerebral malformations and dysplasias
Alpers' cortical degeneration of infancy
Degenerative disease (Gaucher's, Krabbe's lucodystrophy and Niemann Pick disease)

Miscellaneous

Narcotic withdrawal
Compression head injury without haemorrhage
Neoplasm
Ectodermal dysplasia with hyperpyrexia
Exogenous toxins (e.g. hexachlorophane)

are now only likely to be seen in small premature infants, with a low serum albumin and a poor bilirubin binding capacity, who develop septicaemia and acidosis or who suffer from the respiratory distress syndrome. It is important to remember, even with the enormous increase in knowledge of the newborn in recent years, that there still remains a small group of infants (about 3 per cent according to Brown's 1973 review) whose fits have no attributable cause. There is also a rare familial disorder characterized by frequent and often refractory neonatal convulsions for which no cause has been found. If the infants escape hypoxic brain damage recovery is complete and subsequent development is normal (Carton, 1978).

DIAGNOSTIC EVALUATION

The diagnostic evaluation of a newborn with seizures should include a complete prenatal and natal history and a comprehensive physical examination, with emphasis on a neurological examination appropriate to a neonate (Prechtl and Beintema, 1964). The first laboratory tests are directed against the two diseases that are especially dangerous but treatable, i.e. hypoglycaemia and bacterial meningitis. Serum electrolytes, urea, calcium, phosphorus and magnesium should also be measured and a blood culture should be started. The place of the EEG examination will be discussed later. When attempting to make an aetiological diagnosis it should be remembered that several factors may be operating in the same patient, for example hypoxia-ischaemia, hypocalcaemia and infection, so therefore investigation must be detailed.

THERAPY

The treatment of neonatal seizures depends on establishing the cause as quickly as possible and acting appropriately. The question of prevention is of great importance especially in the case of anoxic-ischaemic brain injury. Careful monitoring of the fetus and prompt and skilled intervention at the first signs of fetal distress are critical. Symptomatic hypoglycaemia should also be completely preventable today. Continuous or frequent seizures of themselves can result in brain injury because they are often accompanied by serious hypoventilation and/or apnoea which results in hypoxaemia and hypercapnia. Hypoxaemia may result in cardiovascular collapse and ischaemic injury to the brain. A diminution in cerebral blood flow can also occur with increased intracranial pressure which can be aggravated by hypercapnia. Consequently, vigorous support of ventilation and blood pressure is important in the sick convulsing neonate.

Drugs and other treatment

Many of the established anticonvulsant drugs have been used in the treatment of frequent severe or continuous convulsions in the newborn. At present there is considerable interest in the ability of phenobarbitone in high dosage to decrease the rate of cerebral metabolism. Single doses of 10 mg/(kg BW) have been used intravenously in the full-term baby and this dose may have to be repeated in less than one hour (or sometimes, 20 mg/(kg BW) is given as a single bolus). Therapeutic levels will usually be reached with a dose of 20 mg/(kg BW) on the first day or 10 mg/(kg· day) on the first two days, followed by a maintenance dose of 5 mg/(kg· day) in two divided doses at 12 hourly intervals. Since the plasma half-life of phenobarbitone in the first weeks of life may be twice that of adults (Holden and Freeman, 1975), it is important to watch for signs of respiratory depression because ventilatory support may be necessary. Monitoring of serum levels may be very helpful if available.

Phenytoin is used in high dosage intravenously (10 mg/[kg BW] as a single initial dose (and repeated after a short interval if necessary) but, again, toxic levels may occur and therefore monitoring is important. There is the possibility that toxic levels of this drug may damage the developing cerebellum. Also, intravenous diazepam has been used in a regimen of 0.1 mg every two minutes up to a maximum of 1 mg and repeating this dose at 1–3 hour intervals. However, this drug does not seem to be particularly effective in controlling neonatal seizures, is short acting in its effect, may carry an increased risk of respiratory depression when used with phenobarbitone and has been criticized for use intravenously in the neonate because its vehicle (sodium benzoate) is an effective uncoupler of the bilirubin-albumin complex and may increase the risk of kernicterus. Paraldehyde has been used intravenously in a 3–10 per cent solution injected slowly, but it has the disadvantage that it is excreted through the lungs and may produce a pneumonitis. Gamstorp (1970) has advocated the use of lignocaine (xylocaine) in an intravenous infusion, and recommends 3–4 mg/(kg· h) for 12–24 hours initially and continuing in gradually diminishing doses over the next few days provided the infant is seizure free.

Volpe (1976) has stressed the importance of maintaining an adequate supply of glucose to the brain in asphyxiated infants. He pointed out that work with newborn animals had shown that glucose reduced mortality and brain cell loss and prevented the fall in brain glucose which occurred during continuous seizures. However, as already mentioned, this manoeuvre has to be balanced against the risks of fluid over-load increasing cerebral oedema.

Dexamethasone 0.5 mg/(kg BW) intravenously, followed by the same dose given in four divided doses every 24 hours for approximately three days, has been used to reduce cerebral oedema, but its use is still controversial. Similarly, there is some dispute over the use of hypertonic solutions, such as mannitol, in the treatment of cerebral oedema because of the fear that these hyperosmolar preparations may increase the risk of intracranial haemorrhage, especially in premature infants. It is important to emphasize that infrequent or mild seizures may not need to be treated. Holden and Freeman (1975) stress that, in general, more harm may be done by the side-effects of the anticonvulsants used for the treatment of infrequent 'twitches' than by the seizures themselves. If necessary, they can be treated with oral phenobarbitone in a dosage of 5–7 mg/ (kg· day) or with chloral hydrate 50 mg/(kg· day) in divided doses.

Hypoglycaemia is likely to cause convulsions only if it is severe, which usually means a blood glucose concentration of less than 1.1 mmol/ℓ (20 mg/100 ml). In an emergency situation glucose may be given as a bolus injection of 2 ml/(kg BW) of a 50 per cent solution. However, a bolus injection of this kind is not helpful in the long term because it causes a sudden peaking of blood glucose which leads to insulin release followed by a rapid fall in blood glucose. A suitable regimen is a continuous infusion of 10 per cent dextrose, 65 ml/(kg BW) in the initial 24 hours with increasing amounts subsequently as the infant's fluid needs increase, bearing in mind the danger of water intoxication. Occasionally, stronger concentrations of dextrose (up to 15 per cent) are used by infusion but they carry a risk of producing venous thrombosis. Resistant hypoglycaemia may require treatment with glucagon, steroids or ACTH or even diazoxide.

The treatment of hypocalcaemia is less urgent since neonatal tetany is a more benign condition. Calcium gluconate may be given as a 10 per cent solution before each feed, even though the effect on the serum calcium may be slow. Alternatively 0.2 ml/(kg BW) of 10 per cent calcium gluconate may be given slowly intravenously, but intravenous calcium can be dangerous and its effect is brief. Perhaps the most important therapeutic measure is to reduce the phosphate load by using a low phosphate milk such as breast milk or a humanized dried milk formula (SMA) or a dilute cow's milk formula, e.g. evaporated milk one part and water four parts. Associated hypomagnesaemia may be treated by giving 0.2 mg/(kg BW) of 50 per cent magnesium sulphate intramuscularly and repeating this dose if necessary while monitoring the serum magnesium at the same time.

PROGNOSIS

The prognosis of neonatal convulsions depends on various factors including birth weight and aetiology of the seizures. Fits occurring in the first few days of life in general carry a poor prognosis. Brown,

Cockburn and Forfar (1972) had 11 deaths among 60 babies with seizures commencing 1–4 days after birth. Of these babies 15 subsequently developed severe or moderate handicap, both physical and mental, and 34 babies had a mild handicap or were normal. In contrast, of 60 babies developing seizures from 5–7 days after birth, virtually all were normal subsequently and none died. Many of the earlier surveys of neonatal seizures grouped together early and late-onset seizures and consequently found a better overall prognosis. Knauss and Marshall (1977) have recently reviewed the prognosis for babies in a neonatal intensive therapy unit who developed seizures, and more than half the convulsions occurred in the first 72 hours of life. The type of seizure was predominantly multifocal clonic (50 per cent) but 16 per cent had tonic seizures and half of the babies with this latter type died. Perinatal events were the most prevalent aetiological factors in infants with seizures in the first 72 hours of life, irrespective of birth weight. Hypoglycaemia was an infrequent primary cause but was associated with other aetiologies in approximately a third of the cases. Infections were an important cause of convulsions in babies weighing less than 2500 g at birth. In infants weighing less than 1500 g at birth who developed seizures the mortality was 61 per cent and the morbidity was 43 per cent in the survivors. In those weighing between 1501–2500 g at birth the mortality rate was 44 per cent and the morbidity was 46 per cent in the survivors. In infants whose birth weights were greater than 2500 g the mortality rate was 35 per cent and the morbidity was 40 per cent in the survivors. In other words, low birth weight infants with a short period of gestation had a higher mortality rate, but the rates of morbidity among all the survivors did not vary significantly with birthweight.

However, despite these gloomy figures, it seems likely that the prognosis for neonates with seizures will steadily improve in the future in line with better obstetrical management and intensive therapy of the neonate. As in post-traumatic epilepsy in older children (described in Chapter 13), there is probably a good case for keeping infants who have had significant neonatal seizures on maintenance anticonvulsant therapy for a minimum of 6–12 months, and phenobarbitone, phenytoin or carbamazepine may be used for this purpose. However, it is obvious that convulsions occurring at the end of the first week and due to tetany carry no risk of causing death or neurological sequelae and consequently, prophylaxis is quite unnecessary.

Electroencephalography

The value of the interictal EEG in prognosis has been stressed by some authors, especially Rose and Lombroso (1970). In their series infants with seizures and a normal interictal EEG had an 86 per cent chance for normal development at the age of four years, whereas an EEG with multifocal abnormalities was associated with only a 12 per cent chance for normal development. In 10 per cent of the patients in their series they demonstrated a periodic burst/suppression pattern consisting of alternating periods of flatness in the tracing interrupted by bursts of high-voltage sharp waves and spikes and also slow waves. This pattern was correlated with severe cerebral disease and a poor prognosis in the full-term baby, but a similar pattern can occur normally in young premature infants with a gestational age of less than 34 weeks. It must always be remembered that the interpretation of the EEG in the newborn is difficult and most experienced electroencephalographers are aware that in about a quarter to a third of full-term neonates with seizures doubtful of borderline abnormalities occur which are difficult to relate to either short-term or long-term prognosis.

Computerized tomographic (CT) scanning is being used increasingly in the investigation and prognosis of neonates with seizures, particularly when cerebral haemorrhage is suspected. This method of investigation will undoubtedly add greatly to our knowledge of acute emergencies in the newborn associated with seizures. So far, little definitive information has appeared in the literature, but interested readers are referred to Volpe's (1977b) review of neonatal intracranial haemorrhage where the value of CT scanning in demonstrating subdural haematoma, intraventricular haemorrhage and acute ventricular dilatation due to obstruction of the cerebrospinal pathways by blood is mentioned. CT techniques suitable for use in small babies are described in detail by Harwood—Nash and Fitz (1976), and the use of CT scanning in infants and children is extensively reviewed by Gomez and Reese (1976) and by Day, Thomson and Schutt (1978).

REFERENCES

Brown, J. K. (1973). 'Convulsions in the newborn period.' *Devl Med. child Neurol.* **15**, 823–846

Brown, J. K., Cockburn, F., Forfar, J. O. (1972). 'Clinical and chemical correlates in convulsions of the newborn.' *Lancet*, **1**, 135–139

Carton, D. (1978). 'Benign familial neonatal convulsions.' *Neuropädiatrie*, **9**, 167–171

Cockburn, F., Brown, J. K., Belton, N. R. and Forfar, J. O. (1973). 'Neonatal convulsions associated with primary disturbance of calcium, phosphorus and magnesium metabolism.' *Arch Dis. Childh.* **48**, 99–108

Day, R. E., Thomson, J. L. G. and Schutt, W. H. (1978). 'Computerised axial tomography and acute neurological problems of childhood.' *Arch Dis. Childh.* **53**, 2–11

Desmond, M. M., Schwanecke, R. P., Wilson, G. S., Yatsunaga, S. and Burgdorff, I. (1972). 'Maternal barbiturate utilisation and neonatal withdrawal symptomatology.' *J. Pediat.* **80**, 190–197

Gamstorp, I. (1970). *Pediatric Neurology*, pp. 92–93. New York: Appleton-Century-Crofts, Educational Division/Meredith Corporation

Gomez, M. R. and Reese, D. F. (1976). 'Computed tomography of the head in infants and children.' *Pediat. Clin N. Am.* **23**, (3), 473–498

Harwood-Nash, D. C. and Fitz, C. R. (1976). 'Computer Tomography.' In *Neuroradiology in Infants and Children,* Vol. 2, pp. 462–463. Saint Louis, USA: C. V. Mosby

Holden, K. R. and Freeman, J. M. (1975). 'Neonatal seizures and their treatment.' *Clin. Perinatology*, **2**, (1), 3–13

Knauss, T. A. and Marshall, R. E. (1977). 'Seizures in a neonatal intensive care unit.' *Devel Med. child Neurol.* **19**, 719–728

Prechtl, H. and Beintema, D. (1964). *Clinics in Developmental Medicine, No. 12: The Neurological Examination of the Full-term Newborn Infant.* London: Spastics Society and Heinemann

Purpura, D. P., Shofer, R. J. and Scarff, T. (1967). 'Intracellular study of spike potentials and synaptic activities of neurons in immature neocortex.' In *Regional Development of the Brain in Early Life*, pp. 297–325. Ed A. Minkowski. Philadelphia: F. A. Davis

Purvis, R. J., MacKay, G. S., Cockburn, F., Barrie, W. J. McK., Wilkinson, E. M., Belton, N. R. (19730. 'Enamel hypoplasia of the teeth associated with neonatal tetany: a manifestation of maternal Vitamin-D deficiency.' *Lancet,* **2**, 811–814

Rose, A. L. and Lombroso, C. T. (1970). 'Neonatal seizure states.' *Pediatrics,* **45**, 404–425

Volpe, J. J. (1973). 'Neonatal seizures.' *New Engl. J. Med.* **289**, 413–416

Volpe, J. J. (1976). 'Perinatal hypoxic-ischaemic brain injury.' *Pediat. Clins N. Am.* **23**, (3), 383–397

Volpe, J. J. (1977a). 'Neonatal seizures.' *Clins Perinatology*, **4**, (1), 43–63

Volpe, J. J. (1977b). 'Neonatal intracranial haemorrhage: pathophysiology, neuropathology, and clinical features.' *Clins Perinatology*, **4**, (1), 77–102

CHAPTER 4

Convulsions in Early Infancy and Infantile Spasms

After the neonatal period and up to the age of five or six months convulsions are a relatively uncommon symptom, and this time of life could be called the silent period for epilepsy, particularly when it is remembered that convulsions are commoner during the first five years of life than at any other time. Furthermore, convulsions in the early months are difficult to recognize and are often partial, fragmented and disorganized. There may be only localized jerking movements at irregular intervals. The reasons for these characteristics have already been discussed in Chapter 3 and are connected with the slow transmission of discharges in the brain at this age. There is a high 'convulsive threshold' in early infancy and this is why even clinically trivial epilepsy at this age may, in fact, be symptomatic of a serious underlying brain disorder or abnormality.

In a personal series (O'Donohoe, 1971) of 20 infants presenting with partial seizures between one and three months of age and followed prospectively for eight years, only four patients were later found to be of normal intelligence and 14 patients were mentally handicapped, usually to a moderate or a severe degree. While five patients had probably suffered perinatal brain damage, nine had an apparently normal birth history and it was assumed that the seizures were probably symptomatic of some generalized abnormality of the brain.

Convulsions in this age group should make for a guarded prognosis, particularly when the infant's development is suspect. They are, in fact, a developmental warning sign at this age. The other important point which should be remembered is that infantile spasms are preceded by some other type of convulsive attack in a proportion of cases which varies for 20–30 per cent in different series. Indeed, five patients out of the series quoted went on to develop infantile spasms.

INFANTILE SPASMS (WEST'S SYNDROME)

Inhibitory influences in the brain gradually decline and the conduction of discharges improves so that by five to six months of age generalized epilepsy becomes possible, and the very serious disorder known as *infantile spasms* has its peak time of onset during this period (*Figure 4.1*). The first description of this remarkable condition appeared in *Lancet* in 1841 when Dr W. J. West wrote a letter to the editor under

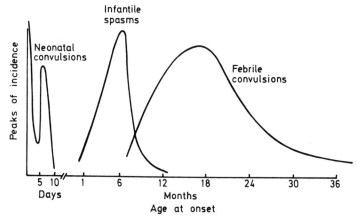

Figure 4.1. Chronology of epilepsy in infancy and early childhood

the heading 'On a peculiar form of infantile convulsions'. He described both the onset of the attacks in his own son at the age of four months and the subsequent intellectual regression in the child who had been developing normally up to the onset of the epilepsy. Over 100 years later Gibbs and Gibbs (1952) described the chaotic EEG pattern in the condition and gave it the title of hypsarrhythmia. The triad of spasms, retardation and hypsarrhythmia is frequently called West's syndrome and appears to be an age-specific convulsive disorder of infancy. In 1958 Sorel and Dusaucy–Bauloye described the results of treatment with ACTH. The *International Classification* of Epileptic Seizures (Gastaut, 1970) recognized infantile spasms as one of the types of generalized epilepsy, i.e. bilaterally symmetrical seizures without focal onset. There is now an increasing tendency to group infantile spasms under the general heading of myoclonic epilepsies of infancy and childhood, giving the alternative title of massive myoclonic seizures of infancy to infantile spasms. This particular problem of classification will be discussed in more detail in the section on the myoclonic epilepsies (*see* Chapter 5).

Clinical aspects

Clinically, infantile spasms involve sudden bilateral symmetrical contraction of muscles. In the commonest type, flexor spasm, simultaneous flexion of neck and trunk occurs. Also, flexion, abduction or adduction of the upper limbs and flexion and adduction of the lower limbs occur simultaneously. The flexor spasm (*Figure 4.2*) may be confused with

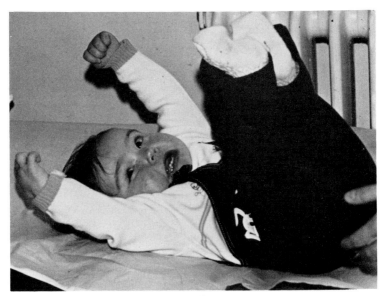

Figure 4.2. A flexor spasm

sudden colic or even with a Moro reflex. In the rarer extensor spasm, the neck and trunk extend and again there may be a resemblance to a Moro reflex. Sometimes, the neck and trunk may flex and the lower limbs extend. There is no relationship between the type of spasm and the seriousness or otherwise of the condition. Perhaps the most characteristic feature of these attacks is their tendency to occur in a repetitive series in which each attack is brief, lasting only seconds or less, and there are probably brief interruptions of consciousness, although this is not certain. A cry or scream is common just after a spasm and the child may be very irritable between series of attacks. At the onset of the illness the attacks may be relatively infrequent becoming very frequent at the height of the illness. Attacks tend to be more frequent during periods of drowsiness, either when dropping off to sleep or on awakening, and may also be provoked by handling the baby. Other types of seizure, including generalized tonic-clonic attacks, may sometimes occur concurrently in patients with infantile spasms.

It is generally agreed that infants who develop spasms demonstrate a cessation of normal psychosocial development and frequently show a marked developmental deterioration as the spasms continue to occur. Motor performance may be affected to a lesser degree than adaptive behaviour. It is, of course, important to realize that a large proportion of infants will already have shown evidence of developmental delay prior to the onset of their illness, but the association between infantile spasms and intellectual dilapidation is irrefutable.

Males preponderate among patients with infantile spasms. In the author's personal series of 100 cases studied from 1960 through to 1975 there were 57 males who presented with this condition (O'Donohoe, 1976). Others have described a male to female ratio of 2:1. A familial occurrence of infantile spasms is rare and the familial incidence of epilepsy is low in patients with infantile spasms.

Cryptogenic and symptomatic infantile spasms

Consideration of any large number of infants with infantile spasms reveals that there are three groups of patients of which two are well defined. The smaller of these, called the cryptogenic group, consists of patients who develop normally before the onset of spasms and in whom there are no clear-cut aetiological factors. These form about a third of most series. The second group, called the symptomatic group, consists of patients in whom a definite predisposing aetiological factor can be identified and these usually form approximately 60 per cent of most series. The onset of spasms is frequently preceded by suspect developmental progress and other types of seizure may often antedate the actual spasms. There is a third group, labelled doubtful, in which the development is abnormal prior to the spasms but no definite aetiology can be established. This usually forms less than 10 per cent of the cases.

Aetiology

The cryptogenic group is particularly important because it is now fully realized that early diagnosis and vigorous treatment of these children may reverse whatever process is causing the illness, and may even bring about subsequent normal intellectual development. On the other hand, treatment of symptomatic cases, even after early diagnosis, is very disappointing. It is now recognized that infantile spasms represent a nonspecific reaction on the part of the brain to a wide variety of insults. *It seems likely that the condition is more age specific than disease specific.* The insult may be prenatal and follow a complication of pregnancy, a congenital cerebral defect, an intrauterine infection or it may occur in an infant who has been small for dates. Perinatal birth injury, particularly anoxic injury, is a frequent forerunner of the disorder. After birth a neonatal meningitis may injure the brain and be followed by infantile spasms. Metabolic disorders, such as untreated phenylketonuria, are not infrequently complicated by infantile spasms and damage produced by neonatal hypoglycaemia can also be causative. The hypoglycaemia resulting from unrecognized leucine sensitivity may cause brain damage in much the same way (Lacy and Penry, 1976).

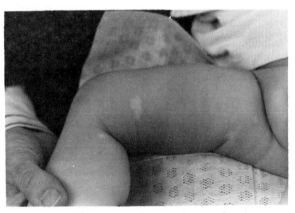

Figure 4.3. 'White patches' in tuberose sclerosis

Two conditions merit special attention, namely, the association with *tuberose sclerosis* and the cases associated with *triple immunization.* Infantile spasms are a common early manifestation of the tuberose sclerosis syndrome, which may be the cause where the infantile spasms are of doubtful aetiology. Clues to the diagnosis may be the presence of poorly pigmented areas on the trunk and limbs, the so-called 'white patches' (*Figure 4.3*), and the later development of the rash of adenoma sebaceum on the face (*Figure 4.4*) (Pampiglione and Moynahan, 1976). Intracranial calcification is rarely seen in infancy, but may occur after the age of four years (*Figure 4.5*). A further reference to tuberose sclerosis will be made in Chapter 14.

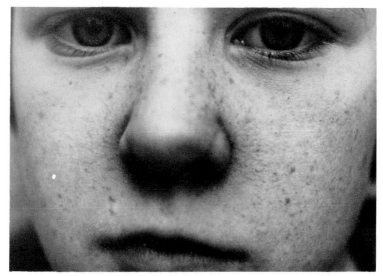

Figure 4.4. The rash of adenoma sebaceum in tuberose sclerosis

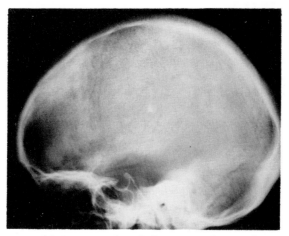

Figure 4.5. Periventricular calcification in tuberose sclerosis.
(Courtesy of Dr J. Toland)

It is not proposed to enter into the controversy concerning the relationship between pertussis immunization and epilepsy. The possibility certainly exists that the connection between the two may be purely coincidental since immunization is normally carried out at the peak time of onset of infantile spasms. However, it must then be admitted, in a small proportion of cases, that there is such a close proximity in time between the immunizing dose and the onset of the epilepsy that the possibility of a causal relationship seems likely. This is especially so where a striking neurological reaction (screaming, irritability and sleeplessness) has quickly followed injection. In such cases early diagnosis and treatment may reverse the reaction which is presumably of an allergic or immunological type (Kulenkamff, Schwartzman and Wilson, 1974).

Finally, before leaving aetiology, the syndrome of infantile spasms, agenesis of the corpus callosum and atrophic areas in the choroid described by Aicardi in 1969 and now bearing his name, must be mentioned. It seems to be confined to females and is usually fatal (Aicardi, Chevrie and Rouselle, 1969).

Diagnosis

The diagnosis of infantile spasms is based on clinical suspicion aided by EEG examination (*Figures 4.6a, b*). The EEG nearly always shows a total disorganization of the record with almost continuous spikes and polyspike discharges present bilaterally forming the general abnormality called hypsarrhythmia. Like infantile spasms, hypsarrhythmia is an age-specific abnormality and may be found in severely abnormal children in the same age group who do not have the clinical syndrome of infantile spasms. The abnormality is usually present during sleeping and waking but may be more marked during sleep in certain cases. Hypsarrhythmia persists for a time and then disappears with advancing age of the child and maturation of the nervous system and is replaced by a less disorganized pattern. An upper age limit for hypsarrhythmia has not been established but it is uncommon beyond the age of three years. The presence of hypsarrhythmia in an infant during his first year of life is a physical sign of grave prognostic significance, whatever the cause, and implies that the later incidence of mental subnormality will be at least 80 per cent (Friedman and Pampiglione, 1971). Some patients with infantile spasms have periods of relatively organized brain activity separating the periods of hypsarrhythmia in their EEGs. This periodic pattern is entitled 'modified hypsarrhythmia'. Very rarely patients with infantile spasms may have normal EEGs. Lombroso and Fejerman (1977) described 16 infants, aged 3–8½ months, with seizures which resembled infantile spasms, but the infants were without arrest or regression in psychomotor development and with normal EEGs. The prognosis was excellent with or without therapy and they called the condition 'benign myoclonus of early infancy'.

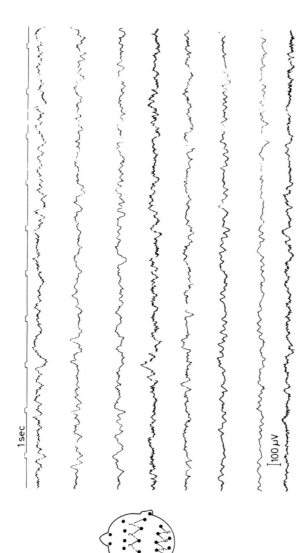

Figure 4.6a. Normal EEG in a five months old male infant who is awake with eyes open

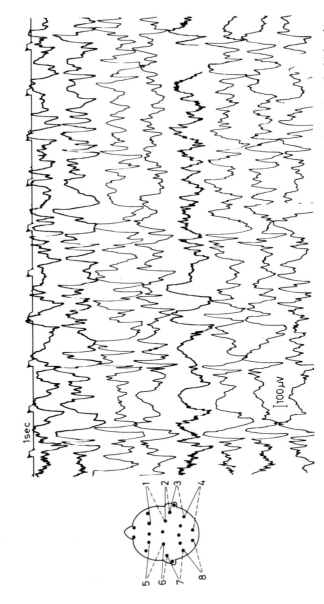

Figure 4.6b. Female infant aged six months and awake with eyes open. EEG shows hypsarrhythmia. Note the high-voltage irregular activity and frequent spike discharges

Mental retardation

The most important feature of infantile spasms is the association with intellectual retardation. The majority of patients in the symptomatic group, apart from the postimmunization cases, will have shown evidence of developmental delay prior to the onset of the spasms. Further intellectual deterioration may occur when the spasms commence, but this may not be particularly marked. Patients in the cryptogenic group, however, will usually have been normal developmentally prior to the onset of spasms and will then, as a rule, show striking developmental regression. It appears that the same process which leads to the occurrence of spasms also halts normal development and then leads to regression. As the spasms are treated or gradually disappear with the passage of time developmental progress picks up again to a greater or lesser degree.

THERAPY

Therapy for infantile spasms was extremely disappointing prior to the apparently successful use of ACTH in 1958. Since then there has been controversy about the efficacy or otherwise of this method of treatment. In the reported series there has been considerable variability in the therapeutic agents employed (ACTH or steroids), the dosages used and the duration of therapy. Most workers have favoured ACTH rather than steroids for initial therapy because it was claimed that a more rapid response was obtained, but some experienced clinicians have advocated steroids as superior agents. The dosage of ACTH has varied from fairly moderate daily dosages (20–40 units) up to very high dosages (80–120 units/day). The initial administration of 40 units/day for one to two weeks, followed by 20 units/day for a further two to three weeks, followed by oral steroid therapy for up to three months, has been a widely recommended regimen. Others have recommended continuing ACTH for three to six months after the initial month of treatment perhaps using 20–40 units on alternate days. Prednisolone in an initial dose of 2 mg/(kg· day) or dexamethasone in a dose of 0.3 mg/(kg· day) have been used with gradual reductions in dosage to a maintenance level for a variable duration of therapy (Lacy and Penry, 1976).

Controversy has centred around the question of whether this form of treatment really benefits the patient. There is fairly general agreement that patients who have normal development up to the onset of spasms, i.e. the cryptogenic group, are most likely to respond to treatment and are least likely to relapse subsequently. The same can also be said about those patients who develop infantile spasms following immunization, assuming that one accepts a cause and effect relationship between the two events. Another point about which there is some agreement concerns the time-lag between onset of spasms and commencement of treatment. The shorter this is, and particularly if it is less than one month, the better the response and the outlook. But again, this mainly applies to the cryptogenic and postimmunization cases. A rapid clinical response to ACTH or steroid therapy is also accepted as another good prognostic indicator. However, in various series nearly 70 per cent of cases responded well initially but over half of those who did subsequently relapsed, and a sustained improvement was reported in just under a third of the total number of patients treated. Furthermore, Jeavons and Bower (1964) in their report on a large series, stressed that patients with relapsing infantile spasms are unlikely to respond to additional courses of treatment, although repeated courses are usually given. Usually EEG improvement parallels clinical improvement, and this usually becomes apparent in the second week of therapy. However, it is important to stress that clinical improvement can occur without EEG improvement and vice versa. Relapses are usually accompanied by a return of the severe EEG abnormality, and the frequency of these relapses has led many to question whether ACTH or steroid therapy has anything other than a transient beneficial effect, and to ask whether they confer any long-term benefit. Despite these doubts most physicians confronted with a patient with infantile spasms, especially if they are of recent onset and occurring in a previously normal or immunized child, would hesitate to withhold ACTH or steroid therapy.

Even if it is accepted that treatment stops the spasms and improves the EEG, there still remains the most important question of intellectual improvement. Again, many would contend that the cryptogenic and postimmunization group, especially if diagnosed and treated early, probably does benefit intellectually in the short term and in the long term from ACTH or steroid therapy. Some would argue that those cases which improve would do so anyway without treatment or with anticonvulsant therapy using a benzodiazepine drug. There is no agreement about the effect on intellectual development in those infants with symptomatic spasms, other than the postimmunization group, and probably the majority would contend that ACTH or steroids do no more than improve the epilepsy and the EEG temporarily. There is a growing feeling that this group should not be given this type of therapy but should have anticonvulsants only. It should be emphasized that ACTH and steroids used in large doses at this age lead to obesity, electrolyte disturbances, fluid retention and increased susceptibility to infection, particularly pneumonia and septicaemia. Death during treatment is not uncommon. One particular hazard, in the author's experience, is profound depletion of body potassium and this can be fatal if unrecognized.

The hazards of hormone therapy have led to a search for alternative methods of treatment. The benzodiazepine drugs, particularly nitrazepam and clonazepam, have been used with some success in controlling the spasms but with no significant beneficial effect on intellectual retardation. Most clinicians would prefer to use ACTH or steroids as primary therapy, particularly in cryptogenic spasms, while reserving the benzodiazepines for the occasional child with cryptogenic spasms but without evidence of psychomotor regression, a clinical situation which is difficult to establish with certainty. These drugs are also used in those children with symptomatic spasms where hormone therapy is considered to be futile, and also as maintenance therapy after treatment with hormones. The reader will notice that this short account of the benzodiazepines seems to imply that ACTH and steroids confer some extra, perhaps physiological, benefit on the patient which cannot be achieved by a chemical medication. This, in fact, has never been proven and the hormones are probably only symptomatic treatment at best. The benzodiazepines will be discussed in greater detail in the section on the drug therapy of epilepsy (see p. 241).

PROGNOSIS

There have been relatively few studies of the long-term prognosis of infantile spasms. Probably the most informative is the study of Jeavons, Bower and Dimitrakoudi (1973) which was concerned with 150 children seen between 1954 and 1970. Just over two-thirds of the cases received hormone therapy. There were 44 cryptogenic cases, 96 symptomatic cases of which 21 were considered to be related to immunization, and 10 doubtful cases. The criterion of normality was considered to be attendance at a normal school. The length of follow-up was 2–12 years.

The study of Jeavons, Bower and Dimitrakoudi (1973) confirmed that the most important factor associated with complete mental recovery was normal development prior to the onset of spasms. This group of patients, which included the cryptogenic and postimmunization cases, had a 37 per cent chance of complete recovery in this series. However, in the total series only 16 per cent achieved complete recovery, and of the rest 34 per cent was severely subnormal, 47 per cent had neurological abnormalities (usually a spastic hemiplegia, diplegia or tetraplegia) and 22 per cent died. The greatest mortality occurred before the age of four years and reference has already been made to the causes of this high death rate.

In the author's series (O'Donohoe, 1976) 100 consecutive cases were seen between 1960 and 1970 and followed-up until 1975. Of these children 21 were found to be normal physically and intellectually on follow-up. When the cryptogenic cases (33) and postimmunization cases (11) were grouped together 47 per cent (21) of these were considered to have recovered fully. Of the 100 children 46 were severely abnormal intellectually, 19 were moderately or mildly subnormal and 27 had cerebral palsy and were usually severely mentally handicapped in addition. In this series 19 children died and a third of the deaths occurred during ACTH therapy. Over 90 patients had received this form of treatment so that a comparison between treated and untreated cases was not possible. However, Jeavons, Bower and Dimitrakoudi (1973) were able to make such a comparison and were not convinced that treatment had influenced the long-term prognosis.

In the light of such gloomy long-term results and despite the evidence that ACTH and corticosteroids have no influence on the ultimate developmental status and only transient effects on the seizures and EEG abnormalities, it must again be asked why these agents continue to be used ? The answer at present appears to be that since ACTH and steroid therapy undoubtedly has a beneficial, although often temporary, effect on the spasms and the EEG and since the prognosis is generally so bad, it seems reasonable to continue to use this form of therapy, particularly in those cases where there may be hope of a successful outcome.

The essential pathological change in this remarkable age-related condition remains a mystery. It has not been possible to find a suitable animal model for study. Investigations using special staining methods and microscopic techniques have suggested that there may be a decreased number of synaptic sites in the brains of these children, particularly at certain cortical levels. Others have suggested that there may be a disturbance of synaptogenesis or in development of neurotransmitter mechanisms at a critical stage of cortical maturation (Kristt, 1976). It is to be hoped that future neuropathological and neurochemical research along these lines will shed more light on this tragic and, as yet, little understood type of generalized epilepsy in early infancy. The new technique of CT scanning is already adding to our knowledge of the structural abnormalities in this syndrome, enabling us to make a more definite distinction between primary and secondary cases and also to give more accurate information about prognosis. Gastaut *et al.* (1978) have emphasized its value in demonstrating the presence of cortical atrophy, malformations such as agenesis of the corpus callosum and calcification in tuberose sclerosis.

REFERENCES

Aicardi, J., Chevrie, J. J. and Rouselle, F. (1969). 'Le syndrome spasmes en flexion, agénésie calleuse, anomalies chorio-rétiniennes.' *Archs fr. Pédiat.* **26**, 1103–1120

Friedman, E. and Pampiglione, G. (1971). 'Prognostic implications of electro-encelphalographic findings of hypsarrhythmia in first year of life.' *Br. med. J.* **4**, 323–325

Gastaut, H. (1970). 'Clinical and electroencephalographical classification of epileptic seizures.' *Epilepsia,* **11**, 102–113

Gastaut, H., Gastaut, J. L., Regis, H., Bernard, R., Pinsard, N., Saint-Jean, M., Roger, J. and Dravet, C. (1978). 'Computerized Tomography in the Study of West's Syndrome.' *Devl Med. child Neurol.* **20**, 21–27

Gibbs, F. A. and Gibbs, E. L. (1952). *Atlas of Electroencephalography, Vol. 2: Epilepsy.* Cambridge, Mass.: Addison–Wesley

Jeavons, P. M. and Bower, B. D. (1964). *Clinics in Developmental Medicine, No. 15: Infantile Spasms: A review of the literature and a study of 112 cases,* pp. 50–63. London: Spastics Society and Heinemann

Jeavons, P. M., Bower, B. D. and Dimitrakoudi, M. (1973). 'Long-term prognosis of 150 cases of "West Syndrome".' *Epilepsia,* **14**, 153–164

Kristt, D. A. (1976). 'Development of neuronal circuitry in cerebral cortex.' In *Infantile Spasms.* Proceedings of the First European Regional Conference on Epilepsy, Warsaw, June, 1976, p. 7. London: Epilepsy International

Kulenkampff, M., Schwartzman, J. S. and Wilson, J. (1974). 'Neurological complications of pertussis immunisation.' *Archs Dis. Child.* **49**, 46–49

Lacy, J. R. and Penry, J. K. (1976). *Infantile Spasms* New York: Raven Press

Lombroso, C. T. and Fejerman, N. (1977). 'Benign myoclonus of early infancy.' *Ann. Neurol.* **1**, 138–143

O'Donohoe, N. V. (1971). Communication to the British Paediatric Neurology Study Group, Brighton, 1971. Unpublished

O'Donohoe, N. V. (1976). 'A 15-year follow up of 100 children with infantile spasms.' *Ir. J. Med. Sci.* **145**, 138

Pampiglione, G. and Moynahan, E. J. (1976). 'Tuberous sclerosis syndrome: clinical and EEG studies in 100 children.' *J. Neurol. Neurosurg. Psychiat.* **39**, 666–673

Sorel, L. and Dusaucy-Bauloye, A. (1958). 'A propos de 21 cas d'hypsarhythmie de Gibbs: Son traitment spectaculaire par L'ACTH.' *Acta neurol. psychiat. belg.* **58**, 130–140

West, W. J. (1841). 'On a peculiar form of infantile convulsions.' *Lancet,* **1**, 724–725

CHAPTER 5

The Myoclonic Epilepsies of Early Childhood

It has been seen in the preceding chapter how infantile spasms represent a nonspecific reaction on the part of the brain to a variety of insults occurring at a particular developmental stage which lead to a severe and often intractable type of generalized epilepsy. Lennox (1960) originally pointed out that the type of epilepsy which occurs in a child represents a confluence of age, heredity and structural brain abnormality. The syndrome of infantile spasms illustrates this concept, even though heredity does not seem to play a significant role. The heterogeneous group of disorders, now usually called the myoclonic epilepsies of childhood, represents another set of age and development-dependent conditions and is one in which various brain insults and heredity may be involved.

The history of the myoclonic epilepsies is a confused one. Lennox (1945) recognized that they were distinct from true petit mal and he described their earlier time of onset as being in the age group of 1–6 years. He noted the male predominance, the common association with structural brain abnormality, the high incidence of mental handicap, the variety of seizures which could occur, the fact that hyperventilation did not provoke attacks and the lack of response to the then specific therapy for petit mal with the dione drugs. He also described their frequent association with an EEG pattern of slow spike-wave discharges occurring at a rate of 1.5–2.5 complexes/second. The term 'petit mal variant' was coined but this has since been abandoned because it tended to compound the confusion about terminology. Gastaut et al. (1966)

reviewed the problem in a classic article and proposed the title 'childhood epileptic encephalopathy with diffuse slow spike waves'. He also proposed an alternative title of the 'Lennox syndrome' which was subsequently altered by others to the 'Lennox-Gastaut syndrome'. These eponymous titles are in wide use but it should be realized that they refer to a heterogeneous group of disorders of diverse aetiology, occurring at different ages in early childhood and with the characteristics described by Lennox (1945) and further amplified by Gastaut et al. (1966). The general title 'myoclonic epilepsies of early childhood' is, in the author's opinion, to be preferred. The term 'minor motor seizures' is also used in the USA and in Europe.

The resemblances between the clinical characteristics as defined by Lennox (1945) and the clinical features of the infantile spasms syndrome will be apparent to the reader. Indeed, infantile spasms are sometimes referred to as infantile myoclonic epilepsy. Furthermore, between one-fifth and one-third of the patients with infantile spasms go on to develop clinical myoclonic epilepsy, with or without a fit-free interval, and they may show the typical slow spike-wave patterns in their EEGs.

PRIMARY AND SECONDARY GROUPS

Myoclonic epilepsies in early childhood are generalized epilepsies and can conveniently be regarded as falling into two groups in much the same way as infantile spasms, namely a primary group (cryptogenic or idiopathic) and a secondary group (symptomatic). As with infantile spasms the secondary group is always the larger group forming at least two-thirds of most series, and, on closer inspection, many apparently primary cases will be found to have had suspect neurodevelopmental history prior to the onset of epilepsy. However, there are certainly primary cases which have a completely normal history up to the time of onset of the epilepsy, and in those one is the same state of puzzlement with regard to aetiology as with cryptogenic infantile spasms, i.e. are they due to a metabolic cause, to an autoimmune reaction to infection or perhaps immunization or to hereditary factors influencing neurological development in some way ? For example, Doose et al (1970), in Germany, have described a group of children with myoclonic epilepsy with onset in the third and fourth years, who have a strong family history of epilepsy in close relatives, who have a normal psychomotor development prior to onset of the epilepsy and in whom organic brain lesions are uncommon. They concluded that a genetically determined susceptibility to convulsions played a highly important aetiological role in these children. The distinction between primary and secondary myoclonic epilepsies is also important in relation to prognosis, as will be seen later.

Varieties of myoclonic seizures

A variety of seizures occurs in the myoclonic epilepsies, the commonest
being the following:

1. Atonic-akinetic attacks in which violent falls occur suddenly with
   immediate recovery and resumption of activity, the duration being
   less than a second (*Figure 5.1*); multiple injuries may occur, particularly to the forehead, lips, teeth and chin

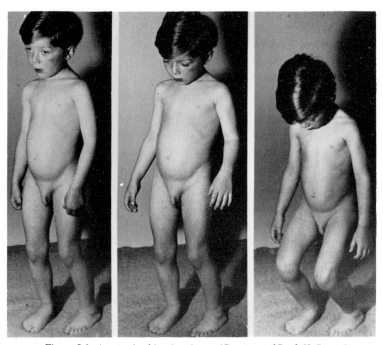

Figure 5.1. An atonic-akinetic seizure. (Courtesy of Prof. H. Doose)

2. Head-dropping or head-nodding attacks, which may be just a partial
   form of the generalized atonic-akinetic attacks
3. Atypical absences, consisting of a brief interruption of consciousness
   which is often incomplete and which has a gradual onset and cessation,
   perhaps accompanied by automatisms; consciousness is usually
   clouded rather than completely lost
4. Myoclonic phenomena, consisting of symmetrical and synchronous
   flexion movements; asymmetrical myoclonic jerks also occur infrequently

5. Major tonic-clonic generalized seizures may occur, as may brief tonic attacks, particularly in sleep

6. Episodes of minor epileptic status (Brett, 1966) in which recurring atypical absences, atonic-akinetic attacks and myoclonic jerks are repeated over hours or days may also be seen.

Sometimes the onset of myoclonic epilepsy may appear in an innocent way with the occurrence of a grand mal seizure, perhaps precipitated by fever. Weeks may then go by before the more serious manifestations of myoclonic epilepsy appear, including the very characteristic atonic-akinetic attacks. Patients frequently manifest a variety of different types of seizure.

With regard to *the aetiology of the secondary or symptomatic group*, the conditions producing the cerebral insult are as diverse as they are in symptomatic infantile spasms, and in a proportion of cases the aetiology may not be obvious. It seems likely that multifocal or diffuse brain damage is at play in all the secondary cases. Perinatal difficulties, intra-uterine infections and acquired brain damage from whatever cause may all precede the condition. Tuberose sclerosis may also be a cause. As with those severely affected by infantile spasms, neurological abnormalities such as spasticity are common in the severely affected cases of myoclonic epilepsy.

Mental retardation

Although mental handicap is very frequently associated with the myoclonic epilepsies, the degree of handicap is variable. There is a definite correlation between the age of onset of the epilepsy and later intelligence. The earlier the onset the more mentally retarded the patient. Those beginning under three years of age do far worse than those at three years or over. The younger age group contains a larger number of definite secondary cases and also those who have previously had infantile spasms, whereas in the older group there are more primary cases. Aicardi (1973) has estimated that the proportion of severely mentally retarded patients may be three times higher in the secondary group when compared with the primary group. In a recent Japanese follow-up of 116 cases of the 'Lennox syndrome' (Ohtahara, Yamatogi and Ohtsuka, 1977) 98 cases (84.5 per cent) were shown to have some degree of mental defect and 71 patients (61.2 per cent) continued to have seizures. Both primary and secondary cases were included. The resemblance to the usual figures quoted for mental defect and epilepsy after infantile spasms should be noted.

PROGNOSIS

The reasons for the differences in prognosis between the primary and secondary groups are not clear. However, in the secondary group an earlier age of onset probably reflects the greater severity of the cerebral insult, whereas in the primary group hereditary factors are probably more important than the underlying brain abnormality. Therefore, one may say with a certain amount of confidence that the later the onset and the more blameless the history antedating the disorder, the better the response to therapy and the better the prognosis for mental development. The term 'Lennox–Gastaut syndrome' might perhaps be reserved for those cases of earlier onset with a poor prognosis, although it must be emphasized that severe cases can occur at any age up to seven years or even later. Whatever the type of case, the long-term outlook for these epilepsies is always uncertain and recovery from the more severe Lennox–Gastaut syndrome is rare. In those who continue to have epilepsy a fluctuating course is characteristic and the pattern of the seizures changes with the years. Diurnal and particularly nocturnal tonic-clonic attacks predominate later on, and brief tonic attacks occurring in slow-wave sleep but not in REM sleep are a characteristic later feature (Gastaut et al., 1966).

DIAGNOSIS

The diagnosis of myoclonic epilepsy is usually not difficult if the characteristic atonic-akinetic attacks occur. However, in the event of the condition beginning with a major generalized seizure in a setting of fever the clinician may be misled. Lennox and Davis (1949) described the slow spike-wave complexes in these epilepsies and emphasized the lack of temporal relationship between the EEG paroxysms and the clinical seizures. In the early stages of myoclonic epilepsy, even in the severe Lennox–Gastaut syndrome, the EEG may be normal but it usually shows diffuse slowing. The characteristic slow spike-wave complexes may not appear for some time, and this abnormality usually occurs in bursts of variable duration and not necessarily in association with clinical seizures (*Figure 5.2*). The abnormality may be continuous for long periods and this EEG status may or may not be associated with clinical minor epileptic status. Polyspikes and slow waves may be present instead of slow spike-wave complexes, and there may even be a pattern resembling hypsarrhythmia in severely affected individuals. The EEG tends to change from examination to examination and occasionally reverts to a nearly normal pattern in good periods, although some diffuse slowing usually persists. The EEG abnormalities may be more marked during sleep, particularly in slow-wave sleep.

49

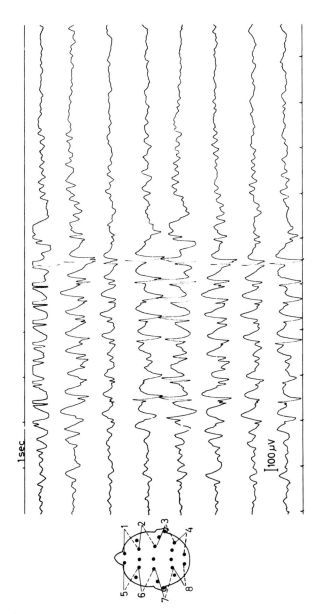

Figure 5.2. Girl aged 10 years and awake with eyes open. EEG shows a short burst of slow spike-wave complexes

Differential diagnosis

There is sometimes another diagnostic difficulty in the myoclonic epilepsies of later onset. In this situation there is a grey area in which it is difficult to differentiate the condition from true or typical petit mal. This diagnostic difficulty may arise when absences are the main clinical seizures present. One should always be wary of a child with apparent petit mal presenting under five years of age who has a history suggesting a structural lesion of the brain, where there is a possibility of associated mental handicap even of mild degree and where the EEG patterns are atypical and irregular. The distinction between primary (petit mal) and secondary (myoclonic) generalized epilepsy is often difficult to determine in the young child. However, it is important to distinguish between them because of the prognostic implications with regard to the control of the epilepsy and to the future intellectual status and also because the drug treatment is different in these two types of epilepsy. Further reference will be made to the differential diagnosis of absences in the chapter on petit mal (*see* Chapter 7).

Mention must also be made of a group of young children who develop *myoclonic jerks* as the main type of seizure but who have no other symptoms to warrant inclusion in the atonic-akinetic group. This particular type of epilepsy may begin around three years of age or even earlier. The EEG usually shows an irregular spike and wave pattern, mainly at three complexes per second and sometimes with multiple spike discharges, in contrast to the slow spike-wave pattern of the conditions already described. The author has recently seen a boy who apparently recovered unscathed from infantile spasms of the cryptogenic type and then developed this type of epilepsy at the age of 3½ years. Jeavons (1977) has entitled it simply 'myoclonic epilepsy of childhood' and it has been called 'cryptogenic myoclonic epilepsy of childhood' and 'true myoclonic epilepsy' (Aicardi and Chevrie, 1971). It may or may not be associated with mental handicap and is particularly resistant to drug therapy.

Heterogeneity of myoclonic epilepsies

It has frequently been stressed (Aicardi, 1973), and the author would also like to emphasize the fact, that the myoclonic epilepsies of early childhood represent a heterogeneous group of disorders and not a single entity. They range from severe so-called 'Lennox—Gastaut syndrome' with its violent and intractable epilepsy to the myoclonic epilepsy appearing in a child of over three years who has been previously normal and the group also includes the so-called 'true myoclonic epilepsy' described above. Mental handicap is also a variable feature as are the EEG patterns. Some of the mentally handicapped children may demonstrate the type of 'autistic' withdrawn behaviour with bizarre mannerisms which is also seen after infantile spasms. Myoclonic attacks may even be a feature of the early stages of degenerative disease of the central nervous system, particularly in subacute sclerosing panencephalitis (SSPE) where sudden head nodding attacks of split second duration may be the presenting feature and are accompanied by the characteristic repetitive EEG complexes.

Ataxia and myoclonic epilepsies

Transient cerebellar syndromes or transient ataxia lasting from a few days to several weeks may occur in the myoclonic epilepsies and may even in the initial presenting complaint (Aicardi and Chevrie, 1971). There is frequently a definite temporal relationship between the episodes of ataxia and temporary worsening of the epileptic disorder. The ataxia later improves if and when the epilepsy responds to treatment. The EEG is particularly useful in identifying myoclonic epilepsy as a cause of the ataxic syndrome and in making the distinction from degenerative disorders with progressive myoclonus such as Lafora body disease (*see* page 97). Another condition which may present with myoclonic attacks and progressive dementia is the late infantile form of neuronal ceroid lipofuscinosis or Batten-Vogt disease. In this disease the EEG usually shows bursts of slow waves and irregular spike-wave complexes and there is an abnormal sensitivity to photic stimulation at a flash frequency of 2–5 flashes/second (Pampiglione and Harden, 1977).

THERAPY

In line with their heterogeneity, one might expect that the treatment of myoclonic seizures would be difficult and indeed it is notoriously so. There is hardly another group of epilepsies in childhood which so often proves as unyielding to medication as do the myoclonic seizures. Drugs used in major generalized epilepsy in older children and adults, for example phenobarbitone, primidone, phenytoin and carbamazepine, are usually ineffective and, indeed, both phenobarbitone and primidone often tend to exacerbate the over-activity and aggressiveness which are common accompaniments of these epilepsies. However, in the author's experience, primidone may be worth a cautious trial in some cases. Occasionally, even ethosuximide may prove surprisingly successful, especially in so-called 'true myoclonic epilepsy'. ACTH has been used in some severe cases of the Lennox–Gastaut syndrome and sometimes brings about a measure of control in much the same rather inexplicable way in which it benefits children with infantile spasms. When this regimen is beneficial it usually has to be continued for many months, and the author has used empirical doses of 40 units on alternate days, gradually lengthening the intervals between doses to twice weekly. The most important recent advances, however, have been the use of the benzodiazepines and sodium valproate in treatment. It is now customary to use one or other of these initially. The two *benzodiazepine drugs* which have been used are nitrazepam, which is not available in the USA, and clonazepam, which is. Diazepam has also been used orally in large doses (betwen 5–30 mg/day) but side effects such as drowsiness, ataxia, diplopia and extrapyramidal movements have largely precluded its widespread use. Nitrazepam has been used more successfully than diazepam and, if it is introduced in a small dose (2.5–5 mg at night, depending on the age of the child) and if increments are made very slowly until attacks cease or until side-effects occur, then it may be quite well tolerated. However, clonazepam is now the benzodiazepine most widely used in the myoclonic epilepsies. Hanson and Menkes (1972) treated 59 patients with 'minor motor seizures', selected because they did not respond to the usual medications. The series included some patients who had had infantile spasms. Of the 59 patients in the series 45 derived significant benefit from clonazepam after a three month trial and 39 continued to receive benefit for periods of 3–18 months. Hanson and Menkes concluded that clonazepam appeared to be the most useful anticonvulsant available in the management of the myoclonic epilepsies. Roussounis and Rudolf (1977), on the basis of their results, also regarded the response to clonazepam as encouraging. In their myoclonic-akinetic group control was achieved in 14 out of 22 patients. O'Donohoe and Paes (1977) also reported good results with the drug (i.e. better than 50 per cent control of attacks) in eight out of 10 patients with myoclonic-akinetic attacks, and good control in three out of seven patients with more severe and intractable myoclonic epilepsy (Lennox–Gastaut syndrome). Many of their patients had previously been taking a variety of other drugs without success. The arbitrary maximum dosage for infants under one year was 0.3 mg/ (kg· day), and for those over a year the dose was 0.25 mg/(kg· day). The drug was introduced extremely slowly, beginning with 0.25 mg at bedtime and increasing by small increments every fifth day until the epilepsy responded or serious side effects were encountered. These included drowsiness, hypersecretion and drooling, ataxia, and, in older children, hyperactivity. Most people using the benzodiazepines as anti-convulsants have noted the development of tolerance to the drugs which develops in 8–25 per cent of those treated (Brown and Penry,

1973) usually 1–6 months after the commencement of treatment. It has been suggested that this is less of a problem with clonazepam than with the other benzodiazepines.

Sodium valproate is a relatively recent addition to the antiepileptic drugs and it will be discussed in greater detail in a later chapter on drug therapy (*see* p. 241). It may act by increasing the level of GABA in the brain by inhibiting the enzyme responsible for its breakdown. GABA is a known inhibitor at certain synapses. Jeavons, Clarke and Maheshwari (1977) have recently reported on its use in the myoclonic epilepsies. They reported good results (control or marked improvement) in 16 of their 32 patients with atonic-akinetic seizures. Similar responses were obtained in 10 of their 11 patients with true myoclonic epilepsy. They concluded that, in their opinion, sodium valproate was superior to all other drugs in the treatment of the myoclonic epilepsies. In the author's experience it has been particularly successful in primary or cryptogenic myoclonic epilepsy, beginning in the child of three years or older, in those with atypical absences, and in true myoclonic epilepsy. However, like most other drugs it is unpredictable in its effects on the secondary myoclonic epilepsies, including the severe Lennox–Gastaut syndrome, and makes some patients worse. It does not appear to be superior to the benzodiazepines in these patients.

The effects of a *ketogenic diet* on intractable epilepsy have been known since the early 1920s, and the diet appears to act by increasing the concentrations of acetoacetate and β-hydroxybutyrate levels in the plasma. It is suggested that the availability and use of ketones by the brain result in certain biochemical changes which reduce the tendency for neurones to discharge and also inhibit the spread of discharges in the brain. The diet has been regarded as expensive, difficult to manage, unpalatable and even nauseating. Huttenlocher, Wilbourn and Signore (1971) brought about a significant practical advance in the use of this dietetic regimen when they used medium-chain triglycerides (MCT) to induce ketosis. This made the diet easier to manage, more palatable and also meant that carbohydrates need not be so rigidly restricted. This modification of the ketogenic diet has been found to be most effective in younger children, but is probably worth considering at any age. The author has had a dramatic success in treating a 12 year old with severe myoclonic epilepsy (Lennox–Gastaut syndrome) and recurrent status epilepticus, the latter being experienced for many years. Similarly a five-year-old patient with very severe atonic-akinetic seizures, which had resisted the established and recently introduced anticonvulsants, has been free of fits for nearly nine months to date on the ketogenic diet with MCT oils. It may be significant that the mothers of both patients are trained nurses. The success of the method depends on both the understanding and co-operation of the mother and on the acceptance of the diet by the child. Strict adherence to the diet and the maintenance of persistent ketosis are essential. Full details of the diet are given in the Appendix (*see also* Gordon, 1977).

Finally, the *general care* of the child with these chronic and disabling epilepsies is of the utmost importance. They present an enormous challenge to the paediatrician or paediatric neurologist dealing with

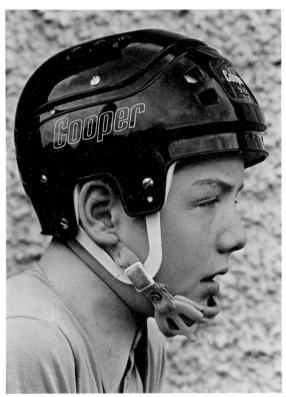

Figure 5.3. The Lennox–Gastaut syndrome. Patient wearing protective headgear and having an absence attack

them. The parents need regular advice and support. Protective headgear is frequently necessary (*Figure 5.3*), particularly when the atonic-akinetic drop seizures are frequent. This particular type of epilepsy, as Lennox (1960) remarked in his classic work on the subject, is surely the charter member of the ancient order of 'Falling Sickness'! Further discussion of the educational and other problems which beset these patients will be found in a later chapter (*see* Chapter 19).

REFERENCES

Aicardi, J. (1973). 'The problem of the Lennox syndrome.' *Devl Med. child Neurol.* **15**, 77–81

Aicardi, J. and Chevrie, J. J. (1971). 'Myoclonic epilepsies of childhood.' *Neuropädiatrie*, **3**, 177–190

Brett, E. M. (1966). 'Minor epileptic status.' *J. neurol. Sci.* **3**, 52–75

Brown, T. R. and Penry, J. K. (1973). 'Benzodiazepines in the treatment of epilepsy: A review.' *Epilepsia*, **14**, 277–310

Doose, H., Gerken, H., Leonhardt, R., Volzke, E. and Volz, C. (1970). 'Centrencephalic myoclonic-astatic petit mal. Clinical and genetic considerations.' *Neuropädiatrie*, **2**, 59–78

Gastaut, H., Roger, J., Soulayrol, R., Tassinari, C. A., Regis, H., Dravet, C., Bernard, R., Pinsard, N. and Saint-Jean, M. (1966). 'Childhood epileptic encephalopathy with diffuse slow spike-waves (otherwise known as petit mal variant or Lennox syndrome).' *Epilepsia*, **7**, 139–179

Gordon, N. S. (1977). 'Medium-chain triglycerides in a ketogenic diet.' *Devl Med. child Neurol.* **19**, 535–538

Hanson, R. A. and Menkes, J. H. (1972). 'A new anticonvulsant in the management of minor motor seizures.' *Devl Med. child Neurol.* **14**, 3–14

Huttenlocher, P. R., Wilbourn, A. J. and Signore, J. M. (1971). 'Medium-chain triglycerides as therapy for intractable childhood epilepsy.' *Neurology, Minneap.* **21**, 1097–1103

Jeavons, P. M. (1977). 'Neurological problems of myoclonic epilepsies in childhood and adolescence.' *Devl Med. child Neurol.* **19**, 3–8

Jeavons, P. M., Clark, J. E. and Maheshwari, M. C. (1977). 'Treatment of generalised epilepsies of childhood and adolescence with sodium valproate ("Epilim").' *Devl Med. child Neurol.* **19**, 9–25

Lennox, W. G. (1945). 'The petit mal epilepsies; their treatment with Tridione.' *J. Am. med. Ass.* **129**, 1069–1074

Lennox, W. G. (1960). *Epilepsy and Related Disorders*, Vol. 1. London: J. and A. Churchill and Boston: Little, Brown

Lennox, W. G. and Davis, J. P. (1949). 'Clinical correlates of the fast and the slow spike-wave electroencephalogram.' *Trans. Am. neurol. Ass.* **74**, 194–197

Ohtahara, S., Yamatogi, Y. and Ohtsuka, Y. (1977). 'Prognosis of the Lennox syndrome. A clinical and electroencephalographic study.' *Epilepsia*, **18**, 130–131

O'Donohoe, N. V. and Paes, B. A. (1977). 'A trial of clonazepam in the treatment of severe epilepsy in infancy and childhood.' In *Epilepsy.* Proceedings of the Eighth International Symposium, pp. 159–162. Ed J. K. Penry. New York: Raven Press

Pampiglione, G. and Harden, A. (1977). 'So-called neuronal ceroid lipofuscinosis. Neurophysiological studies in 60 children.' *J. Neurol. Neurosurg. Psychiat.* **40**, 323–330

Roussounis, S. and Rudolf, N de M. (1977). 'Clonazepam in the treatment of children with intractable seizures.' *Devl Med. child Neurol.* **19**, 326–334

CHAPTER 6

Febrile Convulsions and Status Epilepticus

Aetiology of febrile convulsions

These occur in young children who have an individual susceptibility to convulse in a setting of acute fever. The incidence of these fits is about 3 per cent in the population at risk, they are rare below six months and above five years of age and the peak incidence occurs from 9–20 months. The term 'febrile convulsions' should be confined to those occurring solely with fever and should not be applied to fits which occur in young children with an infection of the nervous system such as meningitis.

The typical febrile convulsion is brief, generalized, tonic-clonic in sequence and the body temperature is high. It occurs more frequently when the child is asleep, and the illness which causes the fever is commonly an acute upper respiratory tract infection (Millichap, 1968). The parents almost invariably find the seizure very frightening if they witness it and are apprehensive that the child may be dying. The convulsion is usually single, but repeated ones can occur in the same illness. The attack is followed by sleep as a rule and parents, when asked about the duration of the episode, may give a false impression about its length by including the postictal sleep. This may be important when the clinician is attempting to judge the seriousness of an attack retrospectively.

Raised temperature and the infective agent

The convulsion is more likely to occur when the temperature is rising rapidly, and this situation is associated with the onset of the illness in about half the cases. However, further convulsions are uncommon even though the temperature remains elevated, and this fact casts doubt on the proposition that the fever is primarily or solely responsible for triggering the seizure. The actual rate of the rise in temperature may be the important factor, but the temperature achieved is not thought to be of primary importance. It is possible that fever causes some other change in the young individual which may then be the triggering factor; for example the increased oxygen demand consequent on fever may over-tax the cerebral oxidative mechanisms.

Viral illnesses causing upper respiratory tract infection are perhaps the commonest cause of fever leading to febrile seizures. Wallace and Zealley (1970), in a careful study of children with proven viral illnesses and febrile convulsions, concluded that seizures associated with viral infections were more likely to be long, repeated or focal than were those associated with nonviral illnesses. However, in a similar investigation Stokes et al. (1977) were unable to confirm this observation.

Age dependency

As with so many types of childhood epilepsy febrile convulsions are highly age dependent. The reasons for their relative rarity under six months of age have been discussed in a preceding chapter.

Genetic influence

Individual susceptibility to febrile seizures appears to depend on the transmission of a specific trait by a single autosomal dominant gene (Ounsted, 1971). Family histories of those affected reveal that one-third to one-half of the patients have a relative who has experienced at least one convulsion. When monozygotic twins were studied there was an 80 per cent concordance for febrile seizures (Lennox—Buchthal, 1971). The incidence of this condition in parents and siblings of children with febrile convulsions is approximately 10 per cent.

Sex

The sex of the individual plays an important role in the incidence of febrile seizures. Boys outnumber girls in most series. There are biological differences between the sexes with regard to incidence and age. Taylor and Ounsted (1971) showed that the decline in incidence in males is smooth over the first four years, whereas in girls the decline is sharp and sudden and occurs mainly in the latter part of the second year of life. They explained this phenomenon by the hypothesis of differential cerebral maturation. This theory was based on the fact that as a rule girls mature faster than boys and that this also applies to the process of cerebral maturation. Because the latter process reduces the liability to convulse in response to fever, and perhaps sustain damage thereby, females will be at an advantage by being exposed to this risk for a shorter period of time than boys. Paradoxically, however, those females who do convulse with fever are relatively more prone to serious sequelae because they convulse more frequently at a younger age.

The chronological age at the time of the first seizure is of critical importance as far as sustaining brain damage is concerned because the brain is more vulnerable in the young. Boys certainly experience more febrile seizures than girls but these are spread out over a longer period of time. It is pertinent also at this point to mention the usual unilaterality of brain damage after febrile seizures. Taylor and Ounsted (1971) stressed that complicated febrile seizures damage those territories which are most rapidly acquiring ordered learning. In the first two years the nondominant (normally right) hemisphere is learning visuospatial skills and at the age of two years the emphasis shifts to the dominant (usually left) hemisphere for learning speech and language.

Severity of attack

The severity of a febrile convulsion is its most important feature as far as causing death or permanent damage is concerned, and the duration of the convulsive attack is the main yardstick by which its severity should be measured. Where the convulsive movements last longer than 30 minutes the attack should certainly be judged as severe, and a duration beyond 20 minutes should probably be similarly judged. It should be realized that the term 'status epilepticus' is normally given to a convulsion lasting more than an hour or to a series of convulsions without return of consciousness for the same period of time. In the young, however, the term should probably be applied when the duration exceeds 30 minutes.

Status epilepticus in childhood has been reviewed by Aicardi and Chevrie (1970) who studied 239 patients who were under 15 years of age at the time of the first status. They found that status was an early event in the history of childhood epilepsy with the first attack occurring before three years of age in 75 per cent of their cases. In nearly half the cases a definite cause was implicated, such as meningitis, encephalitis or a severe electrolyte disturbance; but in just short of a third of the cases, where fever was present at the onset, the clinical picture was indistinguishable from a prolonged febrile seizure and the possibilities for permanent brain damage occurring as a consequence of the status were great. Nearly all the episodes of febrile status reported by these authors were in children of less than 18 months of age and were equally divided between those less than and more than 12 months old.

In the series of children with febrile convulsions studied by Lennox—Buchthal (1973) in Denmark, 29 per cent of the fits occurring in children below 13 months were severe, 15 per cent were severe in the age group of 14–17 months, 12 per cent were severe in the age group of 18–36 months and of those occurring in children over three years of age only 9 per cent were severe. Consequently, age is the crucial factor in determining the severity of a febrile convulsion. Girls with severe febrile convulsions usually outnumber boys in the younger age group because of the reasons already given, namely that the peak age of onset for febrile seizures occurs earlier in girls. Multiple convulsions in the same febrile illness, which are also potentially brain damaging, are also commoner in the younger patient.

Severe, i.e. prolonged, febrile seizures are particularly likely to be unilateral. Gastaut *et al.* (1960) drew special attention to this fact and Aicardi and Chevrie (1970), in their study of status epilepticus, confirmed that severe seizures are unilateral and made the point that the trained observer in hospital was more likely than the parents to note the predominant unilaterality of the attack.

Gastaut *et al.* (1960) described a syndrome associated with febrile status epilepticus which they called *the HHE syndrome (i.e. a condition of hemiconvulsions, hemiplegia and later epilepsy*). They reviewed 150 cases that had severe prolonged and mainly unilateral convulsions in a setting of fever, mainly occurring in children under two years of age. The condition was frequently followed by a permanent hemiplegia and by evidence of more extensive brain damage which manifested itself as mental handicap and later epilepsy. They also described acute pathological findings of venous congestion, vascular thrombosis and massive cerebral oedema with later evidence of cortical atrophy which was demonstrated by pneumoencephalography.

Isler (1971) also studied the HHE syndrome and commented that the incidence of later epilepsy might be reduced considerably by prolonged prophylactic anticonvulsant treatment. This may be an example of the prevention of the so-called 'kindling' effect which is described later in the chapter on post-traumatic epilepsy (Chapter 13).

The increasing use of CT scanning should enable clinicians to learn more about the HHE syndrome. The problems presented by the postictal neurological defect will be discussed later in the section on temporal lobe epilepsy (*see* Chapter 10).

The exact micropathology is still far from clear. Presumably in the milder benign and transitory postictal hemiparesis (*Todd's paralysis*) vasospasm is mainly responsible, while in the irreversible postictal hemiplegic cases compression and occlusion of cerebral arteries by cerebral oedema occur. Once again the duration of the seizure seems to be a crucial factor. The severe febrile seizure is distinguished from the 'benign' febrile seizure by its duration and the consequent brain damage. The evidence is now overwhelming that severe febrile convulsions cause brain damage and various chronic brain syndromes including later epilepsy. The major importance of febrile convulsions in the natural history of childhood epilepsy is evident once this point is grasped. It should be possible to make a major contribution to the prevention of later epilepsy by the effective treatment and prevention of febrile convulsions. One of the problems in this particular area is that the most severe febrile convulsions occur in the very young and the very first seizure is often the most severe. Even when the first attack is mild a subsequent one may be severe. Indeed, as has already been mentioned, convulsions greater than 30 minutes in duration occurred in nearly 30 per cent of Lennox–Buchthal's series when the children were aged 13 months or less at the time of the illness. After any type of initial attack the overall recurrence rate is about 25–50 per cent under the age of three years, and this figure is greater the younger the child. About one in five of subsequent seizures is severe.

Classification

Livingston (1954) distinguished between what he called 'simple febrile convulsions' (by which he meant brief generalized seizures with no clinical or laboratory evidence of cerebral infection or intoxication) and what he termed 'epileptic seizures precipitated by fever' or 'atypical febrile convulsions', which were usually prolonged and often focal or lateralized and were frequently followed by later epilepsy. Livingston (1972) agreed that children with simple febrile convulsions showed strong hereditary tendencies to convulse with fever and cited a family history of 'simple febrile convulsions' in 58 per cent of his series. He also stated that a hereditary factor was found in only 3 per cent of cases of 'epileptic seizures precipitated by fever'. The implication was that the latter group of children had already sustained some brain injury producing an epileptogenic lesion and that they were, in fact, epileptics from the start. Furthermore, in his series, 93 per cent of the atypical febrile seizure patients later developed spontaneous epilepsy while in the benign or simple group the incidence was only 3 per cent. Similarly, of those who developed afebrile seizures later 97 per cent did so by the age of five years.

Livingston's division of febrile seizures in this way is widely accepted in the USA but it has been challenged by others, particularly in Europe. Lennox–Buchthal (1973) maintains that the major difference between febrile convulsions that remain benign and those that presage later epilepsy is related to the severity and the number of convulsions, to the age of onset and antecedent brain injury and possibly to the sex of the patient. Antecedent brain injury, usually perinatal, increases the likelihood of febrile convulsions occurring and also makes severe convulsions more probable and later epilepsy more frequent.

Wallace (1976), who has made major contributions to the understanding of febrile convulsions in recent years, has suggested that the syndrome of febrile convulsions should include more than age, fever and individual susceptibility. She has presented evidence that children who convulse with fever have an increased incidence of factors associated with suboptimal neurological development and has suggested that a convulsion in a febrile child draws attention to a developmental defect. She claims that minor defects or deviations from normal in the acquisition of skills are commonly apparent before the first fit, and most reported series contain a greater number of seriously disabled children than would be expected in the general population. Long-term neurological findings in most cases, she states, probably reflect the preseizure state while about 5 per cent of the total appear to acquire new abnormalities as a result of the illness associated with the fit. She also states that mental retardation is .generally commoner in this particular group of children than one would expect in an unselected group without febrile seizures, while others in the group score unevenly on later psychological testing, even though their intelligence is within the normal range. She feels that such an intellectual deficit may precede rather than result from the initial or subsequent convulsions.

Prognosis

What then is the prognosis for children who suffer febrile convulsions ? They can certainly convulse to death in a febrile status epilepticus but this is relatively rare today. Serious and widespread neurological damage may follow prolonged seizures as in the HHE syndrome. The possibilities for damage to the medial areas of the temporal lobes will be discussed in Chapter 10. The cerebellum and thalamus may also be damaged. The prognosis depends very much on the severity of the individual attack, on the age when it occurs and on the possibility of recurrent seizures of which a fifth will be severe. The child's age, sex and family history can be clues to the possibility of recurrence. If a child is female and under 13 months at the time of the first attack there is a better than 50 per cent chance of a recurrence. However, if the child is male and the same age there is approximately a 30 per cent chance. Between 14 months and three years of age the family history rather than the sex appears to play the important role in determining the rate of recurrence: about 50 per cent will experience recurrence if there is a family history of febrile convulsions, but only 25 per cent will undergo recurrence in the absence of such a history. The severity of the subsequent seizure will depend on the age of the child: the younger the child the greater the chance. A prolonged initial seizure is more likely to be followed by a sustained later seizure. The overall risk that a child who has had one febrile convulsion will have a severe one subsequently is just over 4 per cent, but the risk ranges from nearly 30 per cent in infants of 13 months and younger to 1.4 per cent in children over three years of age (Lennox– Buchthal, 1973).

Most parents will want to know what are the chances of their child developing *later epilepsy*. There are no completely reliable criteria for answering this question. The duration of the seizure is important: long (i.e. over 20–30 minutes) or focal convulsions increase the risk of later epilepsy considerably, and repeated febrile convulsions are also signifi-cant in this respect. A history of antecedent brain injury is also pertinent. An earlier age of onset is important because the chance of a severe seizure is greater the younger the child. The persistence of focal slow waves in the EEG may be followed by the appearance of a persistent spike focus later indicating local brain damage and the possibility, but not the certainty of later epilepsy, because even these later EEG abnor-malities can be transient.

The difficulty in assessing prognosis with respect to later epilepsy is due to the fact that any study which purports to do so must include all the cases of seizures, both mild and severe, occurring at home and in children admitted to hospital. Van der Berg and Yerushalmy (1969), who attempted to do this in California, found a rate of subsequent epilepsy of only 3 per cent of the patients. Frantzen (1971) followed-up 208 children for several years and found an incidence of later epilepsy of less than 2 per cent, but she commented that about a third of the children had behavioural problems, difficulties in concentration and some degree of mental handicap or delayed speech development. These findings are reminiscent of those of Wallace (1976) which are described above. Wallace (1977) reported a series of consecutive hospital admis-sions of children aged between two months and seven years at the time of the initial seizure (a febrile convulsion was defined as any convulsion occurring with any febrile illness). Among the 112 patients successfully followed-up 55 were aged less than 19 months at the time of the first seizure and 75 had had a complicated initial seizure, that is a prolonged or repeated generalized convulsion or one with focal features. At least one spontaneous seizure occurred in 17 per cent of those followed-up for several years and 12 per cent of the patients had recurrent afebrile seizures or epilepsy. Persistent major epilepsy, usually generalized epilepsy of the grand mal type, was commoner in those who had had perinatal problems or a preceding neurodevelopmental abnormality and in those of a lower social class, while prolonged unilateral seizures were more likely to be followed by temporal lobe epilepsy.

Therefore, while all are agreed that children who have had one or more febrile seizure are more likely to become epileptic later, there is disagreement concerning the magnitude of the risk. Perhaps the most important attempt to resolve these apparent differences of opinion has been the prospective study of Nelson and Ellenberg (1976) based on the Collaborative Perinatal Project of the National Institute of Neurological and Communicative Disorders and Stroke in the USA. Out of a total sample of 54 000 children 1706 had had febrile convulsions and were examined for risk factors leading to the development of afebrile seizures, both isolated or recurrent, by the age of seven years (by this time the great majority of the children who were going to develop epilepsy as a consequence of earlier febrile seizures would have done so). In this study a child was considered to have had a febrile convulsion if the first seizure experienced was accompanied by fever, occurred between the ages of one month and seven years and was not symptomatic of a recognized acute neurological illness such as meningitis, encephalitis or encephalopathy. They divided febrile seizures into those that were uncomplicated and those that had complex features. Characteristics referred to as complex features were a seizure of greater duration than 15 minutes, the occurrence of more than a single seizure within 24 hours and focal features. They also compared those children with febrile seizures whose developmental status had been normal prior to the time of the first seizure with those where it had been suspect or definitely abnormal. Later epilepsy was defined as the occurrence of recurrent afebrile seizures, not symptomatic of an acute neurological illness, of which at least one attack occurred after four years of age.

Nelson and Ellenberg (1976) found that of the 39 179 children in the Collaborative Perinatal Project who had never had a febrile seizure and were followed-up until seven years of age, epilepsy developed in 0.5 per cent. Of the sample studied with febrile seizures and followed-up to the same age 65 per cent never had a subsequent seizure after the initial attack, and 32 per cent had one or more attack of febrile convulsions but no afebrile seizures. They also found that at least one asymptomatic afebrile seizure had occurred by the age of seven years in 52 children (3 per cent) and in 34 of these patients (2 per cent of the total) recurrent asymptomatic afebrile seizures developed, that is 2 per cent of the group were epileptic by seven years of age. However, in children whose first or subsequent febrile seizures had any complex features, they found that the risk of developing epilepsy by the age of seven years increased to 4.1 per cent with the greatest risk occurring in those whose febrile seizures had focal features. Children with febrile seizures whose developmental status prior to the occurrence of any seizure was other than normal were found to be three times more likely to be epileptic by the age of seven years when compared with children who were normal on developmental screening prior to the first febrile convulsion. Similarly, children with complex febrile seizures and a previously abnormal developmental status were eight times more likely to develop epilepsy by the age of seven years than were previously normal children with uncomplicated febrile seizures and they were also 18 times more likely to develop epilepsy than were children who had never had any febrile seizure. This study also confirmed the earlier observation that the great majority of afebrile seizures developed within three years of the first febrile seizure. It seems to the author that this outstanding study goes a long way towards resolving many of the controversial problems concerning risk factors and prognosis for later epilepsy in children who have febrile convulsions in infancy and early childhood.

Diagnosis

The diagnosis of a febrile seizure is relatively easy. The importance of not overlooking the possibility of meningitis as a cause does not require emphasis. Occasionally, at least in the author's experience, Reye's syndrome or encephalopathy with fatty degeneration of the viscera can mislead when a convulsion is the presenting feature. The rapid development of coma, hyperpnoea and hyperpyrexia should suggest the correct diagnosis and laboratory evidence of hypoglycaemia, hyperammonaemia and rising liver enzyme levels in the serum will usually help to confirm the diagnosis.

EEG examination is of very limited value in the diagnosis and assessment of the child with a febrile seizure. More than 80 per cent of the children with this condition show marked slowing in the record within the first 24 hours and a third of the children show slowing, usually posteriorly, after five days. The slowing is often asymmetrical, particularly after predominantly unilateral attacks. The significance of persisting abnormalities has already been mentioned. Severe unilateral changes are found in the HHE syndrome and may be followed by a flattening of the EEG on the same side and the appearance of unilateral spike discharges (*Figure 6.1*). Spike-wave paroxysms may also appear in children who have had febrile convulsions, particularly after the age of

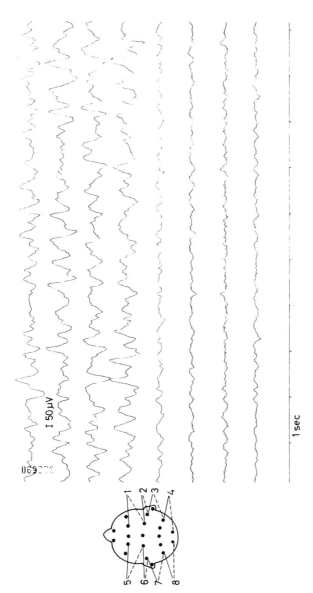

Figure 6.1. Female child aged 19 months and awake with eyes closed. EEG in HHE syndrome showing high-voltage irregular slow-wave activity on the right side

three years and especially in those with a family history of epilepsy and they do not necessarily indicate the later development of epilepsy of the primary generalized (petit mal) type. However, petit mal may follow an earlier history of febrile convulsions in a small number of patients, probably because the two conditions are related on a genetic basis rather than because of any damage resulting from the early seizures. Further reference will be made to the significance of paroxysmal abnormalities in the EEG in Chapter 21.

Therapy

Most febrile convulsions are very brief and are over long before medical help arrives. Repeated convulsions within the same febrile illness are unusual. It is important to remember that sudden vomiting may follow any seizure, however brief, and so the child should be turned on to his side in the recumbent posture in order to prevent aspiration of vomitus. Cooling of the febrile child is of vital importance when seizures threaten or have occurred, and tepid sponging, the use of a fan, if available, and exposing the body so that heat loss can take place are all important. The urge to wrap the child in blankets should be resisted. Antipyretic drugs such as salicylates or paracetamol should be given (e.g. aspirin 60 mg/year of age or paracetamol elixir 62.5–125 mg four hourly). Antibiotics may be required for bacterial infections.

STATUS EPILEPTICUS AND ITS TREATMENT

The treatment of the severe prolonged convulsion is of great importance (*Table 6.1*). A severe continuous seizure or repeated fits with incomplete recovery of consciousness constitute *status epilepticus*. Any such convulsive episode lasting longer than 20–30 minutes may be potentially brain damaging and even life threatening. Young children are at much greater risk of sustaining brain damage in status epilepticus than adults and may do so after a shorter duration of status. During continuous epileptic activity the brain needs a greatly increased supply of oxygen which is not likely to be forthcoming unless the blood flow to the brain increases very significantly. A state of so-called 'consumptive anoxia' then develops in the brain. The increased body temperature, due to the precipitating illness and resulting from the generalized convulsive movements, leads to an increase in the body's metabolism and, in addition, the convulsing muscles utilize increased amounts of oxygen. As the increased demands for oxygen generally outstrip the supply some tissues commence anaerobic respiration. An initial rise in the blood glucose

TABLE 6.1
Treatment of Status Epilepticus

Anticonvulsant treatment

Drug	Mode	Dose
Diazepam	intravenous	initially 0.3–0.5 mg/(kg BW), repeat after 20–30 minutes if necessary, or 1 mg/year of age + 1 mg
	intramuscular	1 mg/(kg BW)
	per rectum	0.5 mg/(kg BW)
Phenobarbitone (see text)	intravenous/intramuscular	5 mg/(kg BW), give half intravenously and half intramuscularly, repeat intramuscular dose in 30 minutes
Phenytoin (see text)	intravenous	10–15 mg/(kg BW) over 30 minutes, not exceeding 20–50 mg/minute
Paraldehyde (see text)	intramuscular	1 ml/year of age up to 5 ml
	per rectum	0.3 ml/(kg BW) in an equal volume of mineral oil
Clonazepam	intravenous or by drip	0.05 mg/(kg BW)
Lignocaine	intravenous	4 mg/(kg BW.hour) for 24–48 hours, then reduce dose

Special care and general measures

Cool patient
Maintain airway
Supply oxygen
Reduce brain swelling: intravenous mannitol 0.5–1.5 g/(kg BW) over 10–30 minutes, repeated 8-hourly (total dose of 6 g/(kg BW.24 hours)
intravenous dexamethasone 2–4 mg initially followed by 1–2 mg six hourly, or 0.5 mg/(kg BW.24 hours)
Treat hypertension/hypotension (see text)
Treat biochemical disturbances (acid-base balance etc.)
Treat infection

level is later followed by a fall. The arterial PO_2 drops, a systemic metabolic acidosis develops and the blood lactate concentration rises. Also, increased levels of lactate and pyruvate may be found in the cerebrospinal fluid (Simpson, Habel and George, 1977). An early sharp rise in systemic blood pressure is later followed by a fall. Circulatory collapse may occur or the child may survive and suffer from permanent brain damage (Brown and Sills, 1977). There may be laminar destruction of neurones in the cortex, the thalamus and cerebellum may suffer damage and, most important of all, the hippocampus may be damaged with extensive neuronal loss followed by later atrophy and gliosis. Falconer, Serafetinides and Corsellis (1964) coined the term 'mesial temporal sclerosis' to describe the last change.

Clinically the effects of a prolonged seizure may be only transient if the convulsion is terminated. A short-lived hemiparesis (Todd's paralysis) may be observed. Irreversible changes in the brain may occasionally manifest themselves in the form of the disastrous HHE syndrome, described above. Acute cerebral oedema may result in acute brain shifts and coning. Also, herniation through the tentorial opening may be clinically evident by the development of decerebrate rigidity and the failure to recover consciousness (Brown and Habel, 1975).

It is mandatory, therefore, to stop the convulsions as soon as possible. There is no excuse for sending the still convulsing child over a long distance to hospital by ambulance. Time is of the essence if brain damage or even death is to be prevented. There is general agreement that diazepam intravenously is the drug of choice in this emergency in children. The initial bolus should not be less than 0.3 mg/(kg BW) (some have used up to 0.5 mg/(kg BW). If the child's weight cannot be measured easily it is safe to give 1 mg/year of age plus 1 mg (e.g. at two years give 3 mg intravenously). The drug should be injected at the rate of 1 mg/minute. The use of a 1-ml tuberculin syringe facilitates the slow administration of small doses. Because free diazepam disappears rapidly from the circulation it may be necessary to repeat the injection after 20–30 minutes if full control is not achieved.

A problem arises when diazepam must be given at home by the general practitioner who, quite reasonably, may not wish to attempt an intravenous injection in a small convulsing child. The drug is, unfortunately, slowly absorbed from the intramuscular site, although intramuscular injections of not less than 1 mg/(kg BW) will produce effective blood levels in 15–30 minutes (Aicardi, 1978). An alternative method of administration is to inject the drug into the rectum using the intravenous preparation and a disposable plastic syringe fitted with a short piece of rubber or plastic tubing. The disposable plastic sheath which normally protects the needle may be conveniently employed after first removing the needle and then snipping off the ends of the sheath with sharp scissors. Rectal injection is easy, harmless to the mucosa and, using a dose of 0.5 mg/(kg BW), produces an effective blood level in a matter of 10 minutes or less (Agurell *et al.*, 1975). Parents can be shown how to perform this manoeuvre in the event of a later febrile seizure and can be provided with a pack containing syringes, ampoules of diazepam and so on for use at home.

The main hazard with intravenous diazepam is the possibility of producing respiratory arrest. This is more likely to happen when the drug is used with phenobarbitone or when the child has previously been on continuous phenobarbitone prophylaxis. However, the risks of producing respiratory arrest in these situations is slight if caution is observed during the intravenous administration of diazepam. If apnoea does occur it is usually only transitory and oxygenation can be maintained by using an Ambu bag or a similar device. Phenobarbitone itself is a poor weapon for treating status epilepticus in children because even when it is given intravenously in a high dosage (5–10 mg/(kg BW), it may take up to one hour to produce an effective therapeutic blood level. When it is given intramuscularly up to four hours may elapse before a satisfactory therapeutic level is attained. There is also the added risk of gradual accumulation of the drug when large doses are used over a period of days. However, many will be tempted to use phenobarbitone in intractable status epilepticus, particularly in the intensive therapy situation when adequate monitoring and ventilatory assistance are available. It may be given in an initial dose of 5 mg/(kg BW), giving half of the dose slowly intravenously and the other half intramuscularly and repeating the intramuscular dose after 30 minutes (Weiner, Bresnan and Levitt, 1977). Blood level monitoring should be employed, if available, and maintenance doses can then be determined by the levels attained.

Phenytoin has also been used intravenously in large doses, particularly in the USA. The dosage employed is 10–15 mg/(kg BW) over approximately 30 minutes at a rate not exceeding 25–50 mg/minute (Weiner, Bresnan and Levitt, 1977). Phenytoin should be used with caution in children with heart disease because there is a possible risk of producing arrhythmias. The maximum intravenous dose at any age in childhood should not exceed 1000 mg. For administration the drug should first be dissolved in its own diluent: this takes a little time and may be hastened by warming the vial. It is then given by slow injection into a saline-containing drip tube. If it is given in dextrose and water it precipitates almost immediately, and if it is placed in a burette of saline it begins to precipitate after 10–15 minutes. Intravenous phenytoin achieves peak blood concentrations in approximately 15 minutes when given intravenously in this manner. Intramuscular phenytoin is not absorbed any faster than by the oral route; moreover, it tends to crystallize in muscle. When the treatment is commenced by the intravenous route maintenance doses may be continued orally (6 mg/(kg· day)). It is important to monitor blood serum levels of the drug when these large intravenous doses are employed.

Paraldehyde, given intramuscularly in a dosage of 1 ml/year of age up to a maximum dose of 5 ml, appears to be achieving a return to favour as it no longer has a deleterious effect on modern plastic syringes. It can, however, produce tissue necrosis if given subcutaneously in error and this can sometimes happen following an intramuscular injection into the lateral thigh muscles, particularly in a thin or wasted child. It should not be given as a bolus intravenously because it can cause phlebitis, but it has been used in very dilute intravenous infusions; however, even this method is not generally recommended. It may also be given rectally in a dosage of 0.3 ml/(kg BW) mixed with an equal volume of mineral oil. The dosage should not exceed 5 ml in a young child and may be repeated after an hour. Paraldehyde should be used with caution in children with pulmonary disease since it is mainly excreted through the lungs.

Therefore, diazepam is still the drug of choice in this emergency. When seizures continue to recur, despite its immediate administration, diazepam may be continued in an intravenous infusion well diluted with dextrose saline. The electrolyte solution containing the drug should be changed at intervals not exceeding six hours because the drug tends to precipitate gradually over a period of time. Another benzodiazepine derivative, clonazepam, has also been used for the emergency treatment of a prolonged seizure in a dosage of 0.05 mg/(kg BW), and it can be given by continuous infusion if required. It probably has no significant advantages over diazepam when used as an emergency medication in this way. Intravenous short-acting barbiturates such as thiopentone have been administered in the treatment of status epilepticus in adults (Brown and Horton, 1967), but they require careful supervision by an anaesthetist. Recently, chlormethiazole, a sedative/hypnotic drug derived from the thiazole part of the vitamin B_1 molecule, has been shown to have an anticonvulsant effect and has been widely used in the treatment of delirium tremens in adults. It is also being tried in the treatment of status epilepticus, but experience in children is very limited. Ingrid Gamstorp advocates the use of lignocaine in the treatment of repeated seizures in the neonate. She uses the intravenous preparation devised for use in cardiology. The usual starting dose is 4 mg/(kg BW·hour) for 24—48 hours, followed by a gradual reduction in dosage over a period of days if and when the convulsions come under control. She claims good results in the newborn and did not experience problems with respiratory depression (Gamstorp, 1970).

Apart from the administration of anticonvulsant drugs, general measures play a most important part in the care of the convulsing child.

It is vital to maintain an adequate airway: the child should be nursed in the semiprone posture, and ideally a simple airway should be inserted and the upper respiratory tract sucked clear of secretions. If an airway is not available extension of the neck and elevation of the jaw will suffice to prevent obstruction by the tongue. It is essential to ensure an adequate supply of well oxygenated blood to the brain and accordingly oxygen should be administed to the patient. If cerebral oedema develops the Cushing effect (a rise in the systemic blood pressure secondary to a rise in the intracranial pressure) may occur and very high levels of systolic and diastolic blood pressure may be recorded. Serious hypertensive changes may develop in the retinae, including haemorrhages. Brown and Habel (1975) recommend reserpine, frusemide or, preferably, intravenous diazoxide for this complication. The later development of hypotension may require the use of drugs to elevate the blood pressure.

Prolonged status epilepticus should ideally be managed in an intensive therapy unit where modern electronic monitoring equipment and special nursing care are available. Cooling of the patient by every means possible is essential since hyperthermia commonly develops as the convulsions continue. The obtundation and coma which characteristically accompany or follow status epilepticus, and which are a consequence of acute cerebral oedema or brain swelling, may be rapidly relieved by the use of intravenous mannitol (0.5–1.5 g/kg over 10–30 minutes and repeated at 8-hourly intervals if necessary). This drug should also be given when the child shows evidence of developing the typical posture of decerebrate rigidity. Simultaneously with the mannitol, which acts rapidly, intravenous dexamethasone may be given in an initial dose of 2–4 mg followed by 1–2 mg intravenously at 6-hourly intervals, depending on the age of the patient. Dexamethasone takes approximately 12 hours to exert an effect in reducing cerebral oedema.

The use of these drugs in status epilepticus may help to prevent or reduce the incidence and severity of brain damage and, by reducing cerebral oedema, they may also act indirectly as anticonvulsants by interrupting the self-perpetuating convulsive mechanism produced by the brain swelling consequent on status epilepticus.

Finally, it is salutary to remember that more deaths have probably been caused by the overtreatment of status epilepticus than by undertreatment, and constant re-evaluation of the regimen being employed and its effects on the patient should be made (see Table 6.1).

Prevention

One of the most controversial questions in paediatrics today is whether further febrile convulsions can be prevented and how this can best be achieved. Unfortunately, the first febrile seizure is often the most severe and damaging and enlightened vigorous treatment of the attack is the best one can hope for at present.

Formerly, intermittent anticonvulsants were advised but they were usually ineffective because the seizure generally occurred during the rapid rise of temperature and not when the fever had been established for some hours. Furthermore, adequate blood levels of circulating anti-convulsants could not be achieved for at least several days when either oral phenobarbitone or phenytoin was prescribed in the usual doses. The alternatives are to give no medication or to use continuous anti-convulsant prophylaxis.

The definitive study in prophylaxis is probably that of Faerø et al. (1972) which demonstrated that phenobarbitone had a significant effect in preventing febrile convulsions provided an adequate serum level was achieved. The dosage schedule employed was 6 mg/(kg BW·day) for two days followed by 3–4 mg/(kg BW·day) in divided doses. Heckmatt et al. (1976), using the same regimen, were unable to show that pheno-barbitone prophylaxis had a significant effect in preventing further febrile convulsions even though the rate of recurrence was lower than in their controls. However, in a very careful 5-year study involving 355 children in Southern California, who were seen after their first febrile convulsion had been experienced, it was found that no significant dif-ference in the recurrence rate occurred in children receiving intermittent phenobarbitone when compared with those receiving no phenobarbitone, but it was found that the recurrence rate in children receiving daily phenobarbitone was significantly decreased when compared with either of the other two groups (Wolf et al., 1977). Severe recurrent febrile seizures did not occur in the children on daily phenobarbitone. Parental resistance, poor compliance and side-effects from the drug were the main problems encountered in the group on continuous prophylaxis.

Unfortunately, phenobarbitone, although cheap and apparently effective, is prone to cause side-effects in approximately a third to a half of the young children taking it regularly. These include irritability, hyperactivity and sleeplessness. Aggressiveness may also occur and is seen with primidone too. There have also been suggestions that pheno-barbitone may interfere with the learning process during critical periods of rapid learning. In an attempt to reduce the incidence of side-effects Lennox–Buchthal recommended the slow introduction of the drug over a period of 3–4 weeks and the administration of a single dose of 5 mg/(kg BW) at bedtime only.

The use of phenytoin in prophylaxis has been studied by Melchior, Buchthal and Lennox–Buchthal (1971), and they found that it was ineffective in preventing recurrences of febrile seizures even though, when used in a dosage of 4–6 mg/(kg BW·day), it made severe recurrences less likely. Primidone (10–20 mg/kg BW· day) has also been used and carbamazepine and sodium valproate are currently on trial as prophylactics.

Although many view with dismay the prospect of large numbers of small children on phenobarbitone, it is generally accepted that prophylaxis works both in the short term and the long term, and that the prevention of long-lasting febrile convulsions is likely to reduce the incidence of serious and chronic epilepsy in later life. Controversy revolves around the question of whether all children with febrile convulsions should have prophylaxis and around the problem of the duration of therapy. The majority would accept that *prophylaxis is indicated for the high-risk groups* which may be defined as follows:

1. All children having their first convulsion at or under 13 months of age, particularly girls
2. All children aged 14–36 months with a positive family history of febrile convulsions in parents and siblings
3. If the initial seizure is prolonged or leads into repeated convulsions
4. Where the initial seizure is lateralized or followed by a Todd's paralysis
5. After more than two febrile seizures have occurred although other factors, such as the child's age, may be relevant
6. Possibly, if the initial febrile seizure was associated with a proven viral illness.

Some would recommend prophylaxis for all, irrespective of age or type of initial attack. Many would give prophylaxis to all those having the initial seizure under two years of age. Over two years of age the risks of a subsequent severe seizure diminish, particularly in girls, and they are negligible over the age of three years.

The *duration of therapy* is also hotly debated. Most authorities would agree on a minimum period of six months after the initial attack and until the age of two years at least in boys and girls. Others advise continuation of therapy until the age of three years, particularly in the high-risk groups. Some even advocate therapy until the age of five years.

It should be realized that the problem of febrile convulsions is central to the whole question of epilepsy in early childhood and that it has very important implications for the problems of epilepsy in later childhood, adolescence and adult life. A major issue at present is whether the prolonged and damaging febrile seizures are really the same as other uncomplicated febrile convulsions, and whether measures to prevent the former should also be used to prevent the latter. There is also the difficult problem that, in the majority of cases, the most severe attack is the initial one and it may reasonably be asked whether prophylaxis should be extended to protect those at risk on the basis of a positive family history. Heckmatt *et al.* (1976) considered that a strong case could be made for improving the organization of emergency medical services to allow early termination of all continuing convulsions and that arguments about prophylaxis should not be allowed to take consideration over the paramount problem of emergency treatment of the initial seizure. In any event the vast amount of detailed thought and study which this very common problem in childhood is currently receiving in many countries will surely provide answers to these questions within the very near future.

REFERENCES

Agurell, S., Berlin, A., Ferngran, H. and Hellstrom, B. (1975). 'Plasma levels of diazepam after parenteral and rectal administration in children.' *Epilepsia*, **16**, 277–283
Aicardi, J. (1978). Personal communication
Aicardi, J. and Chevrie, J. J. (1970). 'Convulsive status epilepticus in infants and children. A study of 239 cases.' *Epilepsia*, **11**, 187–197
Brown, A. S. and Horton, J. M. (1967). 'Status epilepticus treated by intravenous infusions of thiopentone sodium.' *Br. Med. J.* **1**, 27–28
Brown, J. K. and Habel, A. H. (1975). 'Toxic encephalopathy and acute brain-swelling in children.' *Devl Med. child Neurol.* **17**, 659–679
Brown, J. K. and Sills, J. A. (1977). 'Status epilepticus.' *J. Mat. Child Health*, **2**, 383–389
Faerø, O., Kastrup, K. W., Lykkegaard Nielsen, E., Melchior, J. C. and Thorn, I. (1972). 'Successful prophylaxis of febrile convulsions with phenobarbital.' *Epilepsia*, **13**, 279–285
Falconer, M. A., Serafetinides, E. A. and Corsellis, J. A. N. (1964). 'Etiology and pathogenesis of temporal lobe epilepsy.' *Archs Neurol., Chicago*, **10**, 233–248
Frantzen, E. (1971). 'The prognosis of febrile convulsions.' *Epilepsia*, **12**, 192
Gamstorp, I. (1970). *Pediatric Neurology*, pp. 93–94. New York: Appleton-Century-Crofts, Educational Division/Meredith Corporation
Gastaut, H., Poirier, F., Payan, H., Salamon, G., Toga, M. and Vigouroux, M. (1960). 'HHE Syndrome. Hemiconvulsions, hemiplegia, epilepsy.' *Epilepsia*, **1**, 418–447
Heckmatt, J. Z., Houston, A. B., Clow, D. J., Stephenson, J. B. P., Dodd, K. L., Lealman, G. T. and Logan, R. W. (1976). 'Failure of phenobarbitone to prevent febrile convulsions.' *Br. Med. J.* **1**, 559–561
Isler, W. (1971). *Clinics in Developmental Medicine, Nos 41–42: Acute Hemiplegias and Hemisyndromes in Childhood*, p. 132. London: Spastics International and Heinemann
Lennox–Buchthal, M. A. (1971). 'Febrile and nocturnal convulsions in monozygotic twins.' *Epilepsia*, **12**, 147–156
Lennox–Buchthal, M. A. (1973). 'Febrile convulsions: a reappraisal.' *Electroenceph. clin. Neurophysiol.* Suppl. 32
Livingston, S. (1954). *The Diagnosis and Treatment of Convulsive Disorders in Children*. Springfield Illinois: Charles C. Thomas
Livingston, S. (1972). *Comprehensive Management of Epilepsy in Infancy, Childhood and Adolescence*. Springfield Illinois: Charles C. Thomas

Melchior, J. C., Buchthal, F. and Lennox–Buchthal, M. A. (1971). 'The ineffective-ness of diphenylhydantoin in preventing febrile convulsions in the age of greatest risk, under three years.' *Epilepsia*, **12**, 55–62

Millichap, J. G. (1968). *Febrile Convulsions*. New York: Macmillan

Nelson, K. B. and Ellenberg, J. H. (1976). 'Predictors of epilepsy in children who have experienced febrile convulsions.' *New Engl. J. Med.* **295**, 1029–1033

Ounsted, C. (1971). 'Some aspects of seizure disorders.' In *Recent Advances in Paediatrics*, pp. 363–400. Eds D. Gairdner and D. Hull. London: J. and A. Churchill

Simpson, H., Habel, A. H. and George, E. L. (1977). 'Cerebrospinal fluid acid-base status and lactate and pyruvate concentrations after convulsions of varied duration and aetiology in children.' *Archs Dis. Child.* **52**, 844–849

Stokes, M. J., Downham, M. A. P. S., Webb, J. K. G., McQuillin, J. and Gardner, P. S. (1977). 'Viruses and febrile convulsions.' *Archs Dis. Child.* **52**, 129–133

Taylor, D. C. and Ounsted, C. (1971). 'Biological mechanisms influencing the out-come of seizures in response to fever.' *Epilepsia*, **12**, 33–45

Van den Berg, B. J. and Yerushalmy, J. (1969). 'Studies on convulsive disorders in young children, 1: Incidence of febrile and non-febrile convulsion by age and other factors.' *Pediat. Res.* **3**, 298–304

Wallace, S. J. (1976). 'Neurological and intellectual deficits: convulsions with fever viewed as acute indications of life-long developmental defects.' In *Brain Dysfunction in Infantile Febrile Convulsions*, pp. 259–277. Eds M. A. B. Brazier and F. Coceani. New York: Raven Press

Wallace, S. J. (1977). 'Spontaneous fits after convulsions with fever.' *Archs Dis. Child.* **52**, 192–196

Wallace, S. J. and Zealley, H. (1970). 'Neurological, electroencephalographic, and virological findings in febrile children.' *Archs Dis. Child.* **45**, 611–623

Wolf, S. M., Carr, A., Davis, D., Davidson, S., Dale, E. P., Forsythe, A., Goldenberg, E. D., Hanson, R., Lulejian, G. A., Nelson, M. A., Treitman, P. and Weinstein, A. (1977). 'The value of phenobarbital in a child who has had a single febrile seizure: A controlled prospective study.' *Pediatrics*, **59**, 378–385

Weiner, H. L., Bresnan, M. J. and Levitt, L. P. (1977). *Pediatric Neurology for the House Officer*, pp. 47–49. Baltimore: Williams and Wilkins

CHAPTER 7

Primary Generalized Epilepsy (Petit Mal)

As already discussed, the *International Classification* (Gastaut, 1970) recognized primary generalized seizures as being generalized clinically from the start of each individual attack, as usually making their initial appearance during childhood or early adolescence and as not usually being associated with neurological or psychological evidence of cerebral pathology between attacks. The most important members of this group are primary major tonic-clonic epilepsy (grand mal), typical absence attacks (petit mal) and massive bilateral myoclonic epilepsy of the primary type. In all of these there is usually a lack of a clear-cut aetiology, suggesting that they are essentially dependent upon a hereditary predisposition which is sufficiently pronounced to render slight metabolic problems or slight acquired cerebral lesions epileptogenic.

Terminology

The term 'petit mal' is perhaps the most misused in epileptology. Historically this is understandable because it was originally used as a general term and it was only later that it became condensed into a unitary concept of a particular type of attack. Hughlings Jackson, in his many papers on epilepsy written in the last quarter of the nineteenth century, introduced distinguishing terminology for automatisms and seizures of temporal lobe origin, and gradually the term petit mal came to refer to a particular kind of seizure occurring predominantly in children. In recent years the old term 'absence' has regained popularity as a more vivid and precise description of the attack than 'petit mal'. The word 'absence' was used originally to describe brief attacks of intellectual eclipse.

Characteristics of the petit mal absence

This is usually associated with an interruption of consciousness, it is of sudden onset and termination and is commonest in females between 5–12 years of age. The attacks are frequent, are usually precipitated by hyperventilation and are rarely associated with mental retardation or structural brain damage. Petit mal is likely to respond to certain specific drugs and the prognosis is good. As a rule there is a typical EEG pattern.

It is important to realize, however, that the diagnosis of the petit mal absence and its differentiation from other types of absence attacks are not always easy. The absences of the secondary generalized epilepsies of the myoclonic type have been mentioned already and temporal lobe attacks, which give rise to dreamy states or absences of complex symptomatology, are often preceded by unusual or bizarre auras and will be described in Chapter 10. Temporal lobe absences are often associated with or terminate in gestural and oral automatisms including plucking at clothes, chewing, lip smacking and swallowing, and it is a common clinical observation that children having true petit mal absences may have similar motor and oral automatisms. They may, incidentally, also have incontinence of urine which can be extremely embarrassing when attacks are frequent.

EEG patterns

In order to try to understand the reasons for the similarities between the various types of absence attack, it is necessary to say something about both the EEG patterns and the suggested pathophysiology of absences.

Petit mal attacks are associated with bilaterally synchronous and symmetrical paroxysmal activity in the EEG. The paroxysmal activity occurs bilaterally and begins and ends synchronously over both hemispheres. It is symmetrical, that is the discharges have the same shape and amplitude at homologous points in the two hemispheres. The generalized discharges of petit mal (*Figure 7.1*) consist of regular spike and wave complexes occurring at a rate of 3/second (3 Hz). The spike lasts about 100 ms and precedes the wave, but it may only be seen as a small projection on the ascending segment of the wave. During an attack the frequency of the complexes is 3 Hz at the beginning of the discharge and slows to 2.5–2 Hz towards the end. This type of synchronous, symmetrical and rhythmic paroxysmal activity in the EEG is termed

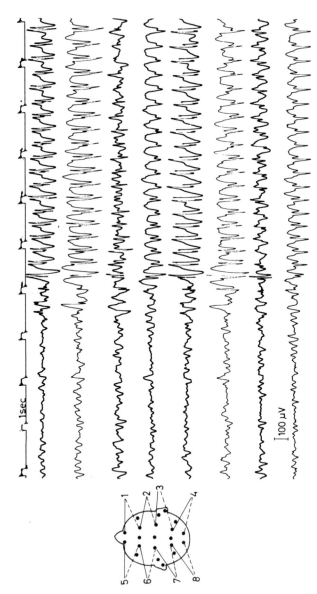

Figure 7.1. Boy aged 11 years and awake with eyes open. EEG shows generalized bilaterally synchronous spike-wave complexes at 3 Hz occurring during hyperventilation

primary bilateral synchrony. In petit mal there is usually a direct temporal relationship between the EEG discharges and the clinical attack, although, of course, the discharges can also occur interictally. It is considered that bursts of spike-wave activity should last at least three seconds to produce some degree of impairment of consciousness or errors in performance, and that automatisms do not usually appear until 20–30 seconds after the onset of the absence.

Theoretical background

The pathogenetic mechanism of the bilaterally synchronous discharges is one of the major problems of epileptology. The classic theory is that of Penfield and Jasper (1954) who proposed that primary bilateral synchrony was produced by a 'pacemaker' situated in the 'centrencephalic system' (by which they meant the central integrating system of the upper part of the brain stem) which is symmetrically connected with both cerebral hemispheres and serves to co-ordinate their function. The alternative hypothesis was that of Gibbs and Gibbs (1952) who proposed that the synchronous discharges primarily arose from the cortex.

The generally accepted theory today derives from the work of Gloor (1968), and in a way it is a composite of the two classic theories described above (*Figure 7.2*). He postulated that the underlying pathophysiological disturbance involved both the cortex and the reticular projection systems of the brain stem and thalamus, and he avoided stressing a primary role for either. He used the term 'disturbance of the cortico-reticular system'. Paroxysmal instability of this system may be genetically determined or result from biochemical upset or may result from diffuse pathological processes involving either the cortex or the brain stem. In pure petit mal absences hereditary factors and biochemical changes (e.g. with hyperventilation) are paramount in causing discharges in the system with primary bilateral synchrony. In diffuse pathological processes involving grey matter in cortical and subcortical structures, Gloor (1968) suggested that a marked focal accentuation of the disease in some area of the cortex, combined perhaps with a hereditary predisposition, may trigger the system leading to what is called 'secondary bilateral synchrony'. Areas of focal disease in the brain may thus assume the role of pacemaker for the system causing secondary generalized epilepsies as a result. Secondary bilateral synchrony may be suspected in the EEG when the paroxysmal activity demonstrates irregular morphology, imperfect symmetry, irregularities of form and synchronization, inconsistencies of frequency and also when the generalized discharges coexist with a focal epileptic abnormality.

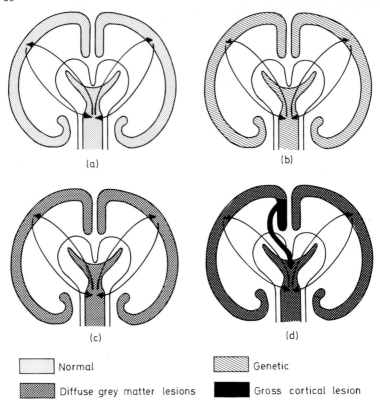

Normal

Genetic

Diffuse grey matter lesions

Gross cortical lesion

Figure 7.2. Diagrammatic representation of conditions that may lead to the appearance of generalized bilaterally synchronous spike and wave discharge.

(a) Normal condition. Stippled areas: the cerebral cortex and the reticular systems of the upper brain stem and thalamus which are mutually interconnected, as indicated by the arrows. It is postulated that under normal conditions controls are operative to prevent the occurrence of generalized paroxysmal discharge within this system.

(b) Genetic form of generalized corticoreticular epilepsy. The hatching of cortex and reticular systems indicates a genetically-determined disturbance in these areas giving rise to generalized spike and wave discharge.

(c) Diffuse organic grey matter disease giving rise to paroxysmal bilaterally synchronous spike and wave discharges. The coarse dots in the cortex and reticular systems signify diffuse lesions of cortical and subcortical grey matter.

(d) 'Secondary bilateral synchrony': a focal cortical lesion in the parasagittal cortex indicated in solid black, present in a brain predisposed to produce paroxysmal bilaterally synchronous discharges, either due to genetic factors (hatching) or due to the presence of diffuse cortical and subcortical grey matter lesions (course dots) may serve as a pacemaker triggering generalized bilaterally synchronous spike and wave discharges. (From Prof. P. Gloor, Epilepsia, 1968, by courtesy of Charles C. Thomas, Publishers, Springfield, Illinois)

The concept of diffuse and/or focal disease triggering the cortico-reticular system (described above) offers an explanation for the similarities and differences that exist between the absences of true petit mal, the absences of the myoclonic epilepsies and the absences with complex symptomatology which occur in temporal lobe epilepsy.

THE PETIT MAL ATTACK

In the petit mal absence there is a suppression of or a decrease in mental functioning which starts and ends abruptly. The duration of the attack is usually 5–15 seconds and occasionally they are longer, but they are rarely longer than 30 seconds. Occasionally, a very prolonged fit or petit mal status may occur. Attacks are usually very frequent throughout the day. The patient is seen to stare, the eyes may drift upwards and the eyelids flicker (*Figure 7.3*).

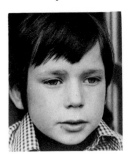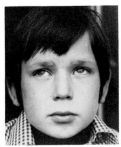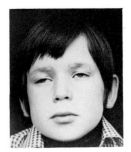

Figure 7.3. Phases of a petit mal attack

The original 'centrencephalic' theory of Penfield and Jasper (1954) postulated that the discharges arose in those parts of the brain regulating consciousness, i.e. the upper brain stem. Consciousness is an awareness of self and environment and depends on more than just the normal functioning of the brain stem, which is primarily concerned with wakefulness. The cortex must also be functioning if one is to be conscious. The mental activity involved in consciousness requires the proper functioning of the cerebral hemispheres. In absence attacks attentiveness, perception, cognition and voluntary motor processes are all impaired and these are all higher cortical functions. However, some automatic motor movements may continue. Children with petit mal attacks have been shown to be impaired on tests of sustained attention (Mirsky and van Buren, 1965), which is an essential part of the learning process. The implications of such impairment are clearly important where school performance is concerned and will be discussed further in Chapter 19.

Gloor (1977) has recently summarized his concept of the petit mal attack by saying that in this condition there is a state of increased excitability of cortical neurones which, for genetic and/or biochemical reasons, makes them, at times, respond to normal thalamocortical volleys by producing spike-wave discharges. On the basis of human experimental evidence, Penry (1977) commented that input or afferent processes appear to be more impaired during spike-wave discharges than are output or efferent processes. There is, as he put it, 'a functional deafferentation', and this may begin a split second before the actual spike-wave complexes start.

No excuses need to be made for dwelling so long on the pathophysiological theories concerning absence attacks. The author is of the opinion that a knowledge of the mechanisms involved is essential for the understanding of many aspects of childhood epilepsy and its problems.

Genetics

The classic studies on the *genetics of petit mal* were those of Lennox (1951, 1960) on twins. Monozygotic twins showed an 84 per cent concordance for spike-wave discharges at 3 Hz in their EEGs and a 75 per cent concordance for petit mal seizures. No dizygotic twins were concordant for petit mal seizures. Approximately one-third of the patients with petit mal had a family history of petit mal or grand mal; the highest incidence (7 per cent and 6 per cent) occurred in siblings and parents (Doose et al., 1973). These authors also found spike waves at rest or during hyperventilation in 20 per cent of the siblings of a large series of patients with petit mal while in controls the incidence did not exceed 3 per cent. They suggested, on the basis of their findings, that several genetic factors were responsible for spike-wave absences. Earlier authors, particularly Metrakos and Metrakos (1961), favoured an autosomal dominant gene with an age-dependent manifestation being responsible.

PROGNOSIS

One of the most controversial questions concerning petit mal is that of prognosis. Gastaut (1954) believed that petit mal epilepsy is seen almost exclusively in children, more rarely in adolescents, and that it should be regarded as a curiosity in both the adult and the aged. Neurologists who study adults tend to disagree with this point of view, but Currier, Kooi and Saidman (1963) maintained that 56 per cent of their patients continued to have attacks beyond the age of 21 years. Most physicians dealing with childhood epilepsy would very strongly disagree with this view. Probably the differences of opinion arise out of the problem of defining what various authors mean by petit mal. True or pure petit mal is rare.

In the series of Livingston et al. (1965) over 15 000 children with epilepsy were studied at the Johns Hopkins Hospital and only 354 or 2.3 per cent fulfilled the true criteria for petit mal. These they defined as paroxysmal periodic attacks of altered consciousness, usually lasting 5–30 seconds, with associated vacant staring. Less frequently they occurred with slight clonic movements of the head and/or upper extremities and even less often they were associated with automatisms such as smacking of the lips, chewing and swallowing movements and, occasionally, mumbling speech. All of their patients commenced symptoms before 15 years of age. Among the 354 patients 117 were followed-up for periods ranging from 5–28 years. Ninety-two patients became free and remained free of both the petit mal attacks and the typical EEG abnormalities, and in 89 of these the attacks stopped before the age of 20 years. In 17 children, who had experienced other forms of epilepsy before petit mal started, epileptic fits continued. Of the 100 patients who started with pure petit mal 54 developed grand mal (major generalized epilepsy) later. Livingston et al. (1965) concluded that although petit mal itself has a good prognosis the later development of major seizures is common. They believed that the incidence of later major epilepsy could be significantly reduced by giving a drug such as phenobarbitone in combination with a specific petit mal drug such as trimethadione or ethosuximide. They conceded that the later the onset of petit mal epilepsy the more likely was the patient to develop other types of seizures, particularly when the onset occurred after 10 years of age. Lennox (1960) shared this opinion precisely and, in the author's view, this is really the kernel of the problem of prognosis and explains why paediatricians and neurologists who study adults differ on the question of prognosis.

Roger (1974) studied 213 patients with petit mal and found that the prognosis was favourable when the onset was from 5–9 years of age, when there was no other form of seizure and when the intelligence was normal. An unfavourable prognosis was seen when the condition developed before five years or after 10 years. The prognosis was good in 48 per cent of the patients he studied. Lugaresi et al. (1974), in an interesting study involving 249 patients from Bologna and Marseilles, were also of the opinion that the condition could be considered benign in 48 per cent of their cases and that it tended towards chronicity in the remaining 52 per cent. However, many of their cases had atypical absences and also atypical EEG findings. They stressed that the late onset of petit mal, the presence of any mental or neurological deficit and the occurrence of other types of seizure were all indicators of a poor prognosis.

To sum up this very difficult problem of prognosis the author considers, looking from the point of view of the paediatric neurologist or the paediatrician, that pure or true petit mal is a relatively uncommon type of childhood epilepsy (2—5 per cent of most large series of children who had epilepsy) and that it is usually very responsive to modern drugs with complete remission occurring in about three-quarters of the cases. Early onset (before 10 years of age), a good initial response to drugs, the absence of other types of seizure, a typical EEG pattern and normal mental and neurological status all indicate an excellent prognosis.

THERAPY

The specific drug therapy of epilepsy first became possible with the successful use of trimethadione by Lennox in 1945. Paramethadione is another member of the oxazolidine-dione group of drugs and it should rarely, if ever, be necessary to use these drugs today. They can cause fatal aplastic anaemia, very often in the first six months of therapy, and the author has had such a tragic experience of this toxic effect in a young patient. This group of drugs was superseded by the succinimide group of drugs after 1958, and *ethosuximide* is by far the most beneficial of these. Ethosuximide can cause side-effects such as nausea, hiccups, headaches, drowsiness, behavioural disturbances and a rash and should be introduced slowly. Toxic blood dyscrasias have been reported but are rare. Complete control of petit mal may be expected in nearly half the patients and significant improvement in a large proportion of the remainder (O'Donohoe, 1964). The maximum dosage of ethosuximide is usually 500 mg/day in those aged six years and under and 750—1000 mg/day in those over six years. It is possible to assay plasma levels of the drug, but these are not often needed because the clinical and EEG responses to the drug are so definite. Ethosuximide still holds its place as the drug of choice in petit mal.

Sodium valproate has now become the leading contender as the drug of choice in petit mal, although it is considerably more expensive than ethosuximide. Simon and Penry (1975) summarized the results of several studies on the efficacy of sodium valproate in petit mal, and reported that of 218 patients approximately 60 per cent achieved a reduction in seizures ranging from 75—100 per cent and a further 25 per cent improved considerably. Jeavons and Clark (1974) claimed that sodium valproate was the most effective drug for typical or atypical absences and that it would control patients not previously controlled by ethosuximide. They emphasized the comparative rarity of side-effects and toxic effects with this drug. Dosage is usually within the range 20–30 mg/(kg BW· day) but up to 50 mg/(kg BW· day) can be used in intractable cases. When doses of 50 mg/(kg BW· day) and over are used plasma levels of the drug should be monitored and platelet counts and bleeding-time tests peformed. Thrombocytopenia has been reported with high doses and the drug may also interfere with blood platelet aggregation thereby prolonging the bleeding times (Sutor and Jesdinsky—Buscher, 1974).

Acetazolamide, a carbonic anhydrase inhibitor and diuretic, was originally tried as an anticonvulsant in the belief that it would cause a metabolic acidosis and possibly produce beneficial effects similar to those of the ketogenic diet. However, it produced only transitory acidosis and dehydration, but it was shown to have anticonvulsant properties, apparently by inhibiting carbonic anhydrase in the brain and thereby interfering with neuronal conduction. Acetazolamide is always worth trying in the refractory case of petit mal although its effect sometimes tends to be transient. It occasionally works well in combination with ethosuximide. An average daily dose of the former is 750 mg. Acetazolamide has also been used in females with major seizures who show an increase in the frequency of fits around the time of menstruation, but the results have been disappointing. The use of acetazolamide in epilepsy has been reviewed by Lombroso and Forsythe (1960).

Clonazepam is a far better drug for refractory petit mal. Lund and Trolle (1973) treated resistant cases with clonazepam and reported results comparable with those obtained when using ethosuximide, and other authors have confirmed these findings. The main problem of using clonazepam in this way is that drowsiness may be troublesome in some patients.

Whatever drug is employed, it is essential that treatment is continued for two years after the absences have been controlled. Some authors recommend combining the drugs used in major generalized epilepsy with the drugs used in petit mal, claiming that this prevents the later emergence of major convulsions. The author does not usually follow this practice, preferring monotherapy with a drug specific for petit mal. It is important to realize that the drugs commonly used in major epilepsy, such as phenobarbitone, phenytoin and carbamazepine have no beneficial effect on true petit mal.

REFERENCES

Currier, R. D., Kooi, K. A. and Saidman, L. J. (1963). 'Prognosis of "pure" petit mal. A follow-up study.' *Neurology, Minneap.* **13**, 959–967

Doose, H., Gerken, H., Horstmann, T. and Völzke, E. (1973). 'Genetic factors in spike-wave absences.' *Epilepsia*, **14**, 57–75

Gastaut, H. (1954). *The Epilepsies: Electro-Clinical Correlations*, p. 86. Springfield, Illinois: Charles C. Thomas

Gastaut, H. (1970). 'Clinical and electroencephalographical classification of epileptic seizures.' *Epilepsia*, **11**, 102–113

Gibbs, F. A. and Gibbs, E. L. (1952). *Atlas of Electroencephalography, Vol. 2: Epilepsy*. Cambridge, Mass.; Addison–Wesley

Gloor, P. (1968). 'Generalised cortico-reticular epilepsies. Some considerations on the pathophysiology of generalised bilaterally synchronous spike and wave discharge.' *Epilepsia*, **9**, 249–263

Gloor, P. (1977). Communication to *Plenary Session of the Joint Meeting of the International League Against Epilepsy and the International Societies for Electroencephalography and Clinical Neurophysiology, Amsterdam, 9th September, 1977*

Jeavons, P. M. and Clark, J. E. (1974). 'Sodium valproate in the treatment of epilepsy. *Br. med. J.* **2**, 584–586

Lennox, W. G. (1945). 'The petit mal epilepsies; their treatment with Tridione.' *J. Am. med. Ass.* **129**, 1069–1073

Lennox, W. G. (1951). 'The heredity of epilepsy as told by relatives and twins.' *J. Am. med. Ass.* **146**, 529–536

Lennox, W. G. (1960). *Epilepsy and Related Disorders*. London: J. and A. Churchill and Boston: Little, Brown

Livingston, S., Torres, I., Pauli, L. L. and Rider, R. V. (1965). 'Petit mal epilepsy; results of a prolonged follow-up of 117 patients.' *J. Am. med. Ass.* **194**, 227–232

Lombroso, C. T. and Forsythe, I. (1960). 'A long-term follow-up of acetazolamide (Diamox) in the treatment of epilepsy.' *Epilepsia*, **1**, 493–500

Lugaresi, E., Pazzaglia, P., Roger, J. and Tassinari, C. A. (1974). 'Evolution and prognosis of petit mal.' In *Epilepsy. Proceedings of the Hans Berger Centenary Symposium*, pp. 151–153. Eds P. Harris and C. Mawdsley. Edinburgh: Churchill Livingstone

Lund, M. and Trolle, E. (1973). 'Clonazepam (Ro 5 - 4023) in the treatment of epilepsy.' *Archs Neurol. Scand.* **49**, Suppl. 53, p. 82

Metrakos, K. and Metrakos, J. D. (1961). 'Genetics of convulsive disorders, Part 2: Genetic and electroencephalographic studies in centrencephalic epilepsy.' *Neurology, Minneap.* **11**, 464–483

Mirsky, A. F. and van Buren, J. (1965). 'On the nature of the "absence" in centrencephalic epilepsy: a study of some behavioural, electroencephalographical and autonomic factors.' *Electroenceph. clin. Neurophysiol.* **18**, 334–348

O'Donohoe, N. V. (1964). 'Treatment of petit mal with ethosuximide.' *Devl Med. child Neurol.* **6**, 498–501

Penfield, W. and Jasper, H. (1954). *Epilepsy and the Functional Anatomy of the Human Brain*. Boston: Little, Brown

Penry, J. K. (1977). Communication to *Plenary Session of the Joint Meeting of the International league Against Epilepsy and the International Societies for Electroencephalography and Clinical Neurophysiology, Amsterdam, 9th September, 1977*

Roger, J. (1974). 'Prognostic features of petit mal absence.' *Epilepsia*, **15**, 433

Simon, D. and Penry, J. K. (1975). 'Sodium di–n–propylacetate (DPA) in the treatment of epilepsy.' *Epilepsia*, **16**, 549–573

Sutor, A. H. and Jesdinsky–Buscher, C. (1974). 'Coagulation changes caused by dipropylacetic acid.' *Medsche Welt, Berl.* **25**, 447–449

CHAPTER 8

Major Generalized Epilepsy (Grand Mal)

At this point it is important to state that despite the many unusual types of seizure which have already been described the major tonic-clonic convulsion or grand mal attack is the commonest epileptic manifestation of childhood. Approximately 75–80 per cent of children with epilepsy have this type of seizure as the only evidence of their epilepsy or in combination with other types of fits. It is this particular type of attack which is associated in the lay mind and, to a lesser extent, in the medical mind with the word 'epilepsy'. This is the archetypal seizure which means total loss of control. Taylor (1973) eloquently described it as an excursion through madness into death. Indeed, as noted already in connection with the first febrile seizure, many parents think that their child has died in the fit. The individual in a major attack appears totally out of control and this frequently fills the observer with fear and revulsion. A great deal of the prejudice about epilepsy arises from this unfortunate feature.

Typical attack

A major seizure may occur without warning or may be preceded by an aura. Sometimes the child may be irritable or show other unusual behaviour for hours or even days before an attack. At the beginning of the ictal phase there is sudden loss of consciousness and if standing the patient may fall. Generalized rigidity (tonic phase) is soon followed by very rapid generalized jerking movements (the clonic phase). During this stage the patient may bite his tongue, although this is unusual in children. Similarly, urinary or faecal incontinence are also less frequent in children during this stage than in adults. Children rarely 'cry out' at the onset of a major attack. In the tonic phase the face is cyanosed when respiration ceases briefly. Breathing becomes jerky and stertorous in the clonic phase and the cyanosis lessens. The clonic movements gradually die away and the patient is left limp and relaxed. The patient may recover swiftly after a short seizure, but after any sort of protracted attack he will usually pass into a deep postictal sleep. When he recovers from this, he may feel weak, complain of headache and fatigue, demonstrate irritability and confusion or vomit persistently. Altered speech and transient paralyses or ataxia may occur. Plantar responses may be extensor for a time. Postictal phenomena may be brief or last for hours or even for days. When a series of tonic-clonic seizures takes place without recovery of consciousness between attacks it constitutes status epilepticus, a serious medical emergency.

Classification and EEG changes

The new *International Classification* (Gastaut, 1969) divides seizures into partial seizures or seizures beginning locally, generalized seizures or bilateral symmetrical seizures without local onset, unilateral seizures and unclassifiable seizures (*see* page 9).

Generalized seizures may be subdivided into primary and secondary generalized attacks. Primary generalized convulsions are generalized from the start and may take the form of tonic-clonic attacks (grand mal), typical petit mal absences or massive bilateral myoclonic jerks. The EEG patterns during the petit mal absence and the myoclonic attack have already been described. During a major generalized attack there are diffuse bursts of multiple spikes which continue during the entire period of the active phase of the convulsion and are followed by diffuse high voltage slow waves in the postconvulsive phase. In the interictal EEGs of patients with major tonic-clonic attacks, one may see a normal background activity on which are superimposed at intervals polyspike and wave discharges or spike and slow-wave discharges without any regular pattern of frequency. One may even see classic spike-wave complexes occurring at 3 Hz. This type of primary grand mal may begin at any age, although the onset is frequently in childhood or adolescence and usually after the age of five years. The patient, as a rule, does not show any neurological or psychiatric evidence of central nervous system disease. There is a good response to the classic anticonvulsants (barbiturates, phenytoin) and the prognosis is usually good.

Theoretical background

Theories concerning the pathogenesis of *primary generalized epilepsy* have already been discussed in the chapter on petit mal (see *Figure 7.2*). In the absence of a clear aetiology it is likely that they derive essentially from a hereditary epileptic predisposition sufficiently marked to render the subject prone to develop epilepsy in the presence of a mild metabolic or other disturbance of body function or in the presence of slight acquired cerebral lesions. In such circumstances the discharges probably originate from the reticular projection systems of the brain stem and thalamus, but there is probably present an additional state of increased excitability of the cortical neurones which make them respond to these volleys from the subcortical system by producing generalized discharges bilaterally and a seizure follows. Similarly, a slight acquired cerebral lesion may make the cortex more excitable in the same way.

Williams (1965) speculated that major epileptic activity always started in the cortex and was rarely, if ever, initiated at the brain stem or subcortical level. He pointed out that studies of large numbers of patients with tumours of the central nervous system had shown that while tumours in certain parts of the cortex were particularly likely to be associated with the occurrence of epilepsy, tumours of the diencephalon and mesencephalon were rarely complicated by epilepsy. Furthermore, diffuse degenerative diseases of the upper brain stem structures were unassociated with epilepsy. He concluded from the clinical evidence that generalized epilepsy did not arise in centrencephalic structures although these structures were probably involved in their propagation, particularly the medial thalamic areas.

Whatever the controversies concerning the initiation of the discharges in primary generalized epilepsy, it seems reasonably certain that a central pacemaker system is involved and this is presumably situated in the upper brain stem or the thalamus. The spike and wave complex of petit mal, which is unassociated with convulsive movements, represents brief excitation followed by slow-wave inhibition which prevents recruitment of excitation and the development of a tonic-clonic attack. In this context primary grand mal seizures may be looked upon as having an initiation identical to that of petit mal attacks, but involving predominantly excitatory pathways or a failure of the inhibitory process. Primary generalized grand mal is the genuine, essential or idiopathic epilepsy of the older writers, and is historically the first type of epilepsy to be recognized as a separate entity, i.e. the original sacred disease or falling sickness.

The second way in which a generalized grand mal seizure may arise is as a secondary phenomenon in the presence of diffuse cerebral disease or multifocal cerebral lesions. This is known as *secondary generalized epilepsy* and is common in childhood. There is usually neurological and psychological evidence of diffuse cerebral involvement with intellectual deficit as a common feature. The attacks are usually generalized from the start and may be major tonic-clonic in type and take the form of generalized tonic seizures or massive bilateral myoclonic jerks. Such a variety of secondary generalized attacks is common in conditions such as infantile spasms, severe myoclonic epilepsy of the Lennox–Gastaut type and in degenerative conditions of the grey matter in childhood. These have been described in previous chapters and it was noted that the EEG tracings showed both considerable disorganization and slowing and the presence of diffuse discharges of the polyspike and slow spike-wave types.

The third way in which a generalized grand mal attack may arise is *when a partial seizure becomes secondarily generalized*. Partial seizures will be dealt with in Chapters 9 and 10, and it is sufficient to say at this point that all forms of partial seizures, whether they have elementary or complex symptomatology, can develop into generalized seizures. Sometimes this occurs so rapidly that the focal features may be unobservable. The generalized seizures which follow may be symmetrical or asymmetrical, tonic or clonic, but most often they are tonic-clonic in type. The focal discharges, which characterize the EEG of those patients with partial seizures, becomes rapidly generalized when the major seizure develops.

Both the occurrence of secondary generalized epilepsy with diffuse cerebral pathology and generalized seizures developing out of partial seizures may be understood from the work of Gloor (1968), which has already been described in detail in Chapter 7. Presumably, in both situations the cortex and the reticular projection systems from brain stem and thalamus are involved and these corticoreticular systems or circuits are utilized to spread the discharges from wherever they originate to all parts of the brain (see *Figure 7.2*).

PROGNOSIS

The prognosis and treatment of grand mal vary depending on the category to which it belongs. In general, grand mal epilepsy is the type most likely to remit in childhood and the one least likely to relapse; pure petit mal is another. Primary generalized epilepsy has an excellent prognosis as a rule but the secondary generalized epilepsies, as emphasized in previous chapters, show a poor response to anticonvulsant medication and generally have a poor prognosis. The prognosis for partial seizures will be considered later but, apart from those of complex symptomatology such as temporal lobe attacks, they respond well to modern therapy.

The time of onset of grand mal is also an important prognostic index. By and large, the later the onset in childhood the better the outlook for seizure control. Major seizures developing in the first three years of life, apart from uncomplicated febrile convulsions, do not have a favourable outlook. Frequently, major epilepsy at this age is a consequence of cerebral injuries sustained in the perinatal period. In contrast, major epilepsy beginning after the age of five years and before puberty has a good prognosis.

The initial response to therapy is important in the prognosis of this condition. Prompt control by medication usually implies a good prognosis and less chance of later relapse. To put this another way, the greater the duration of epilepsy after diagnosis and commencement of therapy the less likely the prospect of permanent remission (Holowach, Thurston and O'Leary, 1972). Livingston (1972) stresses the possibility of relapse during puberty, particularly in females, but Holowach and her colleagues were unable to confirm this observation. In general, those with neurological and intellectual deficits do less well on treatment and this will be discussed later in Chapter 14 which is on mental handicap and epilepsy.

THERAPY

There is now a wide range of drugs available for treating grand mal. These drugs are mainly effective in primary generalized tonic-clonic seizures and partial seizures with secondary generalization. They include phenobarbitone, phenytoin, primidone and carbamazepine. To these have recently been added clonazepam and sodium valproate. The relative advantages and disadvantages of these various drugs will be discussed in detail in the later chapters on drug therapy (*see* Chapters 23 and 24).

The optimal duration of therapy in major generalized epilepsy is also a debatable issue. It is usual to try to maintain remissions in children with epilepsy for four asymptomatic years. Treatment should then be discontinued gradually over a period of several months, and if the child is receiving more than one anticonvulsant the drugs should be discontinued independently. Holowach, Thurston and O'Leary (1972) warned against stopping drug therapy even after four asymptomatic years, where the epilepsy began in later childhood (after nine years of age), where the seizures had resisted initial control for a period of years, where different types of attack were occurring in the same patient, where there were associated neurological and psychological deficits and where the EEG showed paroxysmal abnormalities, was severely abnormal or had changed little over the four-year period of seizure-free observation.

THE SINGLE ATTACK

It is appropriate at this point to consider the child with the isolated epileptic seizure, i.e. the convulsion which occurs only once. These are usually generalized tonic-clonic attacks, and since epilepsy is a chronic recurrent condition these individuals should not be regarded as epileptic. Any person in untoward circumstances may be liable to a convulsion, and it is only when attacks are habitual that a diagnosis of epilepsy should be made. When any convulsion has occurred, and this is particularly true of the single attack, a very careful history should be obtained including a full account of the physical and psychological circumstances surrounding the attack. The more potent the immediate cause the less serious is the convulsion's significance. This is as true in childhood as it is in adult life. The patient who has had a single major fit is in need of careful examination and investigation and does not necessarily need treatment. Indeed, if all investigations are negative prescribing anticonvulsants may not help the patient because it may never be known whether or not he would have had another attack. Isolated fits are not uncommon and treating them may imply a diagnosis of epilepsy without justification. Subsequently, the 'undiagnosis of epilepsy' (a term coined by Jeavons (1975)) may be difficult. It may well be that the child with a single major seizure is suffering from primary generalized epilepsy even though all investigations are entirely negative but, in this particular context, it is better to withhold drugs until further attacks occur, if they ever do. However, it is dangerous to generalize about the problem of the single seizure and each case must be judged on its merits. Livingston (1960) argued that anticonvulsant treatment was mandatory in the child with the single seizure. His reasons were that parents were frightened by the dramatic events of a convulsion and were afraid that injury, death or prolonged unconsciousness might occur in another one. Parents also feared the social stigma attached to their child having a convulsion in public. He felt that parents were happier and more confident about the future when their child was on therapy, and he considered that prevention of recurrent seizures was important because of the known association between prolonged attacks and irreversible organic brain damage.

The only way to reconcile these two opposing views about the problem of the single seizure is to look at each case individually and, particularly, to examine the circumstances in which the convulsion takes place. In the first place the clinician must be sure that an actual epileptic attack has occurred. This matter will be dealt with in detail later in the differential diagnosis of epilepsy (*see* Chapter 20), but, at this point, it should be emphasized that the brief tonic stiffening which so often occurs in a syncopal attack should not be misdiagnosed as epilepsy. It must be realized that anybody can have a fit given the right precipitating circumstances. Convulsions occurring in a setting of intercurrent illness and high fever have been described already and, indeed, severe illness and fever at any time may lead to some degree of encephalopathy and be associated with a seizure. Biochemical and metabolic upset may lead to a single seizure occurring; for instance this may be seen when renal function is compromised either temporarily or permanently. Certainly severe emotional upset can bring about a seizure in an individual with an increased susceptibility to epilepsy (for genetic reasons) and the attack may be an isolated one. For example, the author remembers an 11-year-old boy who witnessed the sudden unexpected death of his father from coronary thrombosis and one week later, while suffering considerable emotional anguish, he had a generalized tonic-clonic seizure which subsequently never recurred. Sometimes, emotional upset and severe fatigue may combine to precipitate a single seizure and particularly in adolescents: chronic fatigue is a well known precipitating cause of habitual epileptic attacks. Similarly, the frustrations and irritations which beset the individual with epilepsy in his daily life may make his epilepsy worse.

Counselling and advising parents

Parents of children who suffer from major epileptic seizures are naturally apprehensive about the attacks and fear that their child may die in one of them. It is important to reassure them that this seldom occurs, provided the attacks are not prolonged. The dangers of sustained and repeated attacks (status epilepticus) have already been discussed in the chapter on febrile convulsions (*see* Chapter 6). It is also important to remember that seizures which are atypical for a particular individual or which last longer than usual may, in fact, sometimes be symptomatic of some other acute disorder, e.g. meningitis.

What to do for a major attack

The parents should be instructed in what they should do during a grand mal attack. If possible, the patient should be allowed to remain where he is ensuring at the same time that he cannot injure himself by knocking against some immovable object or falling off a bed or chair, and he should be prevented from burning himself if he collapses near a fire. The danger of drowning in a bath should be remembered and bathroom doors should never be locked. Moreover, if convulsions are frequent showering is preferable. Tight clothing around the neck should be loosened, and the patient should be turned on his side so that mucus and saliva can flow easily from the mouth. Furthermore, this is a safe posture if vomiting occurs and avoids the danger of aspiration of vomitus. It is not necessary to insert an object between the teeth in children, as a rule, unless the individual habitually bites his tongue or cheeks during the seizure. If something must be inserted, then hard metal objects should be eschewed as they may break the teeth. Firm blunt nondamaging objects such as a well padded tongue depressor or a piece of leather may be used, inserting it anteriorly and then moving it sideways to lie between the posterior teeth. The tongue may fall back and cause respiratory obstruction. With the patient on his side the tongue may be brought forwards by slightly extending the head and neck, inserting one's fingers behind the ramus of the mandible on both sides and drawing the mandible, and with it the tongue, forwards.

The *postictal symptoms* vary in duration depending on the severity of the actual seizure. The postictal period of unconsciousness is something which alarms many parents, and they should be told that this is a recovery phase, that no interference is necessary and that the patient should be allowed to "sleep off" the attack in a comfortable position. This should preferably be on a bed from which the pillows have been removed in order to maintain a horizontal position thus avoiding the risk of respiratory obstruction. It is important that teachers, who may be involved in the care of a child with epilepsy, should also be familiar with the ordinary management of a major convulsion. Hospitalization is rarely necessary unless the particular episode is prolonged or complicated in some way.

REFERENCES

Gastaut, H. (1969). 'Clinical and electroencephalographical classification of epileptic seizures.' *Epilepsia*, 10, Suppl. pp. 2−21

Gloor, P. (1968). 'Generalised cortico-reticular epilepsies. Some considerations on the pathophysiology of generalised bilaterally synchronous spike and wave discharge.' *Epilepsia*, 9, 249−263

Holowach, J., Thurston, D. L. and O'Leary, J. (1972). 'Prognosis in childhood epilepsy. Follow-up study of 148 cases in which therapy had been suspended after prolonged anti-convulsant control.' *New Engl. J. Med.* 286, 169−174

Jeavons, P. M. (1975). *Misdiagnosis of epilepsy*. Reprinted from the Proceedings of the National Seminar on Epilepsy, Bangalore, India. Bangalore, India: Indian Epilepsy Association

Livingston, S. (1960). 'Management of the child with one epilepsy seizure.' *J. Am. med. Ass.* 174, 135−139

Livingston, S. (1972). *Comprehensive Management of Epilepsy in Infancy, Childhood and Adolescence*, p. 585. Springfield, Illinois: Charles C. Thomas

Taylor, D. C. (1973). 'Aspects of seizure disorders II: On prejudice.' *Devl Med. child Neurol.* 15, 91−94

Williams, D. (1965). 'The thalamus and epilepsy.' *Brain*, 88, 539−556

CHAPTER 9

Partial Seizures of Elementary Symptomatology (Focal Epilepsy)

Definitions

Partial epilepsies are disturbances which apparently originate in more or less well defined areas of the brain and produce a variety of symptoms depending on the site of the epileptic focus. At the onset the epileptic episode seems to involve only particular regions of the body, but the attack may spread and become generalized, thereby becoming a secondarily generalized epilepsy, using the terminology of the *International Classification* (Gastaut, 1970). As was pointed out earlier, the word 'focal' may be used synonymously with 'partial' in this context. The partial seizures are further subdivided into those of simple or elementary symptomatology and those of complex symptomatology (temporal lobe or psychomotor seizures). In the former, where the attack remains localized, consciousness is usually retained but in the latter it is usually impaired or lost. Partial seizures, which are focal and/ or lateralized, are common in the neonate and young infant but are relatively uncommon in childhood generally. They become more frequent again in adult life. Some generalized major seizures (grand mal) in later childhood begin as partial or focal attacks in one part of the cortex, but generalization occurs so rapidly that the initial features may not be apparent to the observer, even though the child himself may experience a brief motor or sensory or autonomic aura.

The term *Jacksonian or Rolandic convulsion*, 'a marching spasm or sensation' to quote Lennox (1960), is used to describe an attack which begins in a distal part of a limb and travels proximally. The patient or an observer may see clonic movements beginning, say, in a toe and then travelling to the foot, the knees and to the ipsilateral upper limb. Consciousness is usually lost when the head and neck are reached. In a corresponding sensory attack, feelings of pins and needles or tingling spread proximally and there may be indescribable sensations of heat or cold or other bizarre feelings in the limbs. Mixtures of motor and sensory phenomena may occur. Sometimes, an older patient can abort or limit an attack by applying strong stimuli to the affected limb by the contralateral hand, for example by grasping it firmly, but most patients feel helpless in the face of a 'marching' seizure. As already stated, loss of consciousness occurs when the head and neck are reached and this is usually followed by generalization of the attack. The period of unconsciousness is usually shorter than in a primary generalized major attack but postictal confusion, sleep and transient paralysis (Todd's paralysis) do occur and the period of paralysis may be brief or last up to 12 or even 14 hours. Its resolution may be followed by the persistence of minimal neurological signs on the affected side.

Unfortunately, the term 'Jacksonian', as with so much of the terminology of epilepsy, is used very loosely in the medical literature and is often applied to any attack with a focal motor component. Livingston (1972) strongly emphasized that, in his experience, true Jacksonian seizures, with the characteristic march, were comparatively rare in childhood and this is certainly the author's experience also. A more common type of partial seizure which is seen in children, including young children, is what is known as an adversive attack. There may or may not be prodromal symptoms followed by turning of the eyes and head, and later rotation of the body away from the side of the epileptogenic focus. There is usually a gradual loss of posture and consciousness and the patient may fall to the ground. As he does so the limbs towards which he faces extend and the contralateral limbs flex, much as in the posture associated with the asymmetrical tonic neck reflex in early infancy. There are usually no clonic movements, consciousness is quickly regained and postictal symptoms are short lived. There is debate as to where the epileptogenic focus causing this type of attack is located with some suggesting the frontal lobe anterior to the motor cortex as the site of initiation while others propose a temporal lobe origin. Adversive attacks may be succeeded by generalized major seizures later.

Pathophysiology

The pathophysiology of focal seizures is fairly well understood. Local changes occurring in groups of cortical neurones produce spontaneous and repetitive neuronal discharges. Such discharges are usually recorded as localized spike foci in the EEG.

Periodically, the epileptic disturbances may propagate to the corresponding point in the opposite hemisphere via the corpus callosum forming a 'mirror focus' but without any clinical change. Alternatively, the discharge may spread locally in the brain through short association fibres and involve progressively wider areas of the cortex, or they may extend to the appropriate segment of the thalamus establishing a thalamocortical circuit of impulses. In this case, the patient experiences a focal seizure which may constitute the complete ictal event or may appear as an aura before a secondarily generalized seizure develops.

The discharges may be confined to one area of cortex only, so that jerking of a limb or one side of the body continues for hours or days. This is called *epilepsia partialis continua* and is rare in childhood except in association with serious generalized brain disease such as occurs in degenerative conditions of the central nervous system (Unverricht—Lundborg disease* is a well known cause of this phenomenon). The discharges may advance over the cortex producing a Jacksonian march of symptoms, and they may extend to the medial thalamic nuclei bilaterally and thence to the reticular activating system in the brain stem. When this happens consciousness is lost and the discharges then spread upwards and symmetrically to involve both hemispheres diffusely. At this stage the EEG will show bilateral high voltage high frequency discharges and the pyramidal and extrapyramidal systems then conduct the discharges downwards again to the spinal cord producing the tonic stage of the grand mal attack. After some seconds of tonic contractions, during which the high-frequency discharges continue, the patient relaxes intermittently producing the clonic stage of the seizure. This stage is due to a periodic interruption of the tonic stage and at this point in the EEG the cortical spikes are followed by surface-negative slow waves due to the development of inhibitory postsynaptic potentials acting as a 'brake' on the excitatory postsynaptic potentials characterized by the surface-negative spike discharges. The EEG record then enters a silent or isoelectric flat stage as the convulsive movements cease and this is followed by the appearance of generalized high-voltage irregular slow waves and a gradual return to the resting interseizure EEG pattern with the reappearance of the original focal abnormality.

Unverricht-Lundborg disease (Lafora—body disease or familial myoclonus epilepsy) is characterized by progressive intellectual deterioration and by widespread and frequent myoclonic jerks. The disease presents between the ages of seven and 14 years and is accompanied by a severely abnormal EEG pattern. Concentric cytoplasmic bodies (Lafora bodies) are found in ganglion cells throughout the neuraxis and histochemically these inclusions react as a protein-bound mucopolysaccharide.

Aetiology

The *International Classification* (Gastaut, 1970) defines the aetiology of partial seizures as follows: 'usually related to a wide variety of local brain lesions (cause known, suspected or unknown); constitutional factors may be important.' Constitutional or genetic factors certainly play a much less significant role than in the primary generalized epilepsies, but there are exceptions, for example where an inherited predisposition to convulse with fever is complicated by a prolonged febrile seizure and subsequent focal damage and also in 'benign focal epilepsy' (*see* page 99). It seems likely that *perinatal factors,* particularly anoxic damage, are the commonest cause of partial seizures due to local brain lesions, and it is important to remember that an uneventful birth history does not exclude the possibility of minor brain injury occurring at that time and leaving very slight gliotic scarring of the brain in its wake. Post-traumatic epilepsy may be partial in type. The *severe infections of childhood,* such as meningitis, may cause permanent brain damage and later epilepsy. *Metabolic disturbances* in the dehydrated infant, especially hypernatraemia,may also be responsible.*Prolonged febrile seizures* predominantly damage the temporal lobes, but can also cause damage elsewhere in the cortex. Parents and many doctors often suspect a progressive *space-occupying lesion* when a child develops a partial epilepsy but, in fact, this is a very rare cause and in a series of 114 such children studied by Holowach, Thurston and O'Leary (1958) only one such case was found.

Most people experienced in childhood epilepsy would not perform neuroradiological investigations in partial or focal epilepsy unless there was some evidence present of increased intracranial pressure or perhaps some progressive neurological signs. The advent of the CT scan will probably mean that more children with partial epilepsy will have this painless safe investigation, and this will undoubtedly lead to an increase in the knowledge about the causes of these epilepsies. Routine investigations should include a plain skull X-ray, EEG and blood glucose and serum calcium estimations in case metabolic disorders are triggering the epilepsy. Some writers (Brown, 1976) advocate the use of radioisotope scanning and echoencephalography also, and these investigations have the merit of being painless and safe whereas arteriography and pneumoencephalography carry risks and the latter is painful.

Partial or focal motor seizures are frequent in children with *cerebral palsy*, as are also generalized convulsions. The incidence of epilepsy in cerebral palsy has been variously reported as being from 20—50 per cent. Up to 50 per cent of children with hemiplegia may suffer from epilepsy, often partial in type, and fits are also common in severely tetraplegic children. Some cases of spastic diplegia are associated with epilepsy but it is rare in the athetoid or dystonic variety of cerebral palsy and in ataxic cerebral palsy. Babies with cerebral palsy may develop infantile spasms or one of the myoclonic epilepsies. Epilepsy is a most important complication of cerebral palsy and may be as handicapping as mental retardation as far as the patient's chances of obtaining employment later are concerned.

Partial and secondarily generalized seizures may occur in children in whom *hydrocephalus* has been treated by *ventriculoatrial shunt* procedures. Hosking (1974) studied 200 randomly selected children with hydrocephalus and in half of the cases the condition was associated with spina bifida and in half the hydrocephalus was either primary or secondary to cerebral haemorrhage in the neonate or meningitis in infancy. Children who did not survive for more than six months were not included. Of the 200 cases 197 were treated early by ventriculoatrial or ventriculopleural shunt incorporating a Spitz-Holter valve, and follow-up in the majority exceeded five years. The overall frequency of seizures, either single or recurrent, in the whole group was approximately 30 per cent, 26 per cent in the hydrocephalus-spina bifida group and 35 per cent in the group with hydrocephalus alone. The incidence of seizures was 27 per cent in primary or congenital hydrocephalus, 35 per cent of the posthaemorrhage group and 54 per cent in the postmeningitis group. A small number of patients had fits in relation to valve blockage and two children in the hydrocephalus-spina bifida group developed infantile spasms. Frequent valve revisions appeared to increase the tendency to have fits subsequently. Some authors, notably Graebner and Celesia (1973), have suggested that the ventricular indwelling catheters act to produce an epileptic focus which can then be responsible for a partial epilepsy, and nearly 40 per cent of the shunted patients in their series had focal EEG abnormalities in the neighbourhood of the ventricular catheter.

BENIGN FOCAL EPILEPSY OF CHILDHOOD

Probably the commonest variety of partial epilepsy in childhood is the type first described by Nayrac and Beaussart in 1958 and which is now called by various titles including benign focal epilepsy of childhood, benign centrotemporal epilepsy of childhood, benign epilepsy of childhood with Rolandic (centrotemporal) foci, Sylvian seizures with midtemporal EEG foci and the lingual syndrome! The reader might be forgiven for thinking that this must be an ill-defined condition, to put it mildly, but in fact it is now a well established entity and probably best entitled benign focal epilepsy of childhood. Much of the work on the subject has been from France but Lombroso published an important paper from the United States in 1967 and the subject was reviewed in a leading article in the *British Medical Journal* in 1975.

The characteristics of this syndrome are as follows:

1. It occurs in both sexes with males predominating
2. The commonest time of onset is between seven and 10 years of age
3. It may be uncommonly begin before seven years but rarely presents after 12 years of age
4. The outstanding feature of the attacks is that they occur predominantly during sleep.

In Beaussart's (1972) very large series 51 per cent had attacks in sleep only, 29 per cent had attacks in the waking state only, 13 per cent had seizures while asleep and awake, and in 7 per cent the information was insufficient to place the time of occurrence of the seizures. The nocturnal seizures usually occurred in the middle of the night or towards morning and the distinction as to whether they had generalized or partial characteristics was difficult because they were often unobserved. Recently, Ambrosetto and Gobbi (1975) were able to record an EEG in an affected 10-year-old boy during nocturnal sleep. The spike discharges were activated both in REM sleep and non-REM or slow-wave sleep. The actual attack occurred as the boy appeared to be awakening and while he was still in a drowsy state. Initially the seizure had many of the characteristics of an adversive partial seizure with turning of the head and eyes to the side opposite to that of the resting EEG abnormality and tonic extension of the limbs followed by clonic jerking occurred also on that side. This was followed after about 30 seconds by the head and eyes turning back to the side of the EEG lesion and then by clonic jerking on that side. Cyanosis was a marked feature and postictal sleep followed. It can readily be understood why these attacks have been misinterpreted as primarily generalized seizures in the past rather than partial attacks with secondary generalization. Whether the attacks actually start during sleep and wake the patient as they commence or whether they occur during the drowsy period of waking is debatable, but the former seems more likely on EEG evidence because Blom and Heijbel (1975) have pointed out that EEG discharges show an increase during sleep and in some cases appear only in sleep.

The diurnal attacks, when they occur, are quite remarkable. The patient may show clonic jerking of one side of his face (hemifacial seizures), occasionally with jerking of an ipsilateral limb. Oropharyngeal signs are frequently associated with the hemifacial attack consisting of salivation, gurgling noises, contractions of the jaws and peculiar subjective sensations involving the tongue. One of the author's patients complained that his tongue felt too large and felt as if it was moving in an odd way. Some children may have feelings of suffocation and an inability to swallow, and inability to speak has also been reported in up to 40 per cent of diurnal attacks (Loiseau and Beaussart, 1973). Although these children could not speak, consciousness was retained, as it usually is in this type of partial seizure, and children have said 'I heard my parents speak, I could see them move but I could not answer.' Such arrest of speech may occur irrespective of whether the EEG lesion is located in the speech area or not, and it has been suggested that it is really due to a peripheral aphonia caused by involvement of the articulatory muscles in the seizure movements.

The typical EEG pattern consists of the presence of spike discharges or localized spike-wave discharges situated unilaterally or bilaterally in the lower Rolandic (central) area (*Figure 9.1*), just above the Sylvian fissure or on the upper lateral aspect of the temporal lobe, perhaps in the region of the insula. Loiseau and Beaussart (1973) speculated that the components of the seizures could be explained due to activation of the cortex on either side of the Rolandic fissure. They explained the frequent bilateral oropharyngeal signs and symptoms by the bilateral cortical representation of the mouth, tongue and throat.

Genetic factors appear to play an important role in the causation of this variety of epilepsy. Heijbel, Blom and Rasmuson (1975) in their study of inheritance in this condition, favoured an autosomal dominant manner of inheritance with an age-dependent penetrance which reaches its maximum between the ages of five and 15 years. A previous history of cerebral insult, either at birth or subsequently, is unusual, whereas a positive family history of epilepsy is frequently found. Perhaps the most remarkable statistic given by Heijbel, Blom and Bergfors (1975), based on the Swedish studies, was that this type of epilepsy might account for some 16 per cent of children with epilepsy and that its incidence was nearly four times greater than that of true petit mal in the normal child population. Other findings (Heijbel and Bohman, 1975) were that children with this type of epilepsy were no different from the general population of children with regard to intelligence, behaviour and school adjustment. Furthermore, all those who have studied this condition have emphasized its ready response to therapy and the excellent prognosis for cure of the epilepsy. Most of the children affected become completely free of epilepsy, usually soon after puberty and nearly always by their middle teens (Beaussart and Faou, 1978).

There has been speculation about the aetiology of this particular convulsive disorder, particularly in view of the strong genetic influences present and the excellent prognosis. Beaussart (1972) has suggested that this is a functional disorder of the brain in which both strong genetic factors and minimal cerebral damage may play a part, and that it gradually disappears as maturation of the brain takes place. There are some analogies with the situation in true petit mal.

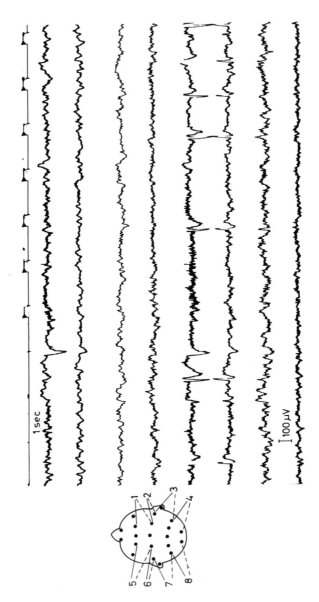

Figure 9.1. Girl aged six years and awake with eyes open. EEG shows spike discharges in the left motor area with phase reveral of these in channels 5 and 6

The clear definition of this variety of epilepsy in childhood has been a most important advance. There are many reasons why children with epilepsy develop behavioural disturbances and not least because of the effect their epilepsy has on both their parents and family. Seizures cause considerable anguish to parents and they may react either by overprotection or rejection of the patient. Their attitudes lead in turn to emotional disturbance in the child. When the parents of children with benign focal epilepsy are given early, exact and repeated information about the nature of the disorder, particularly about its good prognosis, and when this is coupled with the fact that the children usually become seizure free fairly rapidly after initiation of treatment, there is usually a diminution or disappearance of the parents' anxieties and a happier and more optimistic emotional atmosphere is generally created from which the child benefits immeasurably.

THERAPY

In partial seizures of the general type under discussion, i.e. those of simple or elementary symptomatology, the main drugs used in treatment in the past have been phenobarbitone, primidone or phenytoin or combinations of these. In recent years, however, *carbamazepine* has been recognized as being particularly beneficial in the treatment of the partial epilepsies, including those of complex symptomatology (Cereghino *et al.*, 1974). This drug is now frequently the first choice for these epilepsies in adults and children and has the advantages of a marked anticonvulsant action, a possible psychotropic effect and infrequent and mild side-effects. It is now often used as the sole anticonvulsant in the partial epilepsies, using drug level monitoring to achieve a satisfactory therapeutic level in the plasma. The psychotropic effects have been described as improved behaviour with the relaxation of tension and the calming of aggression and an improved learning ability due to increased alertness and concentration (Livingston *et al.*, 1967). The question has been raised as to whether this is a primary effect or whether it is secondary to improved seizure control or withdrawal of other depressant drugs or both. Those who favour a positive primary psychotropic effect claim that the drug also benefits in this way nonepileptic patients who have not received other drugs.

Carbamazepine is particularly valuable in the treatment of benign focal epilepsy of childhood. Since this type of epilepsy mainly occurs during sleep, the hypnotic effects of barbiturates and similar drugs may not only activate seizure discharges in the EEG but may even precipitate clinical seizures. The use of barbiturates in seizures activated by sleep predominantly is probably best avoided. Lerman and Kivity—Ephraim

(1974) studied 40 patients with benign focal epilepsy, ranging in age at the start of treatment from 4½–11 years. All were treated with carbamazepine alone, in most cases with daily dosages ranging from 300–600 mg. The usual maximum recommended daily dose of the drug is 20 mg/(kg BW). Of the 40 patients 38 were fully controlled by treatment and, in the other two regular medication had been neglected. They mentioned three other children, not in the series, who required a combination of carbamazepine and phenytoin to achieve full control. O'Donohoe (1977) also commented on the marked beneficial effect of carbamazepine in this type of epilepsy and on the fact that the drug often worked in apparently subtherapeutic dosages. It may be possible, indeed, to give treatment in a single dose at bedtime. In resistant cases the combination of carbamazepine and phenytoin was found to be particularly effective. The combination of carbamazepine and phenytoin is usually given in a two-to-one dosage ratio, i.e. carbamazepine 200 mg to phenytoin 100 mg. Carbamazepine is particularly useful when given to children insofar as usually a morning hangover effect is not experienced with it and the children may therefore show increased alertness and interest at school.

The importance of not confusing the hemifacial diurnal seizures of benign focal epilepsy with true petit mal has a particular significance in therapy. Carbamazepine has little or no effect on petit mal whereas the succinimides or sodium valproate are highly effective. Finally, it should be remembered that clonazepam may be a very useful drug to try in the treatment of any partial epilepsy which resists control by the other anticonvulsants.

REFERENCES

Ambrosetto, G. and Gobbi, G. (1975). 'Benign epilepsy of childhood with Rolandic spikes, or a lesion?'. EEG during a seizure.' *Epilepsia*, **16**, 793–796
Beaussart, M. (1972). 'Benign epilepsy of children with Rolandic (centro-temporal) paroxysmal foci: A clinical entity. Study of 221 cases.' *Epilepsia*, **13**, 795–811
Beaussart, M. and Faou, R. (1978). 'Evolution of epilepsy with Rolandic paroxysmal foci: A study of 324 cases.' *Epilepsia*, **19**, 337–342
Blom, S. and Heijbel, J. (1976). 'Benign epilepsy of children with centro-temporal EEG foci. Discharge rate during sleep.' *Epilepsia*, **16**, 133–140
Brown, J. K. (1976). 'Fits in childhood.' In *A Textbook of Epilepsy*, pp. 66–108. Eds J. Laidlaw and A. Richens. Edinburgh, London, New York: Churchill Livingston
Cereghino, J. J., Brock, J. T., Van Meter, J. C., Penry, J. K., Smith, L. D. and White, B. G. (1974). 'Carbamazepine for epilepsy. A controlled prospective evaluation.' *Neurology*, **24**, 401–410
Editorial (1975). 'Benign focal epilepsy of childhood.' *Br. med. J.* **3**, 451–452
Gastaut, H. (1970). 'Clinical and electroencephalographical classification of epileptic seizures.' *Epilepsia*, **11**, 102–113

Heijbel, J. and Bohman, M. (1975). 'Benign epilepsy of children with centrotemporal EEG foci: Intelligence, behaviour and school adjustment.' *Epilepsia*, 16, 679–687

Heijbel, J., Blom, S. and Bergfors, P. G. (1975). 'Benign epilepsy of children with centrotemporal EEG foci. A study of incidence rate in outpatient care.' *Epilepsia*, 16, 657–664

Heijbel, J., Blom, S. and Rasmuson, M. (1975). 'Benign epilepsy of childhood with centrotemporal EEG foci. A genetic study.' *Epilepsia*, 16, 285–293

Holowach, J., Thurston, D. L. and O'Leary, J. (1958). 'Jacksonian seizures in infancy and childhood.' *J. Pediat.* 52, 670–686

Hosking, G. P. (1974). 'Fits in hydrocephalic children.' *Archs Dis. Childh.* 49, 633–635

Lennox, W. G. (1960). *Epilepsy and Related Disorders*, pp. 212–220. London: J. and A. Churchill and Boston: Little, Brown and Company

Lerman, P. and Kivity-Ephraim, S. (1974). 'Carbamazepine sole anticonvulsant for focal epilepsy of childhood.' *Epilepsia*, 15, 229–234

Livingston, S. (1972). *Comprehensive Management of Epilepsy in Infancy, Childhood and Adolescence*, p. 49. Springfield, Illinois: Charles C. Thomas

Livingston, S., Villamater, C., Sakata, Y. and Pauli, L. L. (1967). 'Use of carbamazepine in epilepsy.' *J. Am. med. Ass.* 200, 204–208

Loiseau, P. and Beaussart, M. (1973). 'The seizures of benign childhood epilepsy with Rolandic paroxysmal discharges.' *Epilepsia*, 14, 381–389

Lombroso, C. T. (1967). 'Sylvian seizures and midtemporal spike foci in children.' *Archs Neurol., Chicago.* 17, 52–59

Nayrac, P. and Beaussart, M. (1958). 'Les pointes-ondes prérolandiques: Expression EEG tres particuliere. Étude electroclinque de 21 cas.' *Rev. Neurol. (Paris),* 99, 201–206

O'Donohoe, N. V. (1977). 'Tegretol in everyday paediatric practice.' In *Tegretol in Epilepsy: Proceedings of an International Meeting*, pp. 10–12. Ed. F. D. Roberts. Macclesfield, Cheshire: Geigy Pharmaceuticals

CHAPTER 10

Partial Seizures of Complex Symptomatology (Temporal Lobe Epilepsy)

Temporal lobe epilepsy, a partial epilepsy of complex symptomatology in the terms of the *International Classification* (Gastaut, 1970), is also known as psychomotor epilepsy according to the description introduced by Gibbs, Gibbs and Lennox (1937) to encompass its psychic and motor manifestations. It is both one of the most intractable forms of epilepsy and also one of the most commonly encountered seizure types when all age groups are considered. It constitutes 42 per cent of partial seizures and 26 per cent of all seizures (Hauser and Kurland, 1975). Moreover, it frequently presents considerable diagnostic problems.

AETIOLOGY

The condition is of particular interest to paediatricians because of controversy about its causation, whether due to birth injury or to subsequent brain-damaging illnesses. Ounsted, Lindsay and Norman (1966), in their classic monograph, described three aetiological groups of which each formed approximately a third of their series of 100 children with temporal lobe epilepsy. The first group consisted of children who had a known brain-damaging illness or a chronic neurological disease. The conditions included birth injury, head injury, meningitis, encephalitis, tuberose sclerosis and phenylketonuria. The second group consisted of those children who had had an episode of status epilepticus in early life. In the remaining group no definite cause could be identified.

Those who argue in favour of birth injury as an important cause of temporal lobe epilepsy postulate that moulding of the head during birth may lead to herniation of the medial and inferior parts of a temporal lobe into the tentorial opening with consequent occlusion of blood vessels in the area (Earle, Baldwin and Penfield, 1953). It is suggested that the infant may show little or no evidence of damage at the time but that there is later development of an epileptogenic focus. Others have suggested that birth injury is only an indirect cause of temporal lobe epilepsy which acts by producing an epileptogenic focus or foci in the brain which themselves cause prolonged major seizures in early childhood, perhaps triggered by high fever, and resulting in temporal lobe damage due to the status epilepticus (Wallace, 1976). The history of birth injury in temporal lobe epilepsy, however, does not necessarily imply that the presumed temporal lobe lesions occurred at birth.

As has been noted in the section on status epilepticus, this emergency is an early event in the history of childhood epilepsy with three-quarters of the cases occurring in children under three years of age (Aicardi and Chevrie, 1970). Brain swelling, hypoxia, circulatory and metabolic disturbances consequent on status epilepticus lead to neuronal damage and death (particularly in the hippocampal areas of the temporal lobes), and the injurious effects are usually predominantly unilateral. Moreover, apart from epilepsy, diffuse damage may also result in later neurological abnormality and mental retardation. Permanent hemiplegia associated with hemispheric atrophy and later intractable epilepsy and also cerebellar atrophy may follow severe status epilepticus. The role of acute potentially brain-damaging illness, such as meningitis, in causing later epilepsy is also quite complex. Apart from the possibility of the infection itself producing neuronal damage, the prevalence of seizures in children with meningitis aged less than four years is 45 per cent in contrast with an 8 per cent incidence in those children above that age (Ounsted, 1951) and, if the seizures are prolonged, they may produce the serious sequelae of status epilepticus.

Ounsted, Lindsay and Norman (1966) also examined the role of genetic factors in the causation of temporal lobe epilepsy in childhood. Inheritance seemed to play a major role only in children whose epilepsy had followed status epilepticus. In those, the overall risk for any convulsive disorder occurring in brothers and sisters was 30 per cent, and in most cases the particular convulsive disorder was a febrile seizure. In other words, both the patients and their siblings were prone to febrile seizures in early childhood, the difference being that the patient unfortunately had a prolonged and severe attack while his affected siblings had short and mild ones. The genetic factor in temporal lobe epilepsy therefore seems to consist of a predisposition to febrile convulsions and, if the convulsion happens to be prolonged and severe, temporal lobe damage results and an epileptogenic lesion follows later.

There has been increasing awareness in recent years of the early onset of symptoms of temporal lobe epilepsy. Ounsted, Lindsay and Norman, 1966) reported the ages of onset in their series as being widely scattered around a median age of five years four months. Where the epilepsy was related to previous status epilepticus the median age of onset was earlier than this, and where no definite cause could be identified the median age was eight years. Aird, Venturini and Spielman (1967), in a large retrospective survey, noted that 42 per cent of patients with temporal lobe epilepsy reported an onset of some form of convulsive phenomena in the first decade of life. As will be made clear in the discussion on symptomatology, the often bizarre subjective sensations experienced in the attacks are difficult for children to describe, and this makes identification of the time of onset uncertain in many cases.

Anatomy

In order to understand the phenomena of temporal lobe epilepsy it is necessary to know something of the anatomical and pathological substrates of the condition. To anatomists the temporal lobe is that part of the brain below the lateral or Sylvian fissure which extends posteriorly to blend with the occipital lobe. In clinical practice the temporal lobe area is taken to include the hippocampal gyrus lying medially on the undersurface of the cortex and extending forwards as the uncus, and the hippocampus which is a cylindrical grey mass lying in the floor of the inferior horn of the lateral ventricle which extends forwards to fuse with the tail of the caudate nucleus to form the amygdaloid nucleus or amygdala at the tip of the inferior horn. The hippocampus continues posteriorly as the fornix and the hippocampus-fornix complex lies eccentrically round the thalamus in such a way that the hippocampus lies below and lateral to it, while the fornix continues forwards over the dorsal aspect of the thalamus and then extends to lie medial to it, finally ending in the mammillary bodies of the hypothalamus. The anterior thalamic muclei receive afferents from the fornix and the mammillary bodies are also connected by the mammillothalamic tract. The anterior thalamic nuclei also project to the cingulate gyrus, lying above and parallel to the corpus callosum, and to the frontal cortex, and there are returning afferent fibres to the hippocampus via the hippocampal gyrus. There are also connections to the insula and to the homologous areas on the opposite side of the brain. This whole interconnecting system is now usually known as the *'limbic system'* or the 'visceral brain'.

Phylogenetically it represents an old part of the forebrain which has been overlain and surrounded by the larger and more highly differentiated neocortex (*Figure 10.1*).

Functionally, it is now considered that the limbic system is a complex and highly integrated mechanism responsible for the autonomic functions of the individual and the one which is also concerned with emotional expression. The cardiovascular, respiratory and alimentary systems have

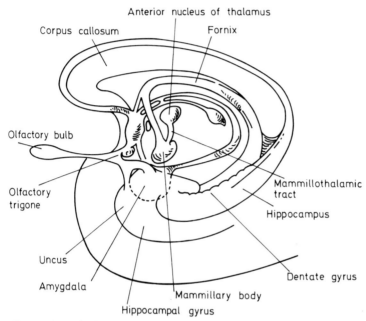

Figure 10.1. The hippocampus and amygdala in the depths of the temporal lobe. (After J. R. Daube and B. A. Sandok, 1978, Medical Neurosciences. Boston: Little, Brown and Co.)

their higher cortical representation in this region. The limbic system influences brain stem function through the reticular system and pituitary function through the hypothalamus, and it is thought to be concerned with the regulation of sleep and with memory. The olfactory input terminates in the uncus and hippocampal gyrus, thereby intimately connecting the sense organs of smell to those parts of the brain which are concerned with memory and also with the hypothalamus. From the evolutionary standpoint, the first parts of the cerebral hemispheres to develop were those connected with olfactory input, and these were evolved to deal with the world of smells and to store the memory of what had been smelt.

Pathology

Our knowledge of the pathology of temporal lobe epilepsy began in the early nineteenth century when at postmortem induration and other changes were observed macroscopically in the hippocampus of affected patients, and this lesion became known as Ammon's horn sclerosis. Renewed interest in this particular finding has been greatly stimulated in the recent past by the examination of material obtained at postmortem and following the operation of temporal lobectomy. Falconer and his co-workers at the Maudsley Hospital, London, have made outstanding contributions in this regard and coined the term 'mesial temporal sclerosis' (Falconer, Serafetinides and Corsellis, 1964) to include the classic Ammon's horn sclerosis and also the more widespread sclerosis extending into neighbouring structures such as the amygdala and the uncus (Figure 10.2). The term is used to embrace both gliosis and neuronal loss. Margerison and Corsellis (1966) in autopsy studies of epileptics, showed that mesial temporal sclerosis was the most common single lesion found in the brains they examined and it occurred in more than half the cases. Furthermore, the lesion was unilateral in 80 per cent of the patients. Taylor and Ounsted (1971) have explained this finding on the basis of differential rates of cerebral

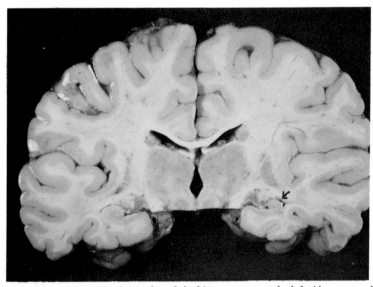

Figure 10.2. Sclerosis and atrophy of the hippocampus on the left side compared with the right, in an adult with a history of a prolonged febrile convulsion in early childhood and subsequent temporal lobe epilepsy. (Courtesy of Dr S. Murphy)

maturation between the hemispheres and between sexes, the right hemisphere suffering damage up to the age of two years and the left hemisphere subsequently. Falconer (1970) cites mesial temporal sclerosis as the example *par excellence* of a lesion of the limbic system and believes that the two most important factors in its causation are prolonged febrile convulsions in early childhood and a genetic predisposition to epilepsy. The latter has already been discussed in detail.

Among the other lesions found in resected material from Falconer's (1970) patients are hamartomas, which constitute about 20 per cent. These are benign indolent lesions which are mainly congenital malformations. They include glial malformations, small angiomas and occasionally areas of tuberose sclerosis. They tend to cluster around the amygdala and in the hippocampal gyrus and so involve the limbic system. Miscellaneous lesions constitute just over 10 per cent of the material and include scars and infarcts. Some of these may be secondary to head injury and others may be consequent on infection. The final 20 per cent of the material includes equivocal or nonspecific lesions, and Falconer points out that in these cases surgery is not so effective therapeutically as it can be when a definite lesion is found. Davidson and Falconer (1975) reviewed their case material with particular reference to children and 24 out of 40 children operated on had mesial temporal sclerosis, included two with hamartomas, and of those with mesial temporal sclerosis only nearly 80 per cent had a history of a prolonged febrile seizure. Finally, Falconer and his co-workers stress that, taking all age groups together, not only do those with mesial temporal sclerosis form the largest pathological group, but also they constitute a group of patients in which the onset of habitual epilepsy occurs in the first decade of life in nearly 60 per cent.

Clinical manifestations related to pathology

The description of temporal lobe seizures in the *International Classification* as partial seizures of complex symptomatology is extremely apt. Epilepsy usually mimics the normal function of the part of the brain involved in the seizure, although it may distort it. The more uncomplicated the function of the area of cortex involved the more accurately will the epileptic event mimic that function. In an area with the elaborate functions of the temporal lobe the epileptic event will necessarily be complex and is more likely to be a travesty of normal activity. Leaving aside its place in the physiology of hearing and speech, the most important function of the temporal lobe is the integration of sensations of all kinds. Williams (1966) has argued that the temporal lobe and limbic system enable an individual to appreciate himself as a unified being because they receive information from the special senses, the viscera and the higher centres. When a person with temporal lobe epilepsy is bombarded with autonomic and indescribable auras he loses this sense of himself, and this leads to emotional disturbance and even terror. Small children with such an aura may fall down wherever they happen to be or run in fear to their mothers. Later, they may avoid the room in which they experienced the frightening sensation. Flor Henry (1969) has written of temporal lobe epilepsy that 'the epileptic patient may experience his aura as weird, terrifying or ominous in its inexplicable foreignness to his personality'. What the patient with a temporal lobe attack feels is unnatural and beyond his normal experience and, in consequence, it is often impossible to describe to his relatives or to his physician.

SYMPTOMATOLOGY

Excessive local neuronal discharge in one or other temporal lobe can give rise to a remarkable variety of minor seizure patterns, many of them with bizarre sensory phenomena. Visceral or special sense experiences include epigastric and olfactory sensations, the latter with peculiar and often unpleasant smells (so-called 'uncinate fits'). The best known distortion of perception is perhaps the sensation of familiarity, of having been there before, known as *déjà vu*. Simple auditory hallucinations include voices or music and there may be complex visual and auditory hallucinations with familiar scenes or people from the past, with or without sounds or voices. Speech disturbances may occur if the dominant hemisphere is involved, and apart from dysphasia the patient may make totally inappropriate remarks in the attack. Emotional sensations of fear or strangeness are common. Occasionally, a feeling of vertigo may be experienced.

Secondary generalized epilepsy and temporal lobe absences

If the seizure discharge spreads to involve the cortex generally a secondary generalized epilepsy occurs (following the terminology of the *International Classification*) and a major tonic-clonic seizure ensues clinically. It is well recognized that epilepsy of temporal lobe origin may present initially with generalized seizures. Because of spread to the limbic system and to the diencephalon absences and automatisms may occur. Automatisms are rather more extended absences. The patient continues to perform familiar actions but in an odd and repetitive way, sometimes with aggressive or difficult behaviour and perhaps with confused mumbling speech.

The differential diagnosis between the absences of primary generalized epilepsy of the petit mal type and absences associated with temporal lobe discharges has already been mentioned in the chapter on petit mal. Penry, Porter and Dreifuss (1975) in a detailed study of 48 children with absence attacks, in which the clinical seizures and the EEGs were recorded simultaneously on video tape, showed that simple absences of the petit mal type with impaired consciousness only were relatively infrequent and usually lasted less than 10 seconds and rarely longer than 45 seconds. They were not preceded by an aura and mental clarity returned abruptly at the end of the attack. On the other hand, absences of the temporal lobe type were rarely less than 30 seconds in duration, frequently lasted from 1–2 minutes and were not uncommonly prolonged for several minutes. The majority of the attacks were preceded by an aura and full consciousness returned slowly rather than abruptly.

Clearly, it is very important to differentiate simple absences of the petit mal type from the complex temporal lobe absences because the treatment and prognosis are quite different for the two conditions.

DIAGNOSIS

The diagnosis of temporal lobe epilepsy is made easier if recognizable epileptic phenomena of a motor kind occur. Difficulties in diagnosis arise where only sensory phenomena or automatisms occur, since these may be difficult to distinguish from behavioural aberrations of one sort or another. In this respect it is important to remember that psychomotor seizures are generally paroxysmal episodes of relatively short duration, usually without any precipitating factor and they start and end abruptly while the reverse is characteristic of psychiatric disturbances. The latter are usually provoked by some disturbing situation. However, the distinction between the two can be blurred by the fact that temporal lobe epileptic attacks are more likely to happen when the subject is emotionally disturbed. Careful history taking should make it possible to recognize the repeated stereotyped epileptic events and distinguish them from the more continuous disturbance associated with a personality disorder. Lennox (1960) said: 'the burden of proof rests on anyone who contends that a given psychic episode, isolated from other evidence of epilepsy, is epileptic.'

There are certain *severe behavioural disturbances,* commonly associated with temporal lobe epilepsy in childhood and adolescence, which are described in detail in the chapter on emotional and psychiatric disorders associated with epilepsy (*see* Chapter 18). The hyperkinetic syndrome occurred in 26 per cent of the cases described by Ounsted, Lindsay and Norman (1966), and these children were most frequently

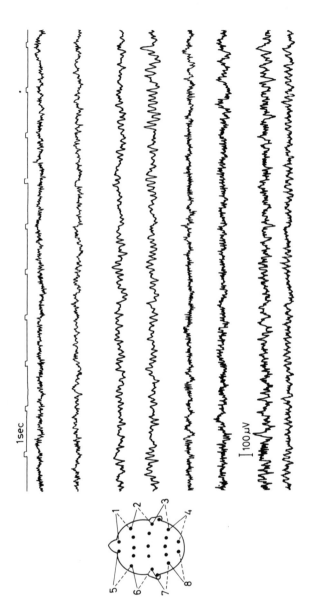

Figure 10.3a. Girl aged 11 years and awake with eyes open. EEG shows irregular slow-wave activity in the left temporal area

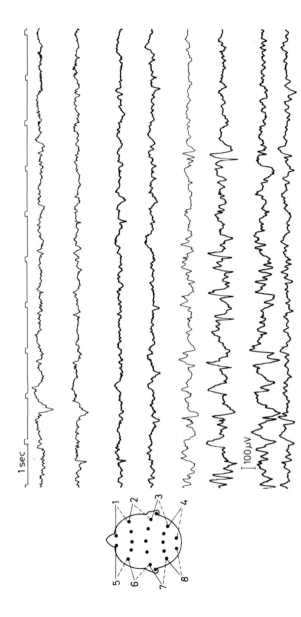

Figure 10.3b. EEG shows spike discharges in the left temporal area in the same patient (as in Figure 10.3a) during light sleep

those who had suffered an early brain insult or who had had status epilepticus, and many of them also showed a significant degree of mental handicap. Ounsted (1970) later postulated that the disruption of exploratory learning in these hyperkinetic children disbarred them from developing the basic mental structures which are the foundation of normal learning and intelligence. He emphasized the importance of remembering that phenobarbitone and related compounds can potentiate hyperkinetic behaviour, and conversely that such behaviour can be alleviated by withdrawing these drugs. Outbursts of catastrophic rage may also be seen in children and adolescents with temporal lobe epilepsy, which is interesting in view of the suggested relationship between limbic dysfunction and aggression. Behavioural disturbances with hyperkinesis or aggressive conduct are much more frequent in children with temporal lobe epilepsy than are the psychoses which are sometimes associated with the condition in adolescent and adult life. In fact it is exceptionally rare to see a psychotic illness in an individual with mesial temporal sclerosis, the commonest single lesion in children with temporal lobe epilepsy. It seems likely that psychosis is a reaction to temporal lobe epilepsy of later onset and this is rarely due to mesial temporal sclerosis. This matter is further amplified in the chapter on emotional and psychiatric aspects of epilepsy (*see* Chapter 18).

The investigation of temporal lobe epilepsy depends particularly on the *EEG examination*. Where the site of origin of an epileptic discharge is on the convexity of one of the cerebral hemispheres, its discovery and localization are relatively easy. In temporal lobe epilepsy, however, the causative lesions usually lie deep in the temporal lobe or on its inferior or medial aspects. Routine recording may fail to reveal the discharging focus, but usually a record during drowsiness or light sleep, either natural or drug induced, will demonstrate the abnormality (*Figures 10.3a* and *10.3b*). Sphenoidal electrodes are infrequently used in children, but nasopharyngeal electrodes, inserted painlessly through the nose, may be helpful in recording from the undersurface of the temporal lobes and electrodes of this type, specially designed for use in children, are now available. As mentioned earlier, if the underlying lesion is mesial temporal sclerosis it is likely to be unilateral in 80 per cent of cases. It has been established that mesial temporal sclerosis is more likely to occur in the right hemisphere if a prolonged febrile seizure occurs under the age of two years while the left hemisphere is more likely to be affected after two years (Taylor and Ounsted, 1971). The hemisphere undergoing more rapid maturational development at the time of the insult is likely to be the more vulnerable. If surgical removal of the affected temporal lobe is being considered at any stage, it is clearly important that the affected side should be detected unequivocally. One of the difficulties in this respect in children is that their EEGs often show generalized abnormalities or bilateral foci which do not crystallize into a clearly defined unilateral temporal lobe focus until adolescence. However, very careful EEG studies in centres skilled in this investigation, coupled with other neuroradiological and psychological investigations, will usually establish the side of the disease with certainty.

CHRONICITY AND PROGNOSIS

Authorities are not agreed on the incidence of temporal lobe epilepsy in childhood. Ounsted, Lindsay and Norman (1966) put it at 10 per cent of all epileptic children referred to hospitals for consultation in the Oxford catchment area. At Yale, Glaser and Dixon (1956) put the figures at 30 per cent. Clearly this variety of epilepsy is common in childhood. Furthermore, chronicity is one of its most characteristic features and in this it contrasts with many other forms of childhood epilepsy which tend to die out as the child gets older and so do not contribute to the adult epileptic population.

THERAPY

Penry (1975) has stated that the treatment of complex partial seizures is one of the greatest challenges in neurology today, and that although many patients with these seizures live successful and happy lives with their attacks completely controlled the proportion is relatively small in comparison with those who are permanently afflicted by the condition. Furthermore, those who do become seizure-free on medical treatment are frequently impaired in their vocational and social adjustments because of the side-effects of medication and such impairment is sometimes compounded by further neurological deficits resulting from the structural lesion of the region of the brain associated with the seizures.

The advent of phenobarbitone in 1912 and of phenytoin in 1938 significantly improved the situation but, because many patients proved refractory to these drugs, the search for new anticonvulsant agents continued with the arrival of primidone in 1954 which brought further benefit to some patients. The availability of carbamazepine since 1963 has undoubtedly been the most significant development in the drug therapy of temporal lobe epilepsy so far. Parsonage (1975), reviewing its use in adults, concluded that it was the best drug available for the treatment of complex partial seizures, and that it should be used as the drug of choice for this type of epilepsy. This view was widely endorsed in discussion at the Ninth International Symposium on Epilepsy held in

Amsterdam in September, 1977, and the relative lack of acute and chronic side-effects from the drug was emphasized (Porter and Penry, 1978).

Gamstorp (1977) reviewed her experience with carbamazepine in the treatment of temporal lobe epilepsy in children and also concluded that it was her drug of choice with phenytoin as her alternative therapeutic agent if carbamazepine failed. Of 101 children (61 boys and 40 girls) studied over five years 44 were seizure free and seven almost seizure free on carbamazepine alone. Fourteen children were seizure free and three almost seizure free on phenytoin alone. Two were relieved of fits on a combination of the two drugs and two others were greatly improved. In cases resistant to these drugs she used primidone, acetazolamide or sodium valproate. She preferred not to use phenobarbitone because of its side-effects. She did not observe any toxic effects from carbamazepine and the side-effects were few. However, she recommended that the drug should be introduced slowly, taking 3—4 weeks to attain the final dose. By this method initial side-effects such as drowsiness and ataxia were avoided. Her daily dosage did not exceed 20 mg/(kg. day) with a maximum total dose of 1200 mg/day. The drug was given in two divided doses in the morning and evening. The author's experience with carbamazepine is similar to that of Gamstorp (O'Donohoe, 1973, 1977).

SURGERY

There is no doubt that surgical removal of the temporal lobe has an important part to play in the treatment of chronic and intractable temporal lobe epilepsy in childhood, provided that the laterality and extent of the disease process can be confidently located before operation (Falconer, 1972). This requires a detailed assessment preoperatively including social and psychometric studies, EEG examination, including sleep and sphenoidal electrode recordings, and air encephalography. Air encephalography will frequently show dilatation of the temporal horn on the side of the lesion (*Figure 10.4*). Indeed, a straight skull X-ray may sometimes show constriction of the middle cranial fossa on the affected side or even calcification in a hamartoma. Electrocorticography will be necessary at the time of operation to confirm the extent of the abnormality. The usual operation is that of anterior temporal lobectomy as devised by Falconer, and the resected specimen includes the major parts of the hippocampus, the amygdala and the uncus. The rationale of the operation is that removal of the affected areas interrupts the neuronal circuits responsible for the propagation of seizure discharges. Falconer's criteria for operation are that the individual should have frequent disabling epilepsy which is resistant to adequate drug therapy, that neuroradiological studies should have ruled out a gross space-occupying lesion, that the EEG studies should have shown a unilateral discharging focus and that the patients should be at least of average intelligence. Davidson and Falconer (1975), in a recent study of 40 children treated surgically, reported that over half of the cases

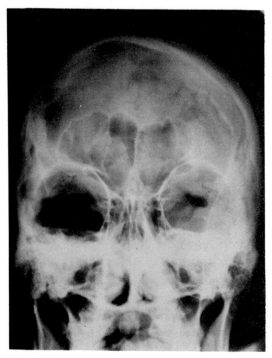

Figure 10.4. Pneumoencephalogram in a patient with temporal lobe epilepsy showing dilatation of the temporal horn of the right lateral ventricle while the appearance of the left temporal horn is normal. (Courtesy of Dr J. Toland)

had mesial temporal sclerosis and that the best long-term results of treatment were obtained when this lesion was present. Of 24 children with mesial temporal sclerosis 14 (58 per cent) became seizure-free in the long term, usually without medication, while eight out of 10 (80 per cent) with hamartomas achieved this goal. Corresponding improvement in behavioural difficulties, notably with regard to aggression, was also achieved.

Clearly, surgery will play an increasingly important part in the treatment of children with temporal lobe epilepsy in the future. In a review of surgery for temporal lobe epilepsy from Denmark (Jensen, 1977), using the criteria for operation of Falconer and his colleagues, the author commented that when the records of age at temporal lobectomy and the eventual results of operation were compared it was clear that the operation should preferably be performed in childhood, adolescence or early adulthood, or at any rate as soon as this particular type of epilepsy proved resistant to medication. The surgical treatment of temporal lobe epilepsy is also considered in Chapter 25.

REFERENCES

Aicardi, J. and Chevrie, J. J. (1970). 'Convulsive status epilepticus in infants and children. A study of 239 cases.' *Epilepsia*, 11, 187–197

Aird, R. B., Venturini, A. M. and Spielman, P. M. (1967). 'Antecedents of temporal lobe epilepsy.' *Archs Neurol., Chicago*, 16, 67–73

Davidson, S. and Falconer, M. A. (1975). 'Outcome of surgery in 40 children with temporal lobe epilepsy.' *Lancet*, 1, 1260–1263

Earle, K. M., Baldwin, M. and Penfield, W. (1953). 'Incisural sclerosis and temporal lobe seizures produced by hippocampal herniation at birth.' *Archs Neurol. Psychiat., Chicago*, 69, 27–42

Falconer, M. A. (1970). 'Historical review: The pathological substrates of temporal lobe epilepsy.' *Guy's Hosp. Rep.* 119, 47–60

Falconer, M. A. (1972). 'Place of surgery for temporal lobe epilepsy during childhood.' *Br. Med. J.* 2, 631–635

Falconer, M. A., Serafetinides, E. A. and Corsellis, J. A. N. (1964). 'Etiology and pathogenesis of temporal lobe epilepsy.' *Archs Neurol., Chicago*, 10, 233–248

Flor Henry, P. (1969). 'Psychosis and temporal lobe epilepsy.' *Epilepsia*, 10, 363–395

Gamstorp, I. (1977). 'A review of children with temporal lobe epilepsy.' In *Tegretol in Epilepsy: Proceedings of an International Meeting*, pp. 1–3. Ed. F. D. Roberts. Macclesfield, Cheshire: Geigy Pharmaceuticals

Gastaut, H. (1970). 'Clinical and electroencephalographical classification of epileptic seizures.' *Epilepsia*, 11, 102–113

Gibbs, F. A., Gibbs, E. L. and Lennox, W. G. (1937). 'Epilepsy: A paroxysmal cerebral dysrhythmia.' *Brain*, 60, 377–388

Glaser, G. H. and Dixon, M. S. (1956). 'Psychomotor seizures in childhood: A clinical study.' *Neurology, Minneap.* 6, 646–655

Hauser, W. A. and Kurland, L. T. (1975). 'The epidemiology of epilepsy in Rochester, Minnesota, 1935 through 1967.' *Epilepsia*, 16, 1–66

Jensen, I. (1977). 'Temporal lobe epilepsy; on whom to operate and when.' In *Epilepsy: The Eighth International Symposium*, pp. 325–330. Ed. J. K. Penry. New York: Raven Press

Lennox, W. G. (1960). *Epilepsy and Related Disorders*. Boston: Little, Brown and Company and London: J. and A. Churchill

Margerison, J. H. and Corsellis, J. A. N. (1966). 'Epilepsy and the temporal lobes: A clinical, electroencephalographic and neuropathological study of the brain in epilepsy, with particular reference to the temporal lobes.' *Brain*, 89, 499–530

O'Donohoe, N. V. (1973). 'A series of epileptic children treated with Tegretol.' In *Tegretol in Epilepsy. Report of an International Clinical Symposium*, pp. 25–29. Ed. C. A. S. Wink. Macclesfield, Cheshire: Geigy Pharmaceuticals

O'Donohoe, N. V. (1977). 'Tegretol in everyday paediatric practice.' In *Tegretol in Epilepsy. Proceedings of an International Meeting*, pp. 10–12. Ed. F. D. Roberts. Macclesfield, Cheshire: Geigy Pharmaceuticals

Ounsted, C. (1951). 'Significance of convulsions in children with purulent meningitis.' *Lancet*, **1**, 1245–1248

Ounsted, C. (1970). 'A biological approach to autistic and hyperkinetic syndromes.' In *Modern Trends in Paediatrics*, pp. 286–316. Ed. J. Apley. London: Butterworths

Ounsted, C., Lindsay, J. and Norman, R. (1966). *Clinics in Developmental Medicine, No. 22: Biological Factors in Temporal Lobe Epilepsy*. London: Spastics International and Heinemann

Parsonage, M. (1975). 'Treatment with carbamazepine: Adults.' In *Advances in Neurology*, Vol. 11, pp. 221–234. Eds J. K. Penry and D. D. Daly. New York: Raven Press

Penry, J. K. (1975). 'Perspectives in complex partial seizures.' In *Advances in Neurology*, Vol. 11, pp. 1–11. Eds J. K. Penry and D. D. Daly. New York: Raven Press

Penry, J. K., Porter, R. J. and Dreifuss, F. E. (1975). 'Simultaneous recording of absence seizures with video-tape and electroencephalography: A study of 374 seizures in 48 patients.' *Brain*, **98**, 427–440

Porter, R. J. and Penry, J. K. (1978). 'Efficacy and choice of antiepileptic drugs.' In *Advances in Epileptology. Proceedings of the Ninth International Symposium on Epilepsy, Amsterdam, 1977*, pp. 220–231. Eds H. Meinardi and A. J. Rowan. Amsterdam and Lisse: Swets and B. V. Zeitlinger

Taylor, D. C. and Ounsted, C. (1971). 'Biological factors influencing the outcome of seizures in response to fever.' *Epilepsia*, **12**, 33–45

Wallace, S. J. (1976). 'Neurological and intellectual deficits. Convulsions with fever viewed as acute indications of life-long developmental defects.' In *Brain Dysfunction in Infantile Febrile Convulsions*, pp. 259–277. Eds M. A. B. Brazier and F. Coceani. New York: Raven Press

Williams, D. (1966). 'Temporal lobe epilepsy.' *Br. Med. J.* **1**, 1439–1442

CHAPTER 11

Reflex Epilepsy

Seizures triggered by a sensory stimulation are sometimes called 'reflex epileptic seizures' since the nerve structure responsible for the seizure is situated between the sensory afferent pathway and the efferent tract responsible for the epileptic phenomena, thus acting as a reflex centre. This concept of reflex epilepsy was very fashionable in the nineteenth century when it was considered that a major cause of epilepsy, particularly in children, was chronic sensory irritation produced by such varied causes as intestinal worms, phimosis, refractive errors and teething. Part of this belief lingers on in the lay mind, and perhaps the association between chronic constipation and epilepsy in the folklore of epilepsy is a part of it.

Criteria

When strict criteria are used for defining 'reflex' epilepsy it is found to be relatively rare. Gastaut and Tassinari (1966) make the point that true 'reflex' epilepsy should be clearly distinguished from the part played by nonsensory epileptogenic factors which seem to act by affecting certain biological constants and modifying the threshold of cerebral excitability. These factors include hyperventilation; hyperthermia; the ingestion of alcohol; metabolic disorders of various kinds including hypocalcaemia and hypoglycaemia; extreme physical or emotional stress, particularly when accompanied by sleep deprivation; and perhaps hormonal changes occurring at menstruation or during puberty.

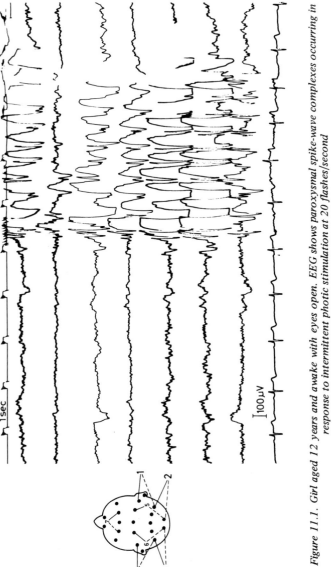

Figure 11.1. Girl aged 12 years and awake with eyes open. EEG shows paroxysmal spike-wave complexes occurring in response to intermittent photic stimulation at 20 flashes/second

PHOTOSENSITIVITY AND TELEVISION–INDUCED EPILEPSY

By far the most frequent of true reflex epileptic seizures are those produced by visual stimuli (i.e. visually-evoked reflex epilepsy), although even those are relatively rare in relation to the overall frequency of epileptic attacks. Photosensitivity can be investigated in the EEG laboratory by applying a very bright rhythmically repeating white flash (intermittent photic stimulation) to the whole of the visual fields of both eyes, open and shut, for short periods. Single visual evoked responses can then be recorded over the occipital areas at slow rates of flicker and continuous rhythmic waveforms occur at faster rates of flicker. These responses do not irradiate anteriorly and cease with the final flash of the stimulating sequence. The most common abnormality following photic stimulation is that induced in the photosensitive epilepsies. This consists of a burst of bilaterally symmetrical generalized multiple spikes (polyspikes) or spike and wave complexes (*Figure 11.1*). These generalized discharges usually appear after very brief stimulation and may sometimes outlast the period of stimulation. This type of response is termed the photoconvulsive response. It may be seen in up to one per cent of normal children (Driver and MacGillivray, 1976) and in a few normal adults. In any individual exhibiting the photoconvulsive response the period of stimulation should be brief in case a seizure is induced.

Some individuals are exquisitely photosensitive and may have a seizure provoked by intermittent light stimulation under natural conditions, for example the play of light through trees or on water or on snow or reflected from a brilliant object. There is a less sensitive group in which clinical seizures can be induced by flickering from a light source of high intensity with relatively darker surroundings. This is the situation which obtains in *television-induced epilepsy* which is by far the commonest type of photosensitive epilepsy today. Gastaut and Tassinari (1966) summarized the characteristic features of television-induced seizures as those occurring essentially but not exclusively in children, being almost always of the primary generalized major tonic-clonic type, being sometimes preceded by generalized myoclonic jerks and almost always showing spike and wave complexes or polyspike and wave discharges during intermittent photic stimulation in the EEG laboratory. An absence, lasting 5–15 seconds, may also be induced by intermittent photic stimulation. Children with photosensitivity are mainly at risk when viewing television while being seated close to a normally functioning set. Neither faulty functioning of the television set producing a flicker effect (as with a faulty line hold) nor the usual play of images on the screen seem to play any significant part in causing seizures, except perhaps in a few very sensitive individuals. The proximity of the screen is of paramount importance in triggering an attack which may occur when the subject approaches the set to adjust it. Some photosensitive children seem compulsively drawn to the screen and may occasionally seem to enjoy the sensation produced, although usually they fear it. Nearness to the screen means that a larger area of the retina is stimulated by flicker and viewing in subdued ambient lighting may also increase the contrast effect produced by the brightly-lit screen. Sensitive subjects are equally at risk from black-and-white television and colour television. There is no convincing evidence that any particular component of the colour spectrum is more epileptogenic than others. Using a portable TV set with a small screen may reduce the risk (*British Medical Journal*, 1978).

Bower (1963) and Troupin (1966) drew attention to the fact that epilepsy induced by television viewing was less commonly encountered in the USA than in Europe. This has been shown to be due to higher frequency of the AC mains supply in the USA which alternates at 60 Hz compared with 50 Hz in Europe. The normally functioning television set produces flicker at the mains frequency and at half that rate, and the slower flicker rates in Europe (50 Hz and 25 Hz) are more likely to produce a photoconvulsive response in photosensitive patients. In the EEG laboratory the great majority of patients with photosensitivity will show photoconvulsive responses (polyspikes, polyspikes and waves or spike-wave complexes at 3 Hz) at flicker frequencies of 15—20 flashes/second. Similar discharges occur on eye closure in the resting EEG in about 20 per cent of sensitive patients, and this finding usually indicates that photoconvulsive responses will follow during photic stimulation.

Photosensitive epilepsy: age of onset and prognosis

Photosensitive epilepsy usually begins in the decade 6—15 years, never earlier and rarely later. It commences most frequently between the ages of 12 and 13 years which suggests a possible link with early puberty. There is a higher incidence of the condition in females. Jeavons and Harding (1975) in their outstanding monograph or photosensitive epilepsy, described the results of a 12-year study of 460 patients. Even after such a comprehensive and lengthy investigation of the problem they were still uncertain about the long-term prognosis for affected patients. Their findings suggested that photosensitivity continued for at least 10 years and disappeared with age, although probably not until well into the third decade of life. They pointed out that it was uncommon in their series to find evidence of photosensitivity in the EEGs of the parents of photosensitive children, even when one or other parent described symptoms associated with flicker at an earlier age. The general experience is that it is unusual to encounter clinical photosensitive epilepsy in adults.

Photosensitivity: genetics

Doose *et al.* (1969) surveyed the hereditary aspects of the EEG abnormalities induced by photic stimulation. They found that 26.2 per cent of the siblings of patients with photosensitive epilepsy showed a photoconvulsive EEG response compared with 6.7 per cent in healthy controls. They concluded that the photoconvulsive response could be a symptom of a very widespread genetically-determined susceptibility to convulsions of the primary generalized type originating from the brain stem, and that the actual morbidity for epilepsy was low. A symptomatic photosensitivity is very rarely associated with organic brain lesions such as brain tumours or after encephalitis, and is a characteristic finding in neuronal ceroid lipofuscinosis (Batten—Vogt syndrome) where discharges occur in the EEG in response to very slow rates of intermittent photic stimulation (Pampiglione and Harden, 1977).

PREVENTION AND TREATMENT

The photosensitive patient should always watch television from a distance of not less than 3 metres and the room should be well lit. He or she should be dissuaded from approaching the set in order to adjust it or to change the channel; however, if this is absolutely necessary one eye should be covered with the palm of the hand as this will usually help to block the photoconvulsive response (Jeavons and Harding, 1970). Polarized sunglasses are helpful outdoors in preventing attacks in bright sunlight. The patient whose seizures are entirely photosensitive will not usually need anticonvulsant therapy, although there are exceptions (particularly where there are epileptic discharges in the resting EEG in addition to those produced by flicker or when clinical seizures are frequent). The patient who has epilepsy other than that produced by flicker (a point difficult to establish with certainty in the very sensitive patient) and who also has definite photosensitive epilepsy will need regular long-term anticonvulsant medication. Although all the commonly used anticonvulsants have been tried for this purpose, there is evidence (Jeavons, Clark and Maheshwari, 1977) that sodium valproate is particularly effective in this regard. Many parents ask whether the images on a cinema screen constitute a risk for a photosensitive patient, but in fact the flickering is at too high a frequency to induce an attack. The flicker effect used in discotheques, on the other hand, may provoke seizures in sensitive individuals, and in 1971 the Greater London Council forbade the use of flicker rates faster than 8 flashes/second; a slow frequency reduces the risk but does not abolish it altogether. Even watching the movement of an escalator may be provocative in some individuals.

Gastaut (1952) was probably the first person to describe *self-induced photosensitive epilepsy* when he wrote: 'One of our young patients provoked his absences voluntarily by placing rhythmically his hand, fingers open, in front of his eyes when he looked at the sun. A little girl took a mischievous pleasure in provoking her absences by moving her head very quickly from right to left behind a window trimmed with stained glass panes brilliantly illuminated by the sun.' The mechanism in this rare form of epilepsy (perhaps commoner, as Gastaut remarks, beneath 'the luminous sky of Provence') consists of the rhythmical interruption of natural or artificial light and is similar to the effects produced by watching sunlight flickering through trees while being driven in a car or by watching the rotation of the blades of a helicopter against a bright sky. Sherwood (1962) collectively reviewed cases of self-induced epilepsy.

Jeavons (1977) differentiates patients with what he terms *'photomyoclonic epilepsy'* from the general body of the patients with photosensitive epilepsy. These are patients, usually adolescents, who show spontaneous spike and wave discharges in their EEGs and also have similar discharges during intermittent photic stimulation. He describes two subgroups comprising first, those patients who have myoclonic jerks of head and arms, occurring spontaneously and during photic stimulation and, secondly, those patients who demonstrate rapid jerking movements of the eyelids immediately after eye closure (associated with bilateral spike and wave activity) and who have brief absences associated with spike wave discharges at 3 Hz which occur both spontaneously and during photic stimulation. The recommended treatment is with sodium valproate.

Before leaving the subject of visually-evoked reflex epilepsy, the condition of *pattern-evoked epilepsy* needs to be mentioned. In this unusual entity seizure discharges are produced in the EEG by looking at certain patterns. Episodes of staring triggered by vertical lines such as striped or corduroy trousers and absences precipitated by other vertical lines such as air vents, tiles or bed spreads have been reported (Chatrian *et al.*, 1970). Pattern-evoked responses probably play a part in reading epilepsy, mentioned below.

NON-VISUAL PRECIPITATING FACTORS

The most common modality of sensory precipitation in reflex epilepsy is visual, but there are rarer sensory precipitants including sound, touch, proprioception and also possibly visceral, olfactory and vestibular stimuli. Seizures may be triggered by a particular mental activity, such as hearing or performing music, reading, writing, specific visual or auditory imagery or mathematical calculation. The term 'startle epilepsy' is sometimes applied to brief clonic or tonic-clonic seizures provoked by auditory stimuli or by touch. Acoustimotor seizures may occur in infants with diffuse brain disease or abnormality, classically in those with G_{M_2} gangliosidosis (Tay-Sachs disease). Similar brief attacks are also seen in older children and are provoked by a violent and unexpected noise, almost always in children with epilepsy due to diffuse organic brain disease. The author has seen them especially in mentally handicapped children who had previously suffered from infantile spasms or who had one of the secondary generalized epilepsies of the myoclonic type. These seizures are particularly resistant to drug therapy in these patients.

A different type of *'startle epilepsy'* may be elicited by touching the patient or by sudden movements which elicit a proprioceptive response. However, such stimuli may prove ineffective unless combined with an element of surprise. This type of startle response may occur following a sudden tap or blow on the head and must be distinguished from vasovagal syncope, a much commoner cause of such an event. Rarely, immersion of the lower parts of the body in water, as when bathing a child, may lead to a reflex epileptic seizure occurring (*immersion epilepsy*). Another type of attack provoked by movement is that usually entitled 'paroxysmal choreoathetosis' (Perez-Borja, Tassinari and Swanson, 1967). These attacks, which can occur either in children or adults, are facilitated by anxiety, tension, sudden movement or a fright. The patient stiffens, stares, adducts the lower limbs and dystonic or writhing movements of trunk and limbs occur accompanied by grimacing. Many authorities have considerable reservations about the genuinely epileptic nature of this curious condition. It is important to remember, however, that persistent choreoathetoid involuntary movements can occur in epileptic patients with chronic phenytoin toxicity (McLellan and Swash, 1974).

The wider one casts the net of reflex epilepsy the more one realizes that the strict distinction between genuine sensory and nonsensory precipitating factors cannot be maintained. For example, *reading epilepsy* (Critchley, 1962) is accompanied by patterned visual and proprioceptive stimuli which could act as triggers, and some patients with reading epilepsy are also photosensitive. Others, however, are affected only by interesting, difficult or emotionally charged reading material. In some, reading is only one of several activities associated with language which induce seizures. In the form of evoked seizures in which the stimuli are complex, such as a particular type of music or a particular type of reading material, part of the response may, in that particular patient, be secondary to emotional factors causing a conditioned response in a Pavlovian sense. In the rare patient whose seizures are precipitated by eating or gustatory sensations, a conditioned reflex is almost certainly responsible. Of interest is the fact that in some of these evoked or reflex epilepsies the patient may be deconditioned to the particular stimulus involved (Forster *et al.*, 1969). A somewhat analogous situation exists in the case of certain partial motor or sensory seizures precipitated by sensory stimuli in which the patient can abort the attack by counter stimulation, for example by vigorously rubbing the hand and arm if the attack has started there.

In conclusion, it must be emphasized that reflex epilepsies, apart from photosensitive epilepsy, are very rare. But, just as their dramatic nature has always intrigued the lay observer their underlying mechanisms have also greatly interested the leading minds in the world of epileptology in efforts to understand the basic pathophysiology of epilepsy. Interested readers are referred to the Symposium on Reflex Mechanisms in the Genesis of Epilepsy, published in *Epilepsia* in 1962.

REFERENCES

Bower, B. D. (1963). 'Television flicker and fits.' *Clin. Pediat.* **2**, 134–138
Chatrian, G. E., Lettich, E., Miller, L. H. and Green, J. R. (1970). 'Pattern-sensitive epilepsy: Part I.' *Epilepsia*, **11**, 125–149
Critchley, M. (1962). 'Reading epilepsy.' *Epilepsia*, **3**, 402–406
Doose, H., Gerken, H., Hien–Volgel, K. F. and Volzke, E. (1969). 'Genetics of photosensitive epilepsy.' *Neuropädiatrie*, **1**, 56–73
Driver, M. V. and MacGillivray, B. B. (1976). 'Electroencephalography.' In *A Textbook of Epilepsy*, pp. 109–144. Eds J. Laidlaw and A. Richens. Edinburgh, London, New York: Churchill Livingstone
Editorial (1978). 'Television-induced epilepsy and its prevention.' *Br. med. J.* **2**, 1301–1302
Forster, F. M., Hanastia, P., Cleeland, C. S. and Ludwig, A. (1969). 'A case of voice induced epilepsy treated by conditioning.' *Neurology, Minneap.* **19**, 325–331
Gastaut, H. (1952). 'Effects de la S.L.I. sur l'activité nerveuse centrale et sur ses composantes somatiques, végétatives et psychiques.' In *Compte Rendus du Bième Congrès Technique National de Sécurité et d'Hygiène du Travail*, pp. 1–10. Paris: Foulon
Gastaut, H. and Tassinari, C. A. (1966). 'Triggering mechanisms in epilepsy. The electroclinical point of view.' *Epilepsia*, **7**, 85–138
Jeavons, P. M. (1977). 'Nosological problems of myoclonic epilepsies in childhood and adolescence.' *Dev. Med. child Neurol.* **19**, 3–8
Jeavons, P. M. and Harding, G. F. A. (1970). 'Television Epilepsy.' (Letter) *Lancet*, **2**, 926
Jeavons, P. M. and Harding, G. F. A. (1975). *Clinics in Developmental Medicine, No. 56: Photosensitive Epilepsy*. London: Spastics International and Heinemann
Jeavons, P. M., Clark, J. E. and Maheshwari, M. C. (1977). 'Treatment of generalised epilepsies of childhood and adolescence with sodium valproate ('Epilim').' *Devl Med. child Neurol.* **19**, 9–25
McLellan, D. L. and Swash, M. (1974). 'Choreo-athetosis and encephalopathy induced by phenytoin.' *Br. med. J.* **2**, 204–205

Pampiglione, G. and Harden, A. (1977). 'So-called neuronal ceroid lipofuscinosis. Neurophysiological studies in 60 children.' *J. Neurol. Neurosurg. Psychiat.* **40**, 323–330

Perez-Borja, C., Tassinari, A. C. and Swanson, A. G. (1967). 'Paroxysmal choreoathetosis and seizures induced by movement (reflex epilepsy).' *Epilepsia*, **8**, 260–270

Sherwood, S. L. (1962). 'Self-induced epilepsy: A collection of self-induced epilepsy cases.' *Archs Neurol., Chicago*, **6**, 49–65

Symposium on Reflex Mechanisms in the Genesis of Epilepsy (1962). *Epilepsia*, **3**, 209–468

Troupin, A. S. (1966). 'Photic activation and experimental data concerning coloured stimuli.' *Neurology, Minneap*, **16**, 269

CHAPTER 12

Epilepsy in the Adolescent

Epilepsy is the most common neurological disorder in adolescence. In one American clinic specifically for adolescent patients, epilepsy accounted for 63 per cent of the neurological problems seen and for 9.9 per cent of the total patients seen (Castle and Fishman, 1973). Cooper (1965), in his large study of children with epilepsy, found a total prevalence rate of 8.2/1000 at the age of 15 years (4.7 new and 3.4 old cases). In Kurland's (1959–60) study the average annual incidence rate for seizures between the ages of 10 and 14 years and between the ages of 15 and 19 years was respectively 24.7/100 000 and 18.6/100 000 population, with higher incidence rates for males occurring with all types of seizures. In a survey of adolescent services in the USA and Canada, Garell (1965) found that convulsive disorders ranked among the five most frequently encountered conditions in most clinics. The frequency with which epilepsy occurs in adolescence and the interaction between the condition and the special problems of adolescence make it necessary to consider the problem and its management in this age group separately. The problem may conveniently be divided into epilepsy beginning before adolescence and epilepsy arising *de novo* during adolescence. The clinical aspects were very well reviewed by Gascon (1974) using this subdivision.

PREPUBERTY EPILEPSY

Epilepsy beginning in childhood may improve or deteriorate with the onset of puberty. In considerably more than 50 per cent of children with true petit mal (primary generalized epilepsy) arrest of the condition or very marked improvement will have taken place. In others, however, primary generalized epilepsy of the grand mal type will complicate their seizure problem. The prognosis of petit mal is discussed in more detail elsewhere (page 82). Benign focal epilepsy of childhood, also described elsewhere (page 99), tends to arrest in early or midadolescence. Any patient with chronic epilepsy who suffers marked deterioration in his symptoms or whose seizure patterns change in adolescence should be suspected of having a slow-growing brain tumour (Kristiansen, Henriksen and Levin, 1970) and should have the appropriate neuroradiological investigations instituted. However, it should be remembered that established temporal lobe epilepsy may be increasingly complicated by behavioural disorders in adolescence and these should be distinguished from genuine seizure patterns.

EPILEPSY STARTING AT PUBERTY

When epilepsy arises *de novo* in this age group it is important to inquire into any previous history of possible seizures which may have been missed or forgotten, for example the brief staring attacks of petit mal or febrile convulsions in early childhood. True primary generalized epilepsy of the petit mal type rarely presents in early adolescence and extremely rarely after the age of 15 years (Livingston, 1972). When it appears to present in adolescence, it is important to remember that the absences may, in fact, be of the temporal lobe type rather than the true petit mal type. Prolonged and/or atypical attacks should suggest this and careful EEG examination, including a sleep record and perhaps telemetry if available, should be performed.

Primary brain tumours, arising in the cortex, are much more likely to present in adolescence than they are in early childhood when subtentorial tumours predominate (*see* Chapter 15). Partial epilepsy may occasionally be the presenting symptom of such a tumour and certainly it looms large in parents' minds when their son or daughter develops epilepsy in adolescence.

Photosensitive epilepsy may present for the first time in adolescence and the mechanism triggering the first attack may be the flashing stroboscopic lights used in the subterranean darkness of a discotheque!

Primary generalized epilepsy of the grand mal type may also present for the first time in adolescence, and the initial attack may be precipitated by lack of adequate sleep, over-indulgence in alcohol or drug abuse or withdrawal.

There is an unusual variety of epilepsy presenting in adolescent patients of normal intelligence about the time of puberty which is variously called *myoclonic epilepsy of adolescence* and *impulsive petit mal* (Aicardi and Chevrie, 1971; Jeavons, 1977). It is rather more common in girls and the attacks may coincide with menstruation. Myoclonic jerks are bilateral and particularly involve the shoulders and the arms. Repeated jerks may occur, usually shortly after awakening. The patient may drop what he or she is holding. Generalized tonic-clonic seizures may also occur but are rare and usually nocturnal. The EEG may be normal or show bilateral irregular spike waves at 3 Hz or poly-spike discharges. Sometimes typical absences of the petit mal type with the typical EEG pattern may occur. This condition is rather unresponsive to drug therapy but the benzodiazepine drugs such as clonazepam may help. An oral contraceptive may work in older patients.

The possibility of *degenerative disease* of the central nervous system should be remembered, particularly SSPE or Van Bogaert's disease, which may present in early adolescence with failing school performance, emotional and personality disturbance and sudden myoclonic movements of the head and limbs which coincide with the characteristic generalized paroxysmal abnormalities in the EEG. High levels of measles antibodies are found in the blood and CSF.

DIFFERENTIAL DIAGNOSIS

Careful history taking and physical examination are as important in adolescence as in any other age group. The differential diagnosis is, however, rather different from that in childhood. Syncope is more common in early adolescence and 'dizzy spells', occurring perhaps under emotional stress, also need to be distinguished from minor epileptic attacks. Malingering and hysterical attacks may also have to be considered, and loss of consciousness provoked by hyperventilation is still seen occasionally in hysterical girls. One should beware of any attack which can be produced 'on request' or before an audience, where the seizure patterns change from attack to attack, where bodily injury never occurs in the seizure, and where recovery is unexpectedly rapid and the usual postictal symptoms of sleep, stupor, confusion and headache do not follow an apparent major tonic-clonic convulsion. The hysterical patient may betray herself by being able to give an account of events which coincided with her actual attack or she may clearly be imitating the genuine seizure patterns of another patient in the same hospital ward.

Investigations

The investigation of epilepsy in adolescence should be limited to the basic tests such as skull X-rays and EEG examination unless there is some specific indication for proceeding to a more detailed study of the patient. EEG examination may show the presence of focal spikes or typical or atypical spike-wave patterns. Interseizure EEG records, both in waking and sleeping, may be quite normal in primary generalized epilepsy (grand mal) of the idiopathic type in which genetic factors are aetiologically predominant. Partial or focal motor convulsions alone are not an indication for extensive neuroradiological investigations unless there are some associated abnormal neurological findings. Careful clinical assessment of the individual patient should remain the essential guide to whether detailed investigation is necessary or not. It must be remember that elaborate often painful investigations are particularly alarming for the adolescent and this includes the performance of a lumbar puncture. Examination of CSF for measles antibodies is, of course, essential in suspected SSPE.

THERAPY

The general problems of anticonvulsant therapy in adolescence are similar to those which obtain in childhood generally, but there are special difficulties peculiar to this age group. *The commonest reason for failure to obtain control or loss of control of seizures in adolescents is the patient's intentional or unintentional failure to take his medication regularly*. The patient should be seen frequently in the early stages of therapy and carefully instructed about the nature of his illness and the need to take his drugs conscientiously.

The use of the word 'drug' in this age group is probably a mistake anyway and the word 'medication' may be preferable. The adolescent is particularly concerned about his appearance, his need to conform with his peers, his sense of personal identity and the need to break away from dependence on his parents; and so the stress of an unpredictable condition such as epilepsy and the need to take regular treatment may place intolerable burdens on him. He will be aware of the social implications of having epilepsy and of the public prejudice about the condition and he may attempt to refute the diagnosis by omitting his drugs. Sudden withdrawal of medication is, of course, a potent cause of status epilepticus at any age. Monitoring of serum levels may be necessary at regular intervals in order to test the patient's compliance with medical advice about treatment (*see* Chapter 25).

The patient will need constant support and encouragement and family counselling and planning regarding vocational aspirations should start at this time. It should be recognized that the earlier one recognizes disabling emotional reactions to epilepsy the easier it will be to alleviate them and to ensure that the patient will maintain a stable personality. The help of a psychiatrist skilled in the management of adolescent problems may be invaluable. The expense of therapy in some countries should also be remembered.

The patient should be encouraged to wear an Medic Alert bracelet indicating the nature of his complaint, especially if his attacks are frequent and major in type, but many adolescents will refuse to do this. In those patients whose epilepsy began before adolescence and who have had some years of remission on treatment, the question of withdrawing treatment will arise. As discussed elsewhere (page 268) there is controversy about whether withdrawing treatment during puberty leads to relapse, but recent evidence suggests that this may not be so (Holowach, Thurston and O'Leary, 1972).

Drugs of choice

If possible, the drugs chosen for treatment should be those which do not interfere with concentration and with academic, social and physical activities. For this reason barbiturates should probably be avoided. Ingesting alcohol with an anticonvulsant such as phenobarbitone will result in a summation of sedative effects, and adolescents with epilepsy should be discouraged from taking alcohol which may in itself provoke a seizure in a susceptible individual. Furthermore, it should be remembered that in depressed adolescents barbiturates are among the most lethal of the common anticonvulsants used in attempted suicide. Carbamazepine is, in the author's experience, an excellent anticonvulsant for general use in adolescence. The problems of using phenytoin at any age are discussed elsewhere but, in the adolescent, thickening of facial tissues, gum hyperplasia and hirsuties may be intolerable side-effects, especially in girls (see Chapter 24). However, there is no evidence that phenytoin exacerbates adolescent acne. The new anticonvulsant, sodium valproate, is being used increasingly in epilepsy generally and is notably free of depressant side-effects.

Withdrawal of therapy

In the author's experience the adolescent with epilepsy lives for the day when treatment is terminated. Withdrawal of therapy should depend on the following considerations:

1. That he has been seizure free for a period of 2–4 years, preferably the latter
2. That his epilepsy was of a type which responded promptly to treatment in the first instance
3. That intelligence is unimpaired and that no underlying neurological disease or serious psychological disorder exists

4. That care is exercised in withdrawing drugs slowly, especially in girls at puberty
5. That EEG abnormalities have not persisted or worsened during therapy.

It should also be remembered, when withdrawing therapy in late adolescence, that even a single seizure may prohibit the patient from obtaining a driving licence or it may cause him to lose the one he has already obtained, thereby perhaps losing him his job also. Therefore, drugs should be withdrawn very slowly (taking 6—18 months for the process), and each drug should be withdrawn independently if two are being used concurrently and, if a relapse occurs, medication should be restarted immediately at the dosage levels which previously controlled the epilepsy.

GENERAL ADVICE

The patient and his parents will be concerned about participation in sports and other physical activities. There is evidence that physical exercise actually raises the seizure threshold (Götze, Munter and Teichmann, 1967) and it is not necessary to place unusual restrictions on the patient which will, in any case, only increase his sense of being different from his peers and draw their attention to the difference. Swimming alone should, however, be prohibited and he should be encouraged to take showers rather than baths.

In late adolescence the patient and his parents will be concerned about vocational training, university education, the prospects of marriage and the genetic risks of epilepsy. The wish to obtain a driving licence will also arise and legal regulations about this vary from country to country and in the USA from state to state.

To sum up, the adolescent patient with epilepsy needs good and regular medical care, an explanation about his illness and constant encouragement. He requires as good an education or vocational training as possible, support and advice to ensure that normal personality development occurs and, perhaps the most important of all, enlightened attitudes about epilepsy from parents, peers, teachers and prospective employers.

REFERENCES

Aicardi, J. and Chevrie, J. J. (1971). 'Myoclonic epilepsies of childhood.' *Neuropädiatrie*, **3**, 177—190
Castle, G. F. and Fishman, L. S. (1973). 'Seizures in adolescent medicine.' *Pediat. Clins N. Am.* **20**, (4), 819—835

Cooper, J. E. (1965). 'Epilepsy in a longitudinal survey of 5000 children.' *Br. med. J.* 1, 1020–1022

Garell, D. C. (1965). 'A survey of adolescent medicine in the US and Canada.' *Am. J. Dis. Child.* 109, 314–317

Gascon, G. G. (1974). 'Epilepsy in the adolescent.' *Postgrad. Med.* 55, 111–117

Götze, W., Munter, St K. M. and Teichmann, J. (1967). 'Effects of physical exercise on seizure threshold: Investigated by electroencephalographic telemetry.' *Dis. nerv. Syst.* 28, 664–667

Holowach, J., Thurston, D. L. and O'Leary, J. L. (1972). 'Prognosis in childhood epilepsy.' *New Engl. J. Med.* 286, 169–174

Jeavons, P. M. (1977). 'Nosological problems of myoclonic epilepsies in childhood and adolescence.' *Devl Med. child Neurol.* 19, 3–8

Kristiansen, K., Henriksen, G. H. and Levin, L. (1970). 'Development of cerebral gliomas in children with chronic epilepsy.' *J. Oslo Cy Hosps,* 20, 97–108

Kurland, L. T. (1959–60). 'The incidence and prevalence of convulsive disorders in a small urban community.' *Epilepsia,* 1, 143–161

Livingston, S. (1972). *Comprehensive Management of Epilepsy in Infancy, Childhood and Adolescence,* p. 58. Springfield, Illionois: Charles C. Thomas

CHAPTER 13

Post-traumatic Epilepsy

The remarkable improvements in modern obstetrics have made brain injury at birth a rarity. The avoidance of breech delivery has been particularly important in this respect. However, the battering of babies (euphemistically called nonaccidental injury) has reached epidemic proportions in many Western societies and injuries to the head and face are all too common. Battering is probably the commonest single cause of subdural haematoma in infancy today. Furthermore, as Caveness (1976) has written: 'accidental death and disability in our time has achieved a magnitude comparable to the plagues of the Middle Ages.' The frequency of post-traumatic epilepsy is increasing, in children as well as adults, because of the larger number and greater severity of head injuries, particularly those caused by traffic accidents. Lesions occur as a result of contusions and lacerations, not only at the actual site of injury but also in distant and opposite regions of the brain. Quite apart from cortical damage, lesions are frequent in the brain stem in many cases of severe head injury. Anoxic damage to the brain and the consequences of cerebral oedema and haemorrhage are additional features. In those who survive, several epileptic foci may develop in different parts of the brain and atrophic changes may also be present.

Children, particularly boys, are at risk of sustaining head injuries as a result of their adventurous play. New and potentially dangerous toys, such as skateboards, may add to the risk unless protective head-gear is worn. Jennett (1973) has estimated that 100 000 patients are admitted to British hospitals with head injuries every year and approximately one-quarter of these are under 16 years of age.

SEIZURES OCCURRING SOON AFTER INJURY

Seizures in the first week after injury are much commoner than those occurring in any of the succeeding weeks. Epilepsy in the first week (early epilepsy) has many differences from that which occurs later. Approximately one-third of early fits occur within an hour of injury, about a third during the rest of the first day and the remainder during the first week. Traumatic epilepsy of this type is most common in young children. The incidence of early seizures is almost twice as great in the under fives as in the over fives. Jennett (1977) emphasizes that any fit in the first week after injury should be taken seriously (particularly in young children) because of the immediate risk of status epilepticus developing, even after relatively mild injuries. The special significance of early epilepsy after a head injury is that it carries four times the risk of the patient developing late epilepsy. Of people who have a fit in the first week after injury 75 per cent never experience another. However, 25 per cent do have a subsequent seizure, and this represents a very significantly increased risk when compared with patients who do not suffer an early convulsion and where the risk of later epilepsy is only 3 per cent. Jennett (1977) found the risk to be exactly the same, even when the injury was trivial, i.e. where no fracture, no unconsciousness or post-traumatic amnesia and no intracranial haematoma occurred. Even a single fit in the first hour signifies a considerable risk, particularly in relation to prophylactic anticonvulsant medication (to be discussed below).

SEIZURES COMMENCING AFTER THE FIRST WEEK

In the case of what is termed late epilepsy (seizures that develop one week or more after an injury has been sustained) the first fit occurs within the first year after injury in more than 50 per cent of cases. However, in about 25 per cent of such patients epilepsy is delayed for more than four years. When can one say that there is no chance of developing post-traumatic epilepsy ? As Jennett says, the answer is never. An individual may have a focal fit directly related to a focal injury 20 or even 40 years later. Late epilepsy is partial in about 40 per cent of cases and is often of complex symptomatology with temporal lobe phenomena of bizarre type which may not easily be recognized as epilepsy. Once late epilepsy develops the seizures persist in about 80 per cent of cases, even though they may be infrequent.

Three conditions contribute to a higher risk of late epilepsy, namely, a fit occurring in the first week, a depressed fracture and an acute intracranial haematoma. Post-traumatic amnesia lasting for more than 24 hours, the presence or absence of both dural tears and focal signs are all of predictive value in estimating the risk of late epilepsy. By using all this information it is possible for the neurosurgeon to identify high risk patients and recommend prophylactic anticonvulsant medication if required (Jennett, 1975). In Jennett's opinion evidence is now available to enable the neurosurgeon to assess the risk of late epilepsy in any individual case of head injury and to offer the patient advice about prophylaxis. How long should prophylaxis be continued ? As already stated the risk of late epilepsy never disappears completely, but of those who are going to develop it nearly three-quarters will do so by the end of the second year after the accident. Several authors, including Jennett and van de Sande (1975) have found EEG studies unhelpful in predicting the possibility of late epilepsy. However, EEG abnormalities are commoner in those who develop late epilepsy and this only reflects the greater degree of brain damage in these patients. Also, there are patients who develop EEG abnormalities but who never have a fit and some who develop post-traumatic epilepsy and have normal EEGs.

PROPHYLAXIS AFTER INJURY

In recent years the question of pharmacological prophylaxis of post-traumatic epilepsy has aroused considerable interest among those dealing with injured adults. This problem arises because of the clinical phenomenon of the latent period, which may be measured in years, between the brain trauma and the appearance of late epilepsy. It has been suggested that a period of 'ripening' of the epileptogenic lesion is required before clinical epilepsy develops. It may be that anticonvulsant drugs can suppress this process long enough for it to disappear, perhaps because damaged neurones die. It is known, from the evidence of experimental neurophysiological research, that the interictal cortical spike may propagate via association tracts to the homologous region of the opposite hemisphere evoking a secondary spike. In chronic preparations in animals such a region of secondary spiking may become independently active, forming a 'mirror' focus, which may persist even after the primary focus becomes inactive or is ablated. Mirror foci are not limited to the cortex, but may also develop in the limbic and other subcortical systems where they are synaptically related to a primary subcortical focus (Proctor, Prince and Morrell, 1966). It seem clear, therefore, that bombardment by neurones of the primary focus alters neurones of the mirror area so that they become independently epileptic.

FACILITATION OF FITS (KINDLING)

The related and remarkable phenomenon called 'kindling', the knowledge of which is based on animal studies (Wada, Sato and Corcoran, 1974; Wada, 1976), is also important in this context. Kindling may be defined as the facilitation of seizure pathways by repeated fits. In the experimental model repeated brain exposures to brief stimuli induce an increasingly pathological response. Initially, the stimulus produces no effect, but later after-discharges occur which gradually increase in severity and duration. Ultimately, spontaneous seizures develop. Many workers now consider the kindling phenomenon to be one of the most convincing animal models of human epilepsy so far discovered. There are obvious lessons for human post-traumatic epilepsy and for the possible suppression of its evolution by prophylactic medication. There may even be lessons for the problem of the brain-injured neonate.

Medicolegal aspects

Paediatricians are sometimes faced with the medicolegal problem of trying to decide whether a child is genuinely experiencing post-traumatic epilepsy or not. Usually, the first question to consider is whether the child is having genuine epilepsy or not, and the case history and the EEG examination are helpful here. Secondly, he should consider whether the type of epilepsy which is occurring is one which is likely to follow trauma. Clearly, a condition such as primary generalized epilepsy of the petit mal type is not a post-traumatic sequela. Thirdly, he should examine the circumstances of the original injury and decide whether it was of sufficient severity to cause brain injury and subsequent epilepsy. A pitfall here has already been mentioned, namely, that even trivial head injuries may be followed by late epilepsy, especially in those who have seizures in the first week after the accident. In any event, head injuries and later epilepsy are closely associated in the lay mind and it may be very difficult to convince juries that a cause and effect situation does not exist in any particular case.

REFERENCES

Caveness, W. F. (1976). 'Epilepsy: A product of trauma in our time.' *Epilepsia*, **17**, 207–215
Jennett, B. (1973). 'Trauma as a cause of epilepsy in childhood.' *Devl. Med. child Neurol.* **15**, 56–62
Jennett, B. (1975). *Epilepsy after Non-missile Head Injuries,* 2nd Edn. London: Heinemann

Jennett, B. (1977). 'Traumatic epilepsy – the scale of the problem'. In *Epilepsy, Trauma and the Family Doctor*, 4–5. Eds B. Jennett and C. W. M. Whitty. Hull: Reckitt and Colman Pharmaceutical Division

Jennett, B. and van de Sande, J. (1975). 'EEG prediction of post-traumatic epilepsy.' *Epilepsia*, 16, 251–256

Proctor, F., Prince, D. and Morrell, F. (1966). 'Primary and secondary spike foci following depth lesions.' *Archs Neurol. , Chicago*, 15, 151–162

Wada, J. A. (1976). (Ed.) *Kindling*. New York: Raven Press

Wada, J. A., Sato, M. and Corcoran, M. E. (1974). 'Persistent seizure susceptibility and recurrent spontaneous seizures in kindled cats.' *Epilepsia*, 15, 465–478

CHAPTER 14

Mental Handicap and Epilepsy

Overall frequency of epilepsy

Epilepsy is one of the most frequently associated handicaps occurring in mentally retarded children, and it is of considerable significance in their management. It is difficult to get a true estimate of the prevalence of epilepsy in the mentally handicapped, but it is certain that the proportion rises steadily as the degree of retardation increases. Tizard and Grad (1961), in a survey of severely retarded children at home and in institutional care, found that 18 per cent suffered from seizures and that the seizures were more frequent among those who were institutionalized. Corbett (1974) reported an epidemiological study of retarded children in Camberwell, London, in which parents were questioned in detail; over 80 per cent of the children had EEGs and all were neurologically assessed. He found that of 155 children with an IQ under 50 or with one of the syndromes associated with severe retardation, 32 per cent had a history of epilepsy at some time during life, while 19 per cent had had at least one seizure during the previous year. In the children with an IQ of less than 50, a quarter under the age of five years had had a fit in the previous year in comparison with an incidence of 18 per cent between the ages of five and 10 years and 5 per cent between the ages of 10 and 15 years. Seizures in the mentally handicapped are therefore a particular problem of early childhood. The frequency of epilepsy in the mildly mentally handicapped is less certain and is probably in the order of 3—6 per cent depending on whether uncomplicated epilepsy or epilepsy associated with other neurological handicaps is considered (Rutter, Graham and Yule, 1970). In the mildly mentally handicapped social and environmental factors are probably as important as organic factors in the aetiology of their condition, and therefore it is not surprising that epilepsy is less frequent in this group.

Variation with different syndromes

The occurrence of epilepsy varies considerably in the different syndromes associated with mental handicap. It is, for example, uncommon in Down's syndrome. In tuberose sclerosis, however, it is very common and, as previously noted, these children may first present with infantile spasms or with isolated and unexplained seizures in the neonatal period or in very early infancy (Gamstorp, 1976). Fits are also frequent in children with cerebral palsy; they occur mainly in those with the spastic variety, but are uncommon in those with choreoathetoid and ataxic forms of cerebral palsy. Similarly, the more severe and generalized the cerebral palsy, and the more profound the mental retardation, the greater will be the incidence of epilepsy. Woods (1957) found that 58 per cent of her 201 cases of cerebral palsy had epilepsy, but lower figures have been reported by others. Acute acquired hemiplegia occurring in a setting of status epilepticus has already been described and is very frequently followed by epilepsy and mental retardation.

Continuing epilepsy as a sequel of infantile spasms, whether cryptogenic or symptomatic in type, has already been discussed. It is significant in this context that preceding perinatal brain damage is the commonest single cause of symptomatic infantile spasms just as perinatal brain damage is also a very important cause of other chronic brain syndromes including cerebral palsy, mental retardation and epilepsy. Indeed, anything which causes widespread structural damage to the developing brain — and this includes inflammatory disorders, metabolic disorders such as hypernatraemia and untreated aminoacidurias, direct trauma and prolonged febrile seizures — is likely to be followed by a moderate or severe degree of mental handicap and by associated epilepsy and neurological deficit. The implications of this as far as preventive paediatrics is concerned will be obvious to the reader.

Behavioural disturbances and epilepsy

The associations between epilepsy and behavioural disturbances in children of normal intellect, and between structural brain lesions, epilepsy and behavioural disorders will be discussed in a separate chapter (*see* Chapter 18). Severely retarded children with epilepsy may also have troublesome behaviour problems, and it is most important to bear in mind that these may be a consequence of over-enthusiastic anti-convulsant medication. Seizures in these children are often refractory to therapy and parents and doctors, especially doctors working with institutionalized children, tend to use excessive doses of drugs or to indulge in gross polypharmacy in attempts to control the attacks. As a result the patient may become overactive, aggressive, destructive and even uncontrollable, or alternatively he may become apathetic and somnolent. Progressive mental deterioration may be suspected as a result. The seizures may even increase in frequency leading to yet more medication. The epilepsy may be blamed for the deterioration in the intellectual level or a condition of minor status epilepticus may be suspected. The EEG is useful in diagnostic differentiation here but it may be difficult to arrange one urgently for children in institutions for the mentally handicapped. Estimating serum levels of anticonvulsants is mandatory in this situation and this service should be available for the severely mentally handicapped with epilepsy. It should also be noted that chronic toxic effects of drugs such as folate deficiency, vitamin D deficiency and the various effects of phenytoin overdosage are commoner in institutionalized mentally handicapped children with epilepsy than they are in normal children with epilepsy living at home (see Chapter 24).

EEG findings

Corbett, Harris and Robinson (1975) summarized their EEG findings of the Camberwell study of 155 children with moderate and severe mental handicap aged from 2–15 years at the time of the survey. They categorized their results as follows. Some records failed to show any abnormality while others showed mild abnormalities only. Clearly abnormal records, including those with unequivocal epileptic abnormalities, occurred twice as frequently in children who had a history of epilepsy. They commented on the difficulties experienced in obtaining satisfactory records in these patients. The recording should preferably be done by a technician experienced in dealing with children and stick-on electrodes are essential if unacceptable movement artefacts are to be avoided.

Drug treatment

The drug treatment of epilepsy in the mentally handicapped should be subject to the same precautions that are applied to normal children with epilepsy. However, it must again be emphasized that children with moderate or severe handicap and those with neurological deficits, such as spastic cerebral palsy, tend to develop troublesome side-effects when treated with phenobarbitone and primidone, particularly abnormal overactivity and irritability.

DOES EPILEPSY LEAD TO MENTAL DETERIORATION?

The parents of any child with epilepsy frequently ask if their child will become mentally subnormal as a consequence of his complaint. Epilepsy and mental abnormality are closely associated in the lay mind, partly because the moderately and severely retarded often have epilepsy as a symptom of their basic brain disease, and partly because the myth of the 'epileptic personality' dies hard and the fear of mental deterioration in the child haunts the parents. The latter problem is discussed fully elsewhere (*see* Chapter 18). However, parents should be assured that although a very small number of children with epilepsy undoubtedly show deterioration of intellect and personality (e.g. some children with infantile spasms and the myoclonic epilepsies and cases of degenerative disease presenting with epilepsy) the vast majority are of normal and often superior intelligence and remain so in spite of their complaint.

REFERENCES

Corbett, J. A. (1974). *Epilepsy in Children with Severe Mental Handicap.* Proceedings of Symposia 16, pp. 27–41. Ed. F. P. Woodford. London: Institute for Research into Mental and Multiple Handicap
Corbett, J. A., Harris, R. and Robinson, R. G. (1975). 'Epilepsy.' In *Mental Retardation and Developmental Disabilities,* Vol. 111, pp. 81–111. Ed. J. Wortis. New York: Brunner, Mazel, Inc.
Gamstorp, I. (1976). In *Epileptic Seizures – Behaviour, Pain,* p. 63. Ed. W. Birkmayer. Bern, Stuttgart, Vienna: Hans Huber
Rutter, M., Graham, P. and Yule, W. (1970). *Clinics in Developmental Medicine, Nos. 35/36: A Neuropsychiatric Study in Childhood.* London: Spastics International and Heinemann
Tizard, J. and Grad, J. C. (1961). *The Mentally Handicapped and their Families.* Maudsley Monograph, No. 7. London: Oxford University Press
Woods, G. E. (1957). *Cerebral Palsy in Childhood.* Bristol: John Wright

CHAPTER 15

Epilepsy and Brain Tumours

Brain tumours have a notorious reputation as a cause of late-onset epilepsy in adults, even though they are responsible for only about 10 per cent of such cases. As the most frequent solid tumours occurring in childhood, brain tumours constitute an important part of paediatric oncology. Brain tumours and epilepsy are inextricably linked in the lay mind and many parents are deeply concerned about this possibility, particularly when their child has his first fit or when the attacks are refractory to treatment. *In fact, brain tumours are a very rare cause of childhood epilepsy.*

In a recent review of tumours in infancy and childhood (edited by Jones and Campbell, 1976), 430 consecutive children with intracranial tumours, the majority treated at the Royal Children's Hospital, Melbourne, were analysed. Tumours occurring in the posterior cranial fossa were the most common and accounted for 51 per cent of their series. Others have put the incidence of subtentorial tumours in childhood as high as two-thirds of all cases (Wilson, 1975). Subtentorial tumours commonly present with signs and symptoms of cerebellar involvement, with evidence of raised intracranial pressure and occasionally with cranial nerve palsies. Fits are almost unknown in such a situation although the intermittent decerebrate posturing of a child with a cerebral tumour compressing the midbrain may be mistaken for an epileptic seizure on occasions. The second most common group of cerebral tumours in children consists of those found in the region of the third ventricle and include craniopharyngiomata, tumours of the optic nerves and chiasma and tumours of the walls and floor of the ventricle. These are nonepileptogenic. Superficial tumours of the cerebral cortex accounted for 10 per cent of the Melbourne series (Jones and

147

Campbell, 1976) and these were usually highly malignant. Nonmalignant tumours such as meningiomata were exceedingly rare, difficult to eradicate and not necessarily associated with seizures, probably because the brain had ample time to adapt to their presence.

Malignant cortical tumours in the Melbourne series (Jones and Campbell, 1976) were evenly distributed over the first three quinquennia of childhood and early adolescence. The commonest locations were in the parietal and frontal lobes and much less frequently they were in the temporal and occipital lobes.

Epilepsy occurred in 26 per cent of those with cortical tumours and was usually focal or partial. Generalized seizures can occur, however, and frontal lobe tumours have a sinister reputation for presenting with status epilepticus in both children and adults (Rowan and Scott, 1970). The other symptoms and signs of cortical tumours in children are headache, vomiting, papilloedema and the occasional development of a hemiparesis. Despite the rarity of this association between brain tumours and epilepsy, fundoscopy should be the rule in all children presenting with their first fit. Unfortunately, complete excision of cortical tumours was possible in only a third of the Melbourne series (Jones and Campbell, 1976) and, indeed, the overall prognosis for cerebral tumours in childhood is tragically bad. The recent monograph by Bell and McCormick (1978) contains an exhaustive review of intracranial tumours in childhood in all their aspects.

REFERENCES

Bell, W. E. and McCormick, W. F. (1978). *Increased Intracranial Pressure in Children*, 2nd Edn, pp. 307–476. Philadelphia, London, Toronto: W. B. Saunders
Jones, P. G. and Campbell, P. E. (1976). *Tumours of Infancy and Childhood*, pp. 231–287. Oxford, London, Edinburgh, Melbourne: Blackwell Scientific
Rowan, A. J. and Scott, D. F. (1970). 'Major status epilepticus. A series of 42 patients.' *Acta Neur. Scand.* **46**, 573–584
Wilson, C. B. (1975). 'Diagnosis and surgical treatment of childhood brain tumours.' *Cancer*, **35**, 950–956

CHAPTER 16

Epilepsy and Sleep

Consideration is given to various non-epileptic paroxysmal nocturnal events in the chapter on the differential diagnosis of epilepsy (page 199– 202). These include nightmares, night-terrors and noctural enuresis. In the author's opinion, neither these nor other phenomena such as sleep-walking should be designated as 'epileptiform' or as 'epileptic equivalents'. However, the close relationship between true epileptic attacks and sleep has been well known since earliest times and the rapidly increasing knowledge of the physiology of sleep in recent years has led to a corresponding interest in the association between sleep and epilepsy.

Since the earliest use of the EEG in clinical research, there has been a close interest in the altered electrophysiological state occurring in sleep and in the relationship between sleep and epilepsy. A very readable account of recent knowledge about sleep is that of Oswald (1974). Janz (1974) has reviewed the available information concerning epilepsy and the sleeping-waking cycle.

SLEEP STAGES, VIGILANCE AND AROUSAL

It is now recognized that sleep may be divided into four stages, called 1 to 4 or, sometimes, A to D (Loomis, Harvey and Hobart, 1937; Dement and Kleitman, 1957). The first stage (stage A) is really not sleep at all but represents drowsiness with eyes closed. The alpha rhythm (8–13 Hz) persists in the EEG but, as drowsiness passes into sleep, it gives way to a flatter wave pattern characterized by slower more irregular theta waves (4–7 Hz) and by low-voltage fast or beta activity (>13 Hz). This is the second stage of sleep or stage B. In the third stage (stage C), the

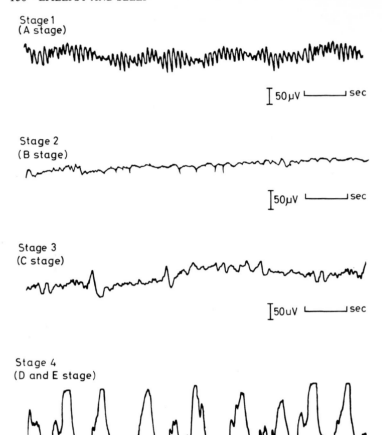

Figure 16.1. The EEG stages of sleep. (1 to 4 or A to D and E). (Courtesy of Roche Products, Ltd., London)

pattern of the second stage gives way to more irregular and slower waves of higher voltage (frequency 1–6 Hz). From time to time spindles of faster waves occur in the anterior areas and are known as sleep spindles. In this stage an appropriate external stimulus, such as a sudden loud noise, will give rise to a characteristic wave pattern known as a 'K' complex. This consists of a small sharp wave succeeded by one or more larger slow waves which are then followed by fast waves. Finally, in stage 4 (stage D) slow irregular high-voltage delta waves (1–3 Hz) replace all other forms of activity and the individual is deeply asleep. Some have distinguished two separate stages (D and E) in deep sleep, depending on whether stimulation elicits 'K' complexes or not. In the understanding of the sleep process, the concept of continuous activity of the cortex as shown by the EEG is essential. Except in the deepest stage of sleep, when stimuli may provoke no reaction, 'cerebral vigilance' remains. This is something quite distinct from normal consciousness. Consciousness depends on a steady activation flow from the reticular formation in the brain stem to the cortex. When this activation flow diminishes or ceases, as it does in sleep, contact with reality, or consciousness as we know it, is lost but cerebral vigilance, although lowered, remains with us until the deepest stages of sleep are reached. Even in the deepest stage of sleep, however, a stimulus with special relevance to the sleeping person may produce arousal as, for example, when a sleeping mother awakens to her baby's faint cry from another room.

The mechanism of *arousal* is centred in the reticular formation of the mid-brain and hind-brain, and with the activation (which the reticular formation gives to the cortex) consciousness would not be possible. In sleep these two parts of the brain behave differently. During the deepest stage of cortical sleep the hind-brain is relatively active, and when cortical sleep lightens the hind-brain sleep deepens producing a situation called 'paradoxical sleep'. During paradoxical sleep, the cortical EEG is characterized by a near wakefulness pattern, and rapid bilateral synchronous eye movements occur. The latter have resulted in paradoxical sleep being called *rapid eye movement or REM sleep*. Cortical vigilance is high in REM sleep and one might also expect consciousness to be present, but the latter is not the case because of the relative inactivity of the reticular formation. The subject is, in fact, difficult to awaken from this type of sleep. During REM sleep there is a suppression of muscle tone and accelerated irregular respiration and heart rates, whereas in non-REM sleep (stages 1–4) muscle tone is present because of the activity of the reticular formation, and heart and respiration rates are slow and regular. Dreaming is generally believed to take place during REM sleep. The pattern of a normal night's sleep is to pass initially into stage 4 sleep and, during the rest of the night, to rise and fall through progressively lighter stages until finally awakening. Superimposed on this pattern are periods of REM sleep which occupy 15–25 per cent of the total sleep time of adults. In the newborn, however, REM sleep occupies 45–50 per cent of total sleep time, but with increasing age the proportion of quiet non-REM sleep soon increases and adult sleep patterns are reached in later childhood.

Non-epileptic disorders

Disorders other than epilepsy which are associated with sleep and which may be confused with epileptic events are well reviewed by Anders and Weinstein (1972). Noctural enuresis, sleep walking, sleep talking and night terrors are associated with the emergence from stage 3 and/or 4 non-REM sleep and are defined as disorders of arousal. Narcolepsy, on the other hand, is associated with the abnormal occurrence of REM sleep and is regarded as a disorder of sleep. The disorders of arousal appear to be associated especially with the presence of normal neurological immaturity in young children.

Stages of sleep and waking related to seizures

Gibbs and Gibbs (1952), in their classic atlas of the EEG, were among the first investigators to emphasize the fact that seizure discharges were much more frequent in sleep than in the waking state and that such discharges were particularly frequent in symptomatic epilepsy. They showed that a sleep EEG was much more likely to demonstrate a temporal lobe epileptic focus than was a waking record. This is not invariable, however, and Matthes (1961) has stressed that sleep may not activate the epileptic focus but may actually cause a decrease in temporal lobe activity in a proportion of children. In using sleep as an initiator of epileptic activity in children, it is important not to be misled by the occurrence of sharp waves and rhythmic spike waves over the vertex during drowsiness and light sleep, findings which many consider normal phenomena.

When the times at which seizures occur in the context of the sleeping-waking cycle are recorded, it will be found that they tend to occur as follows:

1. Within the first or second hour after going to sleep, i.e. during deep sleep
2. One to two hours before the usual time of awakening, i.e. during lighter sleep
3. Within the period of a few minutes to two hours after awakening (early morning seizures).

Epilepsy occurring exclusively during sleep is uncommon at all ages (Gibberd and Bateson, 1974).

When the chronological approach is applied to the various types of childhood epilepsy, both generalized and partial, it will be found that these epilepsies often have fairly clear relationships to the sleeping-waking cycle. Infantile spasms are frequent during drowsiness and just after awakening and may be repeated. Although the EEG pattern of hypsarrhythmia is generally present in both the sleeping and waking states, it may be apparent only during sleep in certain cases. A sleep record should therefore be performed in all patients who shów a normal or non-hypsarrhythmic record at the onset of the illness and it is also useful in monitoring therapy with ACTH or steroids (Jeavons and Bower, 1964).

The sudden bodily jerks of the whole or part of the body upon falling asleep are a very familiar experience and are often accompanied by sudden and violent sensations, particularly by a feeling of falling. The individual usually awakens in an alarmed state. *Sleep jerks* occur at the stage of disappearance of the alpha rhythm and the appearance of low voltage slow waves in the EEG. They are certainly not an epileptic phenomenon and, indeed, there is no evidence for the existence of any type of epilepsy having as its sole symptom the occurrence of epileptic myoclonias on falling asleep or during sleep (Lugaresi *et al.*, 1970).

In the *primary and secondary generalized myoclonic epilepsies* of late infancy and early childhood, including those preceded by infantile spasms, nocturnal fits are common and, as Janz (1974) says: 'when the parents take their ailing child into bed with them, the child's myoclonic jerking throughout the night may give them not a moment's rest.' Short generalized tonic flexion spasms may occur in the severe varieties of myoclonic epilepsy, such as the Lennox-Gastaut syndrome (Gastaut *et al.*, 1966), particularly during the deeper stages of sleep. Drop seizures of the akinetic type often occur following arising, both after awakening from nocturnal and from afternoon sleep. Myoclonic absences are also frequent at these times. In the EEG diagnosis of these epilepsies it is important to remember that the slow spike-wave pattern may be activated by sleep.

The *less serious varieties* of childhood epilepsy also have a close relationship to the sleeping-waking cycle. Lennox—Buchthal (1973), in her monograph on febrile convulsions, emphasized that the attacks occurred during sleep in half the cases studied and that they were related to sleep (on going to sleep or on awakening) in another quarter. Any family doctor or paediatric hospital resident will be only too well aware of this association!

Primary generalized epilepsy of the petit mal type, on the other hand, occurs most frequently after children have awakened, and attacks are particularly common after arising in the early morning although they may occur at any time of the day. The attacks do not, as a rule, occur during sleep, although the EEG discharges may be recorded in sleep. Lack of sleep for any reason may result in an increased number of absences the next day. Where petit mal and grand mal are combined the major attacks tend to occur in the waking state, often after awakening (Janz, 1974).

In the so-called myoclonic epilepsy of adolescence, also known as generalized epilepsy of adolescence with myoclonic jerks (Aicardi and Chevrie, 1971), bilateral myoclonic jerks, especially of shoulders and arms, are frequent after awakening and major seizures may occur during sleep. In some photosensitive individuals the spike and wave activity which occurs after eye closure and which may be accompanied by eyelid flicker and brief absences, is not usually a problem in the dark when the person retires to bed, according to Jeavons (1977). However, Tassinari *et al.* (1977) reported myoclonic jerks which were related to eye closure and occurred at bedtime in five children, four of whom showed photosensitivity. These jerks were noted before actual sleep ensued and so could be distinguished from the normal sleep jerks. In doubtful cases the EEG helps to make the distinction. Children and adolescents with marked photosensitivity may also suffer from myoclonic jerks after awakening in the morning, particularly when sunlight shines into bedrooms as curtains are drawn or when natural or artificial light is reflected from bathroom tiles or mirrors. One of the author's patients, with discharges occurring after eye closure, experienced absences when he dipped his head towards a wash-basin to wash his face.

Primary generalized epilepsy of the grand mal type is relatively uncommon during sleep in childhood. When attacks do occur they tend to exhibit two peaks, either soon after falling asleep or during early morning sleep. Secondarily generalized tonic-clonic seizures in patients with partial epilepsy are much commoner than primary generalized epilepsy of the grand mal type but they are difficult to distinguish from generalized tonic-clonic attacks without focal onset because sleep conceals their initial motor phenomena, such as versive movements or unilateral clonic movements which may be easily observed during wakefulness. By far the commonest epilepsy of this type manifesting itself in sleep is that known as benign focal epilepsy, which is fully described elsewhere (*see* Chapter 9). In one large series (Beaussart, 1972), 51 per cent of the cases had their attacks exclusively during sleep. Ambrosetto and Gobbi (1975) were able to record an EEG during nocturnal sleep in a 10-year-old boy and noted that the spike discharges were activated both in REM sleep and in slow-wave sleep. The actual attack occurred as the boy appeared to be awakening and while he was still in a drowsy state. Adverse movements of the head and eyes away from the side of the EEG abnormality were noted initially and these were followed, on the contralateral side, by tonic extension of the limbs and by clonic jerking. Subsequently, the head and eyes turned back to the side of the EEG lesion and clonic jerking developed on that side also. It can readily be understood why these attacks may be misinterpreted as primary generalized seizures rather than partial attacks with secondary generalization. The EEG discharges are activated by sleep in benign focal epilepsy, making it likely that the attacks actually start during sleep and wake the patient rather than commencing during the drowsy period of awakening.

Partial seizures with complex symptomatology are uncommon during drug-induced or natural sleep despite the fact that sleep is usually a potent activator of focal EEG discharges in this type of epilepsy. Temporal lobe attacks, when occurring in sleep, tend to do so after the patient has fallen asleep rather than in the second half of the night, and they may also occur during an afternoon nap. Tassinari *et al.* (1974) make the important point that they have never observed exclusively nocturnal temporal lobe seizures. Similar attacks are always experienced in the daytime also. The practical importance of this observation is that one should have a very cautious attitude towards diagnosing complex nocturnal behavioural manifestations as being epileptic in nature, even when the interictal EEG records show abnormalities, unless similar diurnal episodes are experienced. Sophisticated methods of continuous EEG recording throughout the night may be necessary in difficult cases in order to establish a firm diagnosis.

Tassinari *et al.* (1977) describe a very rare type of *epileptic encephalopathy* occurring during slow-wave sleep and associated with subclinical status epilepticus. EEG sleep recordings are essential for diagnosis. Continuous high-voltage diffuse slow spike-wave discharges appear as soon as the patient falls asleep and persist throughout non-REM sleep. This makes it impossible to distinguish the stages of sleep. The electrical status disappears in REM sleep phases. The syndrome begins in childhood between the ages of four and 10 years. Infrequent nocturnal seizures, diurnal absences, behavioural disorders and deterioration in intellectual capacity and social performance may occur. The behavioural disorders may be prepsychotic in type and associated with a relative lack of interest in the environment and in normal activities. The condition slowly but never completely remits. It has been suggested that there is a close relationship between the presence of the electrical status in sleep and the psychic syndrome. Tassinari and his co-authors (1977) suggest that the substitution of the continuous spike and wave discharges for the normal physiological sleep pattern of non-REM sleep could be the cause of the psychic disturbances.

Effects of drug treatment

How may these considerations regarding epilepsy and sleep affect general management and treatment ? Since over-fatigue and insufficient sleep may affect fit frequency in some childhood epilepsies, it follows that an ordered life with a regular bedtime and hour for rising should be beneficial. There has long been considerable interest in the effects of drugs on sleep patterns. Barbiturates and related drugs increase the amount of deep sleep. In deep sleep, as already described, the hind-brain and its reticular formation are active and this may facilitate the genesis and propagation of discharges in primary and secondary generalized epilepsies, including those originating in the temporal lobes. Phenobarbitone has long been considered by many as unsuitable for the treatment of epilepsy during sleep (Janz, 1974). In paradoxical or REM sleep, although cortical vigilance is high, there is relative inactivity of the reticular formation and a consequent reduction in epileptogenesis may take place. Drugs with a reduced hynotic effect, such as phenytoin and carbamazepine, and drugs which increase the amount of REM sleep, such as the benzodiazepines, may be more effective in sleep epilepsies than those drugs with a marked hynotic effect.

Finally, it must be admitted that there is a great deal which is unknown concerning sleep and epilepsy. The factors involved may include endocrine and metabolic phenomena because some hormones show circadian rhythms and there are changes in body temperature and in water and electrolyte balances in sleep. There are also alterations in neurotransmitter mechanisms in the brain during sleep (Jouvet, 1972). The intense worldwide interest in the physiology of sleep will surely contribute further to the understanding and alleviation of epilepsy in the future.

REFERENCES

Aicardi, J. and Chevrie, J. J. (1971). 'Myoclonic epilepsies of childhood.' *Neuropädiatrie*, **3**, 177–190
Ambrosetto, G. and Gobbi, G. (1975). 'Benign epilepsy of childhood with Rolandic spikes, or a lesion? EEG during a seizure.' *Epilepsia*, **16**, 793–796
Anders, T. F. and Weinstein, P. (1972). 'Sleep and its disorders in infants and children: A review.' *Pediatrics*, **50**, 312–324
Beaussart, M. (1972). 'Benign epilepsy of childhood with Rolandic (centrotemporal) paroxysmal foci: A clinical entity. Study of 221 cases.' *Epilepsia*, **13**, 795–811
Dement, W. and Kleitman, N. (1957). 'Cyclic variations in EEG during sleep and their relation to eye movements, body motility and dreaming.' *Electroenceph. clin. Neurophysiol.* **9**, 673–690
Gastaut, H., Tassinari, C. A., Regis, H., Dravet, C., Bernard, R., Pinsard, N. and Saint-Jean, M. (1966). 'Childhood epileptic encephalopathy with diffuse slow spike waves (otherwise knows as 'petit mal variant or Lennox syndrome').' *Epilepsia*, **7**, 139–179
Gibberd, F. B. and Bateson, M. C. (1974). 'Sleep epilepsy: Its pattern and prognosis.' *Br. med. J.* **2**, 403–405
Gibbs, F. A. and Gibbs, E. L. (1952). *Atlas of Electroencephalography, Vol. 2: Epilepsy*. Cambridge, Massachusetts: Addison–Wesley

Janz, D. (1974). 'Epilepsy and the sleeping-waking cycle.' In *Handbook of Clinical Neurology, Vol. 15: The Epilepsies*, pp. 457–490. Eds P. J. Vinken and G. W. Bruyn. Amsterdam: North-Holland

Jeavons, P. M. (1977). 'Nosological problems of myoclonic epilepsies in childhood and adolescence.' *Devl. Med. child Neurol.* 19, 3–8

Jeavons, P. M. and Bower, B. D. (1964). *Clinics in Developmental Medicine, No. 15: Infantile spasms. A review of the literature and a study of 112 cases.* London: Spastics Society and Heinemann

Jouvet, M. (1972). 'The role of monoamines and acetylcholine-containing neurones in the regulation of the sleep-waking cycle.' *Ergebn. Physiol.* 64, 166–307

Lennox–Buchthal, M. A. (1973). 'Febrile convulsions: a reappraisal.' *Electroenceph. clin. Neurophysiol.* Suppl. 32, pp. 38–40

Loomis, A. L., Harvey, E. N. and Hobart, G. A. (1937). 'Cerebral states during sleep, as studied by human brain potentials.' *J. exp. Psychol.* 21, 127–144

Lugaresi, E., Coccagna, G., Mantovani, M., Berti-Ceroni, G., Pazzaglia, P. and Tassinari, C. A. (1970). 'The evolution of different types of myoclonus during sleep: A polygraphic study.' *Eur. Neurol.* 4, 321–331

Matthes, A. (1961). 'Die psychomotorische Epilepsie in Kindesalter.' II Mitteilung. *Z. Kinderheilk,* 85, 472–492

Oswald, I. (1974). *Sleep* 3rd Edn. London: Penguin

Tassinari, C. A., Terzano, G., Capocchi, G., Dalla Bernardina, B., Vigevano, F., Daniele, O., Valladier, C., Dravet, C. and Roger, J. (1977). 'Epileptic seizures during sleep in children.' In *Epilepsy. The Eighth International Symposium,* pp. 345–354. Ed. J. K. Penry. New York: Raven Press

CHAPTER 17

Unusual Manifestations of Childhood Epilepsy

References to the less usual varieties of childhood epilepsy are made elsewhere in this book. These include the syndrome of acquired aphasia associated with a convulsive disorder, the unusual types of nocturnal epilepsy and psychotic behaviour and also so-called abdominal epilepsy. Neurologists have always been fascinated by the desire to classify and categorize the many clinical fragments of an epileptic attack. A peculiar or unusual clinical manifestation may be either a facet of a complex seizure or may represent the patient's only presenting symptom.

Laughter and other emotional expressions

The latter situation may be present when uncontrollable pathological laughter occurs as an epileptic phenomenon, a condition termed gelastic epilepsy (gelos = mirth). There is usually a subjective experience of merriment and complex co-ordinate movements with grinning, giggling or joyful weeping may occur. Gascon and Lombroso (1971) have written of this unusual complaint in children and adolescents, and they adopted strict criteria for its diagnosis. These are as follows:

1. Stereotyped recurrence of the attack
2. The absence of external precipitating factors
3. Concomitance of other manifestations generally accepted as epileptic, e.g. tonic and clonic movements, disturbance of consciousness and/or automatisms
4. Interictal and/or ictal discharges being present in the EEG

In four of their 10 patients they observed bursts of uncontrollable laughter occurring simultaneously with discharges in the EEG. They were careful to distinguish between the ictal laughter and the postictal laughter which may occur after seizures of various types. Half of their patients had interictal discharges of the generalized spike-wave type while the rest had discharges located over one or other temporal lobe.

It has been suggested that there is a motor centre for laughter in or near the hypothalamus. Laughing attacks may occur with hypothalamic lesions causing precocious puberty (Williams, Schutt and Savage, 1978). Similarly, involuntary laughter may be associated with lesions involving frontal or temporal lobes and with many other different types of pathology (*British Medical Journal*, 1977). Gascon and Lombroso (1971), however, thought that gelastic epilepsy should be considered as being due to pathological discharges traversing complex neuronal circuits subserving laughter, and arising at quite different levels in different cases. Most authors agree that possible subcortical sites for emotional epilepsy are the limbic system and the hypothalamus. Parts of the limbic system, notably the hippocampus and the amygdala, lie within the temporal lobe and are frequently involved in the pathogenesis of epilepsy. Quite apart from gelastic epilepsy, crying epilepsy (quiritarian or dacrocystic) and running epilepsy (cursive) have been described with temporal lobe lesions, including tumours. Turning of the head may occur with these types of temporal lobe epilepsy, and epigastric auras may precede the attacks indicating juxtaposition in the temporal lobe of brain centres for visceral and affective functions. In 'epilepsia cursiva' or 'running fits' the patient becomes confused, out of contact with his surroundings and thus starts running (Walsh, 1974). In certain cases the patient may be exteriorizing inner feelings of fear or terror as attempts at flight. A generalized seizure may follow if there is diffuse spread of the epileptic discharge. Alternatively, the patient may become combative and violent. Usually, however, any acts of aggression which may occur in temporal lobe attacks are brief and nonpurposeful and are responses to attempted restraint during an automatism.

Changes in mood, attitude and social behaviour

Williams (1966) has written about the dilemma of recognizing what is truly ictal or epileptic in nature and of avoiding the ambiguity of phrases such as *epileptic equivalent states* and *epileptiform attacks* in relation to temporal lobe epilepsy. Patients with this type of epilepsy usually have a structural abnormality and disordered function of the temporal lobe or lobes, i.e. those parts of the brain which are responsible for the integration of all sensation into total experience. Since such experience

TABLE 17.1
Temporal Lobe Seizures Categorized According to their Initial Symptoms

With disturbance of thought

Dreamy states with clouding of consciousness
Illusional or hallucinatory experiences resembling a dream
Feelings of familiarity in strange surroundings (déjà vu)
Visual illusions in which objects appear smaller (micropsia) or larger (macropsia)
Auditory illusions in which sounds become fainter (microacusia) or louder
(macroacusia)
Illusions of depersonalization and unreality, e.g. the illusion of observing oneself
from outside the body
Sudden compulsive thoughts, often of an unpleasant or bizarre nature

With disturbance of langauge

Episodes of dysphasia where seizure discharge involves the dominant hemisphere
Speech automatisms with utterance of identifiable words

With complex motor behaviour

Motor automatisms with confusion, incoherent mumbling, repetitive actions and
inappropriate behaviour
Prolonged 'fugue states' − largely confined to adults

With antisocial behaviour

Moodiness, irritability and anger may occur periodically as epileptic manifestations

With affective disturbances

Feelings of fear which may be intense
Sensations of pleasure or well being
Gelastic epilepsy

With olfactory disturbances

Hallucinations of smell which may be intense and unpleasant (uncinate fits)
Licking and smacking of lips may occur

With visual symptoms

Simple visual hallucinations − lights, stars
Complex visual hallucinations of familiar scenes

With vertiginous symptoms

Sensations of spinning, usually on a vertical axis
Sensations of falling

Abdominal and alimentary sensations

Epigastric sensations which are difficult to describe
A desire to defaecate

With cardiovascular symptoms

Precordial discomfort
Fluttering sensations in the left chest
Tachycardia

is primarily responsible for behaviour, it is not surprising that such epilepsy is associated with psychological disorders reflected in disturbance of mood or attitude or evident in disturbed social behaviour. Williams (1966) recommends that the clinician should keep clearly before him the distinction between what happens in the attack and what results from the postictal confusional state, and that he should divorce these events from the total behaviour of the patient. He notes that many people with aggressive psychopathic behaviour also have disturbance in the temporal lobe areas reflected in the EEG or in morbid anatomical studies, even though they may never suffer from epilepsy. The importance of these observations resides in the fact that frequently a diagnosis of temporal lobe epilepsy is made in individuals, including children, who demonstrate disturbed behaviour and who may have an EEG abnormality over a temporal lobe, without any clinical evidence that they suffer from the paroxysmal disorder of epilepsy.

Bizarre manifestations

It is difficult to list all the unusual, bizarre and often baffling clinical manifestations of epilepsy. In this section, one has merely tried to indicate some of the more dramatic possibilities and a more comprehensive list is provided in *Table 17.1*. The interested reader who desires more information on the subject is earnestly requested to consult William Lennox's marvellous book with its numerous case histories, particularly in the chapter on psychomotor epilepsy.

REFERENCES

Gascon, G. G. and Lombroso, C. T. (1971). 'Epileptic (gelastic) laughter.' *Epilepsia*, **12**, 63–76
Leading article (1977). 'Less usual forms of epilepsy.' *Br. med. J.* **1**, 127–128
Lennox, W. G. (1960). *Epilepsy and Related Disorders*, Vol. 1, pp. 227–321. London: J and A. Churchill and Boston: Little Brown and Company
Walsh, G. O. (1974). 'Unusual presentations of epilepsies.' *Pediatrics*, **53**, 548–551
Williams, D. (1966). 'Temporal lobe epilepsy.' *Br. med. J.* **1**, 1439–1442
Williams, M., Schutt, W. and Savage, D. (1978). 'Epileptic laughter with precocious puberty.' *Archs Dis. Child.* **53**, 965–966

CHAPTER 18

Emotional and Psychiatric Aspects of Epilepsy

'The good physician is concerned not only with turbulent brain waves but with disturbed emotions and with social injustice, for the epileptic is not just a nerve-muscle preparation; he is a person, in health an integrated combination of the physical, the mental, the social and the spiritual. Disruption of any part can cause or aggravate illness' (Lennox and Markham, 1953).

Many writers have suggested that the main handicap associated with epilepsy is of the psychological kind. Observations of the mental peculiarities of epileptic persons extend across recorded medical history (Temkin, 1971). While some individuals with epilepsy may have behavioural disorders as a concomitant of underlying brain disorders, it is of first importance to realize that they may also have psychological morbidity as a result of their failure to adapt to their milieu and as a consequence of the failure of society to encompass them and their disabilities. The impact of chronic epilepsy on a child's emotional and personality development will vary at different ages and it should be clearly understood that *there is no single or characteristic mental state or behaviour pattern consequent on chronic epilepsy*. The factors which tend to increase psychiatric morbidity are as follows:

1. Early age of onset and chronicity
2. Adverse environmental circumstances, including a disturbed family background
3. The occurrence of certain specific varieties of epilepsy such as temporal lobe epilepsy
4. The presence of structural or organic brain disorders.

It is highly improbable that any single form of personality disturbance could emerge in persons with different degrees and types of cerebral damage or with no evidence of damage, with different genetic endowments and environmental circumstances, and who are differently affected by epilepsy. Nevertheless, there persists in the lay mind, and even in the medical mind, a mistaken concept of what has been called 'the epileptic personality'. This was described by Aretaeus of Cappodocia (Temkin, 1971) as follows: 'They became languid, spiritless, stupid, inhuman, unsociable, and not disposed to hold intercourse, nor to be sociable, at any period of life; sleepless, subject to many horrid dreams, without appetite, and with bad digestion; pale, of a leaden color; slow to learn from torpidity of the understanding and of the senses . . .'. Since this first description there have been many other equally pejorative accounts of the sufferer from epilepsy, right up to the present century. Happily, however, this century has seen the abandonment of such an unscientific and prejudiced view of the person with epilepsy. It has been replaced by both concern for the predicament in which the patient finds himself and by increased understanding of the disadvantages which his condition and society have placed on him.

Accounts of the emotional and psychiatric disorders associated with epilepsy in general and with childhood epilepsy in particular are complex and often confusing. In an attempt to give an orderly account it is proposed to discuss the problem under the following headings:

1. Environmental influences including the attitudes of society
2. The influences of age and development
3. The role played by specific varieties of epilepsy
4. The factor of structural or organic brain abnormality
5. The influence of drugs
6. The relationship to serious psychiatric disorders, particularly psychosis.

ENVIRONMENTAL INFLUENCES INCLUDING THE ATTITUDES OF SOCIETY

The psychological effects of seizures on the patient's family have already been discussed in the chapter on the general management of childhood epilepsy (*see* Chapter 22) and are well described by Lindsay (1972). She points out that when parents first see their child having a fit their immediate reaction is often 'I thought he was dead'. This shock to the parents can then set up long-lasting reverberations in their relationships not only with the child himself but also between themselves and with those who care for him and teach him. Even though the child recovers in a few minutes, the parents are often left with an abiding fear that at any time and without warning they could lose their child. Prompt attention to the child and careful explanation to the parents at the time of the first seizure may be very important in preventing later abnormal relationships.

If, following the first seizure, the child is left with a chronic physical handicap, such as a hemiplegia, or if the epilepsy becomes recurrent and chronic then a change in parental attitudes is inevitable. They tend to adopt attitudes of either rejection or over-protection, more commonly the latter. The child is over-indulged and carefully protected from stress. The extent of the handicap is denied and the child is treated as if he were still a baby. This is, of course, more likely to happen when the epilepsy begins in early childhood and if the attacks are severe and/or frequent and if they are associated with mental or physical handicap. The early age of onset, chronicity and associated structural or organic brain abnormality have constantly been shown to increase psychiatric morbidity in the individual with epilepsy.

Rejection is a less common response by parents, but some react in this way because, as Lindsay (1972) points out, the child has a disorder which makes him untrustworthy in the sense that cataclysmic breakdowns in his behaviour may happen without warning. His whole existence as a person may then be denied. The cataclysmic nature of the seizure and its effect on observers will be discussed again shortly (*see* pages 167, 168 and 229), but its critical importance in developing attitudes to the affected individual cannot be over-emphasized. The fear of the child's death may concern the parents and this is not unreasonable.

Sillanpaa (1973), in his lengthy review from Finland of the medico-social prognosis of children with epilepsy, found that deaths were unexpectedly high with a loss of one per cent per year from status epilepticus, chest infections and other complications. Five children among 245 studied drowned, emphasizing the need for some restrictions even with the benefits of modern therapy. Sillanpaa (1973) also found a higher incidence of marital breakdown and divorce among the parents and guardians of the epileptic children studied when compared with the normal population. He stressed that chronic tension within the family and the effects of uncertainty and the restrictions imposed on the child might actually make the epilepsy worse, thereby creating a vicious circle. Lindsay (1972) stresses the contagious nature of the breakdowns which can have their origins in the patient's epilepsy, and it is in such a situation that there may be a need to place the child in a calm and orderly environment and institute psychotherapy for the child and the family. This ideal is not easy to achieve but a model example is to be found at the Park Hospital, Oxford, from where Lindsay writes.

Social aspects

One should enquire into why seizures constitute socially unacceptable behaviour and why, in consequence, there is so much prejudice in the public mind concerning epilepsy. Why it is necessary constantly to prove that it is possible to suffer epilepsy and still be of sound mind ? To some extent it is connected with the fact that epilepsy is not a trivial matter. Many people with multiple handicaps suffer from epilepsy as a secondary effect of the initial brain disease or damage which caused their handicaps. There are also some sufferers from epilepsy who, even though of normal intelligence and free from other handicaps, may nevertheless have their whole lives marred by epilepsy. On the other hand, there are many whose seizure disorder is trouble free. As Ann Hackney (1976) puts it: 'Any single encounter with epilepsy will tell only part of the tale and may lead to unfair generalizations. The condition is too complex, with its wide variety of causes, manifestations and effects. Unfortunately, there are still stereotyped images of epileptic personalities and mentalities which may be true, in part, of some, but are inadequate and unjust to most.' The very complexity and diversity of epilepsy, therefore, is the first reason for public misunderstanding and prejudice.

What is the nature of this innate *prejudice against epilepsy* ? There is evidence of its pervasiveness in different kinds of cultures, both pre-technological and technological, and even among otherwise rational individuals, including physicians. Bagley (1972), in his very perceptive analysis of the problem, felt that the basis of the prejudice was: 'fear, of the sudden loss of physical and emotional control.' He found evidence of social prejudice at all levels – in the field of employment, education and even in medical care – and also found that people with epilepsy were regarded with more hostility than the mentally ill or people with cerebral palsy. He found significant correlations between a scale measuring racial prejudice and one measuring attitudes to the handicapped, the latter being dominated by hostile attitudes towards epilepsy. In addition, he remarked that there were affinities between the two insofar as racial prejudice also involved a fear of the unknown and the unpredictable. Bagley (1972) felt that people with epilepsy are seen in hostile terms which are as great as or greater than those in which ethnic minorities are viewed. 'The man with epilepsy is feared and hated because he does what we are afraid we will do ourselves. He loses control – basic control of his motor movements. He reverts to the 'primitive', so that the punishment of him (by social rejection and ostracism) appears to be justified.' Bagley (1972) goes on to say that widespread social rejection of people with epilepsy may well be largely responsible for the increased prevalence of behaviour disorders among them.

Taylor (1969), discussing prejudice against epilepsy, wrote that the social structure survives through its experience of the value of control, order and reason, and that the two things which most threaten our control over the environment are madness and death. To an observer without medical knowledge an epileptic fit appears as 'a brief excursion through madness into death'. Society has developed mechanisms for coping with these two eventualities, but the psychological difficulty in accepting epilepsy is that having severed human relationships briefly in a similar fashion to madness or death the seizure is then followed by recovery. Every recurring seizure subsequently reinforces the view of witnesses that the epileptic cannot be relied upon to participate fully in society because he is liable, at any time, to go out of control. Therefore, unless he can be cured he must be set apart: he must be reformed or else rejected. Furthermore, every seizure with its humiliations reinforces for the epileptic the failure of society to help him, and this accentuates his feeling of being different. Taylor (1969) also points out that, because epilepsy has its greatest incidence in early childhood, the young child with chronic epilepsy has no experience of normality. His experience of epilepsy is his experience of life. If the epileptic tendency passes away he is left unable to take up normality again, as he might do after a transient illness, because he has to build it for the first time. He is then in danger to the epilepsy becoming a way of life and of relying on the fact of his being different as a protection from the demands of good social behaviour.

In a further analysis of the problem of prejudice and epilepsy Taylor (1973a) considered the stigmas of epilepsy. (A stigma may be defined as a blemish or a token of disgrace or a mark of infamy.) The clearest stigma of epilepsy is the seizure itself with its overt implications of total loss of control. There are other more subtle stigmas too, including the need to take medication regularly, the restrictions on activity, the days off school or work, the periods of hospitalization in some cases and the mysterious injuries that may occur. Consider, for example, the stigma of having to wear a protective helmet. Taylor (1973a) concludes that the only way to combat prejudice is by diminishing ignorance through education, and that we should teach people to tolerate uncertainty and to try to control ancient prejudices by an effort of will.

Livingston (1972) emphasizes that a teacher should explain to a class in which there is a child with epilepsy that it is not contagious, and he must not convey prejudice and must give a simple explanation to the other children about the nature of the fits. It is notable how well other children will accept epilepsy if the general attitude is sensible. It is essential, however, that the same discipline should apply to the child with epilepsy as to the rest of the class. The child will rapidly learn to dominate the class situation if he knows that he will not be punished like the other children. Unfortunately, some doctors still make the excuse that the child cannot help his behaviour because he is an epileptic. This particular attitude is very likely to lead to a personality disturbance and to the development of behavioural disorders in the child.

THE INFLUENCES OF AGE AND DEVELOPMENT

Normal personality development takes place by intimate interaction of the individual with the environment. The environment will have a generally consistent component, either 'good' or 'bad', in the case of a normal child. Where the child has a chronic illness, such as epilepsy, a new variable component is introduced depending on the ways in which the illness of the individual is perceived by various people around him at different times. Taylor (1971a) has adapted a scheme or model of normal personality development devised by Erikson (1966, 1977) in order to illustrate the effects of chronic epilepsy on personality development during the various stages of the child's development.

Infancy

During infancy it is normal for the parents to love their child and for the child to feel loved. Seizures during the neonatal period and during infancy frequently have an ominous prognosis. Death, neurological disability, intellectual impairment and later chronic epilepsy are common. For a mother, an infantile convulsion means that her child is manifestly abnormal. The child may be deprived of mothering through special nursing requirements, through separation or through rejection. The very existence of the child is threatened by the possibility of death and, as we have seen, the parallels between an epileptic seizure and sudden unexpected death are very close. The violence of infantile spasms and the appearance of the child in an attack often give the impression of great and inexplicable pain and anguish for the child. The parents feel cut off from their normal response of giving comfort to the child in his predicament. Furthermore, this very serious disorder is likely to be followed by gross mental defect or by what Ounsted (1970) has called 'a phenocopy of infantile autism' or by both. In these circumstances the mother's trust and the infant's autonomy are threatened. She is afraid to leave her child alone and imposes limitations on his movements. For a child of unimpaired intelligence who is struggling to establish independence this may lead to conflict and humiliation. As Taylor (1971a) says, psychological difficulties are grafted on to a disordered neurological substrate and they impose their own limitations on growth and development. The child's developing sense of separation from the mother and his sense of personal identity may be affected adversely.

Later infancy and early childhood

In later infancy and early childhood the development of the myoclonic epilepsies may have equally disturbing effects on the mother-child relationship. Catastrophic falls to the ground, so characteristic of these epilepsies, may make the erect posture unreliable and dangerous. This leads to great parental anxiety with increased restrictions on a child who is in the exploratory phase of learning and is actively using walking and climbing for that purpose. Febrile convulsions, commonest between six months and four years of age, frequently lead the parents to believe that their child has died. Green and Solnit (1964) described what they called the 'vulnerable child' syndrome in which the parents, having so powerfully experienced the belief that their child was dead or going to die, regard their child quite differently in the event of his recovery. They may feel that the child is on loan and that he might be snatched away at any time. In recurrent epilepsy this proximity to death may regularly occur, constantly reinforcing the parents' beliefs concerning the eventual loss of their child. Thus, although parents often display considerable devotion and withdraw from social pleasures in order to protect the child, the basis of trust is seriously disrupted. The children themselves experience years of treatment with drugs for a condition which they cannot remember experiencing and which is not freely discussed with them. However, their parents' anxiety is communicated to them, in fact so much so that, as Livingston (1972) points out, some children may express a fear of dying during or as a result of a seizure. Children with epilepsy are significantly more anxious, inattentive, overactive and socially isolated than normal children, and boys appear to suffer more in this respect than girls (Stores, 1977). Maladjustment may show itself as feelings of insecurity, inadequacy, various degrees of nervous tension, anxiety and irritability. The child may become withdrawn and defeatist in his attitude or, on the other hand, hostile, aggressive and antisocial in his behaviour. Enuresis, encopresis, temper tantrums, nail-biting and so on may all occur.

Taylor (1971a), again using Erikson's model, points out that the development of petit mal absences may often coincide with what Erikson called the 'phase of initiative'. Children with petit mal have been found to be more neurotic and less antisocial than children with other forms of epilepsy. The inception of petit mal is usually preceded by some years of normal development so that trust and autonomy will already have been established. Petit mal absences then make frequent breaks in consciousness disrupting the child's awareness of what is happening around him. Children with petit mal tend to become compliant and non-assertive, uniformly quiet and well behaved. They tend to fade into the background and these personality traits may persist into adult life.

Later childhood

The inception of new cases of epilepsy falls off sharply from the age of five or six years and probably amounts to 2–4/1000 children of school age per annum (DHSS, 1969). Even those children who have had severe epilepsy in the early years of childhood may show improvement during the school years. However, as Taylor (1971a) emphasizes, the school years are also the period in which the child with epilepsy is exposed to society and its expectations for the first time. The limitations on activity and intelligence, the need for continuing medical care, the effects of drug therapy and of clinical and subclinical seizures on the child's ability to learn all begin to influence the extent to which the child can learn to live with and master his environment. Behaviour problems, formerly latent and private, become public and sometimes intolerable. Normal schooling may become impossible or, at least, severely disrupted.

Adolescence

Adolescence brings its own share of emotional difficulties and readjustments under normal circumstances. When the extra burden of epilepsy is present, it may be difficult to know whether the moodiness, aggressiveness, irritability and emotional changeability are normal adolescent phenomena or largely due to the predicament of having epilepsy. If the epilepsy is not functionally disabling, it is more likely that the behavioural difficulties are due to adolescent turmoil. Temporal lobe epilepsy becomes increasingly more common during adolescence and may be associated with particular behavioural difficulties (*see* Chapters 10 and 12). Taylor (1971a) points out that adolescents with temporal lobe epilepsy, in addition to the normal identity crisis associated with adolescence, may also have problems of personal identity deriving from the temporal lobe abnormality itself. Williams (1969) has written that the most important function of the temporal lobe is the integration of sensations of all kinds. The temporal lobe enables an individual to appreciate himself as a unified being (i.e. the sense of 'I am') because it receives information from the special senses, the viscera and the higher centres. Disruption of this function may have serious psychological consequences. Surgical removal of the temporal lobe for epilepsy may be followed later by lonely, withdrawn, apathetic and passive behaviour and by the presence of hyposexuality (Taylor and Falconer, 1968).

THE ROLE PLAYED BY SPECIFIC VARIETIES OF EPILEPSY

This particular aspect of the emotional disorders connected with epilepsy has already been discussed to some extent and the importance of temporal lobe epilepsy has been alluded to in the previous section (*see* Chapter 10). The way in which any child reacts to having a seizure disorder varies considerably depending on the personality of the child, the family psychopathology and the extent to which the epilepsy responds to medical treatment. There are, however, certain specific syndromes of abnormal behaviour which need description.

The hyperkinetic syndrome

This is probably the best known of the abnormal behaviour syndromes, and may be defined as a pathological excess of energy found in young children with mental defect and brain injury, particularly when epilepsy is present as an additional handicap. Ounsted (1955) used the term 'hyperkinetic syndrome in epileptic children' to describe such patients and found an incidence of 8 per cent in a consecutive personal series of 830 children presenting with epilepsy. Apart from overactivity, the majority of the children showed evidence of distractability, short attention span, wide scatter on test results when given formal intelligence tests, fluctuations of mood with euphoria as the abiding background, aggressive outbursts, diminution or absence of spontaneously affectionate behaviour, lack of shyness and lack of fear. The intelligence level in his patients ranged from high normal to severe mental handicap. These abnormalities, combined with overactivity sustained over months or years, made these children intolerable in both ordinary schools and hospitals and created for their parents and siblings emotional and practical problems of a serious and intractable nature.

The term 'hyperkinetic syndrome' has, in fact, been in use for over a 100 years (Hoffman, 1945) and has been applied to a syndrome which begins early in life, is more common in boys than girls and is characterized by hyperactivity, impulsivity, distractability and excitability. Aggressive and antisocial behaviour, specific learning difficulties and emotional lability are often included as features of this syndrome. Terms such as 'brain damage syndrome', 'minimal brain damage' and 'minimal brain dysfunction' are often used synonomously with the term hyperkinetic syndrome with unfortunate consequences. If the term brain damage is used in its literal sense meaning structural abnormality of the brain, then 'brain damage syndrome' is an inaccurate and misleading term since the majority of overactive children do not suffer from frank brain damage and most brain damaged children do not present with the hyperkinetic syndrome (Rutter, Graham and Yule, 1970). The term 'minimal cerebral dysfunction' has been used to describe children with subtle defects in co-ordination, perception or language development, but here again the symptoms and signs may only occasionally be associated with actual damage to the brain (Rutter, 1968). Moreover, many hyperkinetic children do not demonstrate these subtle neurological signs.

If we return to a consideration of hyperkinesis as a behavioural syndrome only, it should be realized that it has many different causes and that it always requires careful evaluation. Present evidence suggests that the term hyperkinetic syndrome describes a heterogeneous group of children with different aetiologies. In some cases the disorder may be due to structural abnormality of the brain, in others there may be an abnormality of physiological arousal of the nervous system, in others there may be a genetic basis for the disorder while in many others no cause will be found. The reader is referred to the excellent review by Cantwell (1977).

It is important to remember that, apart from the behavioural abnormality, learning difficulties are of major importance as an associated problem, whatever the cause of the overactivity. It has been suggested by Ounsted (1971) that there is a disruption of exploratory learning in hyperkinetic children which disbars them from developing the basic mental structures which are the foundation of normal learning and intelligence. It should be remembered, as Bax (1972) stressed, that the overactive child, particularly the overactive schoolchild, may simply be reacting to stresses in his environment or may be suffering exposure to an inappropriate educational milieu. Children with neurotic or antisocial psychiatric disturbances or who have specific learning difficulties may also demonstrate overactivity, and much of it may be reaction to the predicament in which they find themselves. Furthermore, there are normal children (and adults) who are temperamentally restless, unable to sit still, and who become excited easily over minor matters demonstrating their emotion by the use of motor activity.

Returning to the question of hyperkinesis in children with epilepsy, it is now realized that its incidence in epileptic children generally is much lower than the 8 per cent mentioned by Ounsted (1955). The reason for this is that it has now become clearly apparent that overactivity can be produced or potentiated by related drugs such as phenobarbitone and primidone, and that other drugs such as clonazepam may have a similar effect. Withdrawal of these drugs should always be the initial treatment when a patient taking them for epilepsy becomes overactive. Another important point which should be emphasized is that in a child with epilepsy, of whatever kind, the overactivity may be generated by anxiety, which in turn may be related to a frightening aura or may be a reflection of parental anxiety about the child's epilepsy.

There is no doubt that hyperkinetic behaviour can occur in children with temporal lobe epilepsy. Ounsted, Lindsay and Norman (1966) found it present in one-quarter of their sample of 100 children. It was commoner in males and in those who had suffered an early brain insult or who had had status epilepticus. They concluded that cerebral damage acquired in the course of an initiating illness may be more important in the causation of the hyperkinetic behaviour than is the temporal lobe epilepsy itself. They also found that age was a critical factor, and very early onset of the epilepsy was a feature of their hyperactive children. They also found that the intellectual development of their hyperactive children was significantly retarded compared with other groups of children with only temporal lobe epilepsy. Pond (1961) showed that the behavioural syndrome of overactivity occurred in brain-injured children of low intelligence, particularly males, who did not also have epilepsy. Again, however, he stressed that many of these children did not come from normal homes and, of course, the possible adverse effects of drugs must always be remembered in the mentally handicapped with or without epilepsy.

Rage and temper outbursts

Ounsted, Lindsay and Norman (1966) reported outbursts of catastrophic rage in approximately one-third of their children with temporal lobe epilepsy. However, these rage outbursts are not peculiar to children with temporal lobe epilepsy but seem to represent a general biological reaction, of an intermittent kind, to frustrating situations in brain-damaged people. The Oxford workers suggested that these rage outbursts, although occurring in many different kinds of brain sydrome, might nevertheless be released from specific centres in the hypothalamus. Lindsay (1972) regarded the outbursts as a form of 'fail-safe' device, i.e. the rage occurred when the child had been overloaded with emotional stimuli of one sort and another. She gave as an example a child who had been confined in an overcrowded room or school or hospital from which there was no escape route away from the ambient circumstances. She pointed out that phenobarbitone and related compounds might potentiate the rage phenomenon. Unlike the hyperkinetic syndrome, which is limited to the early years of life, children with temporal lobe epilepsy may manifest rage outbursts at any age and unexpectedly. This can lead to complications in older patients and may take the form of murderous assaults and the infliction of bodily injury on others. Those children in the Oxford series (Ounsted, Lindsay and Norman, 1966) who had had an early brain insult were most likely to develop the rage phenomenon, and those who had had an episode of status epilepticus were the next group most likely to do so. The age of onset of seizures was earlier in the group manifesting rage outbursts, and this phenomenon occurred in children of both high and low intelligence and equally in both sexes. There was an overlap between rage outbursts and the hyperkinetic syndrome, but the two could occur independently of each other. The combination of the two in an individual child virtually guaranteed his or her exclusion from a normal school.

Reference is made in the next chapter to the study by Stores (1977) on behaviour disturbance and on the type of epilepsy in children attending ordinary school. In this study he found that, in general, the children were significantly more anxious, inattentive, overactive and socially isolated than were normal children, and also that boys appeared to be more affected than girls. His EEG investigations showed that anxiety, inattentiveness and (with the exception of the 3 Hz spike-wave subgroup) social isolation particularly characterized each male subgroup, but the left temporal spike subgroup of boys emerged as the most disturbed of all and were also significantly more active when compared with normal boys. Neither the sex nor the subgroup differences were explicable on the basis of seizure frequently or type of drug therapy.

THE FACTOR OF STRUCTURAL OR ORGANIC BRAIN ABNORMALITY

The factors that tend to increase psychiatric morbidity in epilepsy are an early age of onset and chronicity, a disturbed family background, specific kinds of epilepsy such as temporal lobe epilepsy and evidence of structural or organic brain abnormality. The classic study on the part played by the last in causing psychiatric disorders in children with epilepys is that organized by Rutter in the Isle of Wight (Graham and Rutter, 1968; Rutter, Graham and Yule, 1970). The total population of children of compulsory school age (total 11 865) was studied to determine the prevalence of epilepsy, cerebral palsy and other neurological disorders. The association between organic brain dysfunction and psychiatric disorder was examined by comparing the neurological and psychiatric findings in the children with epilepsy or with lesions above the brain stem (cerebral palsy and similar disorders) with those in the following:

1. A random sample of the general population
2. Children with lesions below the brain stem such as muscular dystrophy and paralyses following poliomyelitis
3. Children with other chronic physical handicaps not involving the nervous system such as asthma, heart disease, or diabetes.

The prevalence of psychiatric disorder in the general population of children aged 10 and 11 years was 6.8 per cent. Psychiatric disorder was nearly twice as common (11.5 per cent) among children with chronic physical disorders not involving the brain, including those due to disease or damage at or below the brain stem. However, the rate of psychiatric disorder among children with neuroepileptic disorders was very much higher; in fact over a third (34 per cent) showed psychiatric disorder – a rate five times that in the general population sample. The rate was highest in children with neurological disorders accompanied by fits (58.3 per cent) and lowest in those with uncomplicated epilepsy (28.6 per cent). In those with neurological lesions above the brain stem but no seizures the rate was 37.5 per cent. It was concluded, on the basis of a study of factors associated with psychiatric disorders, that the high rate of psychiatric disorder in the neuroepileptic children was due to the presence of organic brain dysfunction rather than just to the existence of a physical handicap, although the latter also played a part. Moreover, organic brain dysfunction was not associated with any specific type of psychiatric disorder thereby dispelling any lingering doubts about the existence of a specific 'epileptic personality' disorder. Within the neuroepileptic group the neurological features and the type of seizure, intellectual and educational factors and sociofamilial factors all interacted in the development of the psychiatric disorder.

The implication of these findings is that an organic brain disorder puts the individual at special risk of developing psychiatric disorders, both directly as a result of the brain disorder and indirectly as a result of the failure to adapt to the handicap, and that the psychiatric disorders are no different in kind from those of the population at large whether physically handicapped or not. Epilepsy is associated not only with high rates of psychiatric disorder but also, as we have already seen, with many other interrelated indicators of personal and social handicap which are likely to set individuals apart as a disadvantaged group.

THE INFLUENCE OF DRUGS

The effects of various anticonvulsant drugs in causing behavioural disturbances in children with epilepsy have already been referred to on several occasions, and the adverse effects of anticonvulsant drugs generally are dealt with in detail in a separate chapter (*see* Chapter 24). The possibility that behavioural and personality disorders may be due to the chronic toxic effects of the patient's medication should constantly be in the physician's mind. Some drugs, and particularly phenytoin, may cause a progressive encephalopathy due to chronic drug intoxication (Vallarta, Bell and Reichert, 1974). Patients may demonstrate progressive psychomotor deterioration which is indistinguishable from that due to a degenerative disease of the central nervous system. Behavioural abnormalities have also been reported including stubborness, agressiveness, destructiveness, confused withdrawn behaviour, and an abnormal degree of lethargy and inattention to personal needs. Psychotic manifestations, including hallucinations, abnormal inter-personal relationships and thought disorders may also occur. Bizarre gestures and choreoathetoid movements may be observed. All these disorders may be further complicated by impaired intellectual performance. Paradoxically, an increased frequency of seizures and even status epilepticus may be associated with chronic drug intoxication with phenytoin. This may lead to yet another increase in dosage by the unwary physician. Recognition of the problem and the monitoring of blood serum levels of drugs are essential to detect it because this type of encephalopathy is usually reversible if the drugs are withdrawn. Since some of the symptoms, and especially the psychomotor regression, are probably related to interference with folic acid metabolism, measurement of blood serum folate levels is mandatory and should lead to the prescription of folic acid supplements if low levels are detected.

THE RELATIONSHIP TO SERIOUS PSYCHIATRIC DISORDERS, PARTICULARLY PSYCHOSIS

It will be evident from the preceding sections of this chapter that while children with epilepsy are more prone to neurotic or behavioural disorders than normal children, the clinical manifestations of these disorders are no different from those occurring in other disturbed children who do not have epilepsy. However, children with epilepsy may have ictal experiences peculiar to their complaint and some of these resemble transient adult psychotic states, for example hallucinations, depersonalization, derealization, delusions, nameless dread, confused speech and interference with rational thought processes. In the nineteenth century writers on epilepsy liked to categorize the mental peculiarities of people with epilepsy into peri-ictal disorders, interictal disorders and long-term psychoses, and it is still valid to look at epilepsy in this way today (Taylor, 1973b). The peri-ictal disorders can include prodromal mood changes (e.g. sullenness, listlessness, irritability and aggressiveness) preceding an attack and can last for hours, or even days; various aurae may occur including some so bizarre that they resemble the phenomena of schizophrenic psychosis; some epileptic attacks include automatic behaviour with wandering and apparently purposeful but inappropriate actions; and confusional states often coloured by vivid hallucinations may complicate the postictal period, especially after a series of attacks. Changes of mood, often reversing the pre-ictal mood and including feelings of extraordinary well being and relaxation, may be noticed by parents after a major attack.

The interictal disorders have already been dealt with in detail in this chapter and, in this respect, modern writers have abandoned the pejorative concept of an 'epileptic personality'. They have realized that no particular single form of personality could emerge from different degrees and types of cerebral damage occurring at different ages and stages of development in individuals with dissimilar genetic endowments, suffering from different types of epilepsy of varying severity and raised in contrasting environments.

A *psychotic breakdown* in a child with epilepsy is rare before puberty. Conversely, epilepsy is very rare in the syndrome of early infantile autism. Creak and Pampiglione (1969), in a carefully selected group of 35 autistic and withdrawn children who were followed-up for between five and 19 years, found a rate of EEG abnormalities which was above that found in the general population. However, no evidence of any specific abnormality was detected. There may be an increased incidence of epilepsy developing during adolescence in autistic children (Rutter, 1977). In the phenocopy of autistic behaviour which occurs in some children who have had infantile spasms and who are subsequently mentally handicapped and often hyperkinetic, chronic epilepsy and an abnormal (and epileptic) EEG are usual (Ounsted, 1970).

The word psychosis implies a qualitative change from normal behaviour which is neither understandable in ordinary human terms nor in terms of the patient's life experience and environmental circumstances. The classic study of Slater, Beard and Glithero (1963) confirmed that there was an association between epilepsy and a paranoid-schizophrenia state, and that it was greater than that predicted by chance association through the 'frequency of each condition independently; it was shown that the psychosis occurred in individuals with temporal lobe epilepsy. Flor Henry (1969) demonstrated that there was a relationship between the hemisphere affected by temporal lobe epilepsy and the psychological and social sequelae. Left temporal lobe lesions tended to be associated with psychopathic behaviour and psychosis, including a schizophrenia-like state, whereas right temporal lobe lesions were associated with neuroses and depressive psychoses. Although mesial temporal sclerosis was found in half of the material obtained at the operation of temporal lobectomy, Falconer and Taylor (1968) reported that temporal lobe epilepsy due to this neuropathological lesion was rarely accompanied by chronic psychosis. This observation was further elaborated by Taylor (1971b) when he showed that, in individuals with temporal lobe epilepsy who did not develop psychosis, the period of maximum inception of the epilepsy was largely located in early childhood, whereas in those with temporal lobe epilepsy who developed psychosis the period of maximum inception of the epilepsy was around puberty. He also found a general relationship between the onset of epilepsies which lead to psychosis and the adolescent growth spurt in each sex, and that these epilepsies tended to begin earlier in the growth spurt period in girls than in boys. The occurrence of psychosis in relation to lesions of the temporal lobes is not surprising when one remembers the significance of the integrative functions of these parts of the brain in achieving the essential sense of personal identity or 'I am'. Another important factor is the close association between the temporal lobes and the limbic system — that phylogenetically old ring of cortex which loops under the corpus callosum and which has connections with the cerebral cortex, the brain stem and the hypothalamus (see Chapter 10, page 108). It has been argued (Taylor, 1977) that schizophrenic symptomatology may result from disorganization of the structures subserving language and thought (and hence also socialization) which are normally compactly located in the left side of the brain. In the brains of some individuals a tenuous and precarious balance may be temporarily disrupted by a variety of stresses, of which epilepsy is one, and in others this disruption may be more or less total and irreversible.

SUMMARY

In this chapter an attempt has been made to provide an orderly and coherent account of the emotional and psychiatric aspects of epilepsy in childhood and adolescence. It is hoped that it is apparent to the reader that this is a difficult and often confusing subject and that the physician confronted with these problems in the epileptic individual will need help from several different disciplines if he is to evaluate the situation successfully. For example, the findings by Rutter, Graham and Yule (1970) that children with epilepsy and an organic or structural disorder above the brain stem have a one in three chance of having an additional psychiatric disability and an equal likelihood of intellectual or educational retardation makes it clear that paediatricians and neurologists dealing with such children need to have considerable expertise in these related subjects. Despite the frequent need for a multidisciplinary approach, there is no substitute for the interested and concerned physician who is both experienced and skilled in the care of children and sympathetic towards the problems of children with epilepsy especially. He should be prepared to give time, encouragement, advice, education and support to the patient and his family, if necessary for many years. This is real preventative psychiatry in action and the reward will be a family which is well adjusted to the predicaments occasioned by having a child with epilepsy, and able to look forward to a stable and rewarding adult life for the patient in the future.

REFERENCES

Bagley, C. (1972). 'Social prejudice and the adjustment of people with epilepsy.' *Epilepsia*, **13**, 33–45
Bax, M. (1972). 'The active and the over-active school child.' *Devl Med. child Neurol.* **14**, 83–86
Cantwell, D. (1977). 'Hyperkinetic syndrome.' In *Child Psychiatry: Modern Approaches*, pp. 524–555. Eds M. Rutter and L. Hersov. Oxford, London, Edinburgh: Blackwell Scientific
Creak, M. and Pampiglione, G. (1969). 'Clinical and EEG studies on a group of 35 psychotic children.' *Devl Med. child Neurol.* **11**, 218–227
DHSS (1969). *People with Epilepsy. Report of a Joint Sub-Committee of the Standing Medical Advisory Committee on the Health and Welfare of Handicapped Persons.* London: HMSO
Erikson, E. (1966). *Childhood and Society.* London: Penguin
Erikson, E. (1977). *Childhood and Society.* London: Triad/Paladin
Falconer, M. A. and Taylor, D. C. (1968). 'Surgical treatment of drug resistant temporal lobe epilepsy due to mesial temporal sclerosis: etiology and significance.' *Archs Neurol., Chicago,* **19**, 353–361
Flor Henry, P. (1969). 'Psychosis and temporal lobe epilepsy – a controlled investigation.' *Epilepsia*, **10**, 363–395
Graham, P. and Rutter, M. (1968). 'Organic brain dysfunction and child psychiatric disorder.' *Br. med. J.* **2**, 695–700
Green, M. and Solnit, A. J. (1964). 'Reactions to the threatened loss of a child: a vulnerable child syndrome.' *Pediatrics*, **34**, 58–66
Hackney, A. (1976). 'Child epilepsy: The first against prejudice.' London: *The Sunday Times*, January 11th
Hoffman, H. (1845). *Der Struwwelpeter: Oder lustige Geschichten und drollige Bilder.* Leipzig: Insel Verlag
Lennox, W. G. and Markham, C. H. (1953). 'The sociopsychological treatment of epilepsy.' *J. Am. med. Ass.* **152**, 1690–1694
Lindsay, J. (1972). 'The difficult epileptic child.' *Br. med. J.* **2**, 283–285
Livingston, S. (1972). *Comprehensive Management of Epilepsy in Infancy, Childhood, and Adolescence.* Springfield, Illinois: Charles C. Thomas

Ounsted, C. (1955). 'The hyperkinetic syndrome in epileptic children.' *Lancet*, **2**, 303–311

Ounsted, C. (1970). 'A biological approach to autistic and hyperkinetic syndromes.' In *Modern Trends in Paediatrics*, pp. 286–316. Ed. J. Apley. London: Butterworths

Ounsted, C. (1971). 'Some aspects of seizure disorders.' In *Recent Advances in Paediatrics*, pp. 363-399. Eds D. Gairdner and D. Hull. London: J. and A. Churchill

Ounsted, C., Lindsay, J. and Norman, R. (1966). *Clinics in Developmental Medicine, No. 22: Biological Factors in Temporal Lobe Epilepsy*. London: Spastics Society and Heinemann

Pond, D. (1961). 'Psychiatric aspects of epileptic and brain-damaged children.' *Br. med. J.* **2**, 1377–1382, 1454–1459

Rutter, M. (1968). 'Lésion cérébrale organique, hyperkinésie et retard mental.' *Psychiat. Enfant*, **11**, 475–492

Rutter, M. (1977). 'Infantile autism and other child psychoses.' In *Child Psychiatry: Modern Approaches*, pp. 717–747. Eds M. Rutter and L. Hersov. Oxford, London, Edinburgh, Melbourne: Blackwell Scientific

Rutter, M., Graham, P. and Yule, W. (1970). *Clinics in Developmental Medicine, Nos. 35/36: A Neuropsychiatric Study in Childhood* London: Spastics International and Heinemann

Sillanpaa, M. (1973). 'Medico-social prognosis of children with epilepsy.' *Acta paediat. Scand.* Suppl. 237

Slater, E., Beard, A. W. and Glithero, E. (1963). 'The schizophrenia-like psychoses of epilepsy.' *Br. J. Psychiat.* **109**, 95–150

Stores, G. (1977). 'Behaviour disturbance and type of epilepsy in children attending ordinary school.' In *Epilepsy: The Eighth International Symposium*, pp. 245–249. Ed J. K. Penry. New York: Raven Press

Taylor, D. C. (1969). 'Some psychiatric aspects of epilepsy.' In *Current Problems in Neuropsychiatry*. Special publication No. 4. *Br. J. Psychiat.*

Taylor, D. C. (1971a). 'Psychiatry and sociology in the understanding of epilepsy.' In *Psychiatric Aspects of Medical Practice*, pp. 161–186. Eds M. G. Gelder and B. M. Mandlebrote. London: Staples Press

Taylor, D. C. (1971b). 'The ontogenesis of chronic epilepsy psychosis: a re-analysis.' *Psychol. Med.* **1**, 247

Taylor, D. C. (1973a). 'Aspects of seizure disorders, II: On prejudice.' *Devl Med. child Neurol.* **15**, 91–94

Taylor, D. C. (1973b). 'Epilepsy, brain and mind.' *Br. J. Hosp. Med.* 187–191

Taylor, D. C. (1977). 'Epilepsy and the sinister side of schizophrenia.' *Devl Med. child Neurol.* **19**, 403–407

Taylor, D. C. and Falconer, M. A. (1968). 'Clinical, socio-economic and psychological changes after temporal lobectomy for epilepsy.' *Br. J. Psychiat.* **114**, 1247–1261

Temkin, O. (1971). *The Falling Sickness*, p. 44. Baltimore and London: Johns Hopkins Press

Vallarta, J. M., Bell, D. B. and Reichert, A. (1974). 'Progressive encephalopathy due to chronic hydantoin intoxication.' *Am. J. Dis. child.* **128**, 27–34

Williams, D. (1969). 'Man's temporal lobe.' *Brain*, **91**, 639–654

CHAPTER 19

Learning Disorders in Children with Epilepsy: The Acquired Aphasia Syndrome

LEARNING DISORDERS

The problem of learning disorders in children with epilepsy is a confused and controversial one and the author is particularly indebted to the work of Stores (1971, 1973, 1975, 1978; Stores and Hart, 1976) in trying to clarify the various issues involved. Many of the early writers were pessimistic about cognitive function in children with epilepsy and up to the 1940s and even beyond, the concept of progressive 'epileptic dementia' was popular and was attributed by some to the cerebral dysfunction itself and by others to brain damage sustained during attacks. However, as Stores (1971) pointed out, the groups studied were often heterogeneous with respect to age, type and duration of attacks, treatment and associated physical handicaps, and assessment was almost exclusively restricted to 'IQ testing' (*see* Chapter 22), the educational bias of which put many epileptic patients at a disadvantage, especially epileptic children who had lost time at school. However, in recent times psychologists have moved away from the assessment of global intelligence towards the assessment of specific cognitive functions, and groups of children with well-defined types of epilepsy and with other factors in common have been studied.

Poor school progress

The fact that a problem does exist is beyond doubt. Holdsworth and Whitmore (1974a) studied a random group of children with epilepsy attending normal schools. They found that barely one-third were making wholly satisfactory progress. Half the children were achieving a very indifferent performance in the classroom (holding their own at a below-average level), one in six was falling appreciably behind in work and one in five presented with a behaviour problem. These authors emphasized that, even in ordinary schools, children with epilepsy were an educationally vulnerable group. In an earlier survey (Whitmore and Holdsworth, 1971) of children with epilepsy attending normal schools, 42 per cent of them were described by their teachers as being 'markedly inattentive'. The children were described as lethargic, absent-minded, sleepy, lacking in concentration or otherwise unresponsive to what was happening in class. Inattentiveness was found to be associated with unsatisfactory educational progress and with difficult behaviour. In their important monograph on temporal lobe epilepsy, Ounsted, Lindsay and Norman (1966) had asked why so many children with seizure disorders who had at least normal overall intelligence and good control of attacks failed to come up to academic expectations. There are probably many reasons for this failure but at least one of them could be the effects of medication.

Effects of anticonvulsants

Anticonvulsant drugs have been shown to affect attention as well as other aspects of cognitive function. Stores (1975) reviewed the possible harmful effects of anticonvulsant drugs on learning and emphasized that there is a widespread belief among teachers that children treated with these drugs are inevitably handicapped and that this belief contributes to the underexpectations which teachers generally have about children with epilepsy, underexpectations which, unfortunately, parents may also share. Phenobarbitone and primidone have often been incriminated in the learning difficulties of children with epilepsy and Hutt et al. (1968) found that phenobarbitone had an adverse effect on intellectual tasks involving sustained effort. The paradoxical effect of phenobarbitone in young children which results in over-excitement and overactivity may also interfere with any sort of sustained attention and concentration.

Chronic intoxication with phenytoin can lead to intellectual deterioration and this is discussed in Chapter 24. Stores and Hart (1976), in a study of factors associated with the progress of children with epilepsy attending normal schools, found that the reading skills of those children who had taken phenytoin for at least two years were significantly inferior to those who had taken other antiepileptic drugs over a similar period.

Ethosuximide has been linked occasionally with adverse effects on learning in children, mainly as a cause of global mental impairment, but this has not been confirmed in controlled studies. Similar conflicting reports have appeared about sulthiame. However, as Stores (1975) points out, many of the reports about the adverse effects of drugs on learning are difficult to evaluate because they do not clearly distinguish between side-effects, toxic effects and individual idiosyncrasy and because they do not give details of dosage and blood serum levels. Furthermore, the social circumstances of the patients studied are rarely documented.

Male preponderance

Many authors, including Holdsworth and Whitmore (1974), have commented on the preponderance of males among the educationally retarded with epilepsy. Stores (1977), in a survey in which children with epilepsy attending normal schools were compared with nonepileptic children attending normal schools, found that epileptic boys were significantly more inattentive and overactive than nonepileptic boys according to their teachers and parents, and that they performed significantly less well on tests of sustained attention and perceptual accuracy. No such differences were found between epileptic and nonepileptic girls. This contrast between the epileptic groups was not attributable to drug effects or EEG abnormalities. In this context, of course, it should be remembered that epilepsy may coexist with mental subnormality of varying degree which, in its own right, may frequently be associated with defects of attention. Distractibility and overactivity may be other features of the mentally subnormal.

Clues from EEG

The results of several investigations have suggested that certain features characterize the type of seizure discharge which is most disruptive of performance on tests of attention or of cognitive motor abilities. The more generalized, bilaterally synchronous and symmetrical the seizure discharge, the more regular and organized the spike-wave complexes (as exemplified by the 3 Hz pattern of true petit mal), and the longer the duration of the burst the greater is the effect on attention.

Browne *et al.* (1974) studied responsiveness before, during and after spike-wave paroxysms using an auditory stimulus (a sharp whistling noise), a response unit (a telegraph key) and a digital clock that measured time from the onset of stimulation to the closing of the circuit in the response unit. The 26 patients studied ranged in age from 5–20 years with a median age of 12 years and all were suffering from 'absence seizures'. They found that the reaction times during the one second before a paroxysm were within normal limits but only 43 per cent of the reaction times were normal at the onset of a paroxysm. Responsiveness was recovered quickly after a paroxysm. They found that the degree of maximal impairment of auditory responsiveness was the same in paroxysms of both long and short duration, and they concluded that, if possible, therapy for absence seizures should aim at controlling all spike-wave paroxysms.

Hutt (1967) showed that both clinical and subclinical generalized spike-wave bursts could disrupt not only the registration of information but also its storage and recall, and that these effects depended upon the amount and complexity of the information as well as on the rate at which the child worked. The headmaster of the school at the Park Hospital for Children in Oxford, Mr Stedman, has commented that petit mal makes holes in the mind like a paper doyley (Ounsted, 1978)!

Absences and defects of attention

The position with regard to absence seizures generally is a little more complicated when other types of absence seizure, apart from those due to true petit mal, are considered. Mirsky and van Buren (1965) reported a significant decrease in responsiveness to a visual and auditory continuous performance test in the seconds preceding a seizure. Their patients, however, had a mean age of 22 years, and studies were made during a number of types of EEG abnormality, including spike-wave, polyspike and wave and other forms. The defects of attention which occur with paroxysmal discharges of the spike-wave type may be less obvious in the absences seen in children with myoclonic epilepsy and in those occurring in some children with temporal lobe epilepsy. Furthermore, there may be a specific perceptual deficit present in each of these varieties. Another complicating factor is that some children with absences of various kinds may show attention defects between overt attacks and in the absence of EEG abnormalities, possibly because of a persistent disturbance of subcortical mechanisms (Stores, 1973).

Concentration and attention factors: orientation reaction

Clinical experience shows that the occurrence of seizures is sometimes related to particular activities or experiences. Lennox, Gibbs and Gibbs pointed out, as long ago as 1936, that the frequency of seizures was lessened by tasks requiring some degree of concentration or arousal.

Ounsted and Hutt (1964) demonstrated that seizure discharges occurred less frequently in circumstances which were neither boring nor excessively stressful. If the degree of attention required became too stressful the seizure discharges increased and performance declined.

Although defects of attention are usually associated with subcortical seizure discharges, there is reason to suppose that frequently occurring localized cortical discharges may adversely affect some aspects of attention and learning. Studies of focal epilepsy suggest that when a part of the brain is occupied by an electrical discharge it cannot perform its normal functions. In general, it has been found that temporal lobe lesions in the hemisphere dominant for speech cause impairment of verbal abilities, including defects of retention and learning of verbal material, while lesions of the temporal lobe on the nondominant side tend to impair visuospatial skills and to cause perceptual difficulties (Fedio and Mirsky, 1969; Ounsted, Lindsay and Norman, 1966).

It may be that a chronically discharging cortical focus, at least in some areas, disturbs the 'orientation reaction' by either increasing excitation of corticoreticular connections and maintaining a heightened arousal state or by interfering with the normal reactivity to novel stimuli and causing inattentiveness. The orientation reaction is defined as the total action of paying attention to important stimuli, and consists of a variety of physiological changes which increase the sensitivity of the sense organs and prepare the organism to deal with the situation. Characteristics of stimuli which elicit the orientation reaction include novelty, intensity, complexity, uncertainty and surprise (Lynn, 1966).

Perceptual difficulties

Gastaut (1965), using comprehensive psychological testing on children with epilepsy, showed that as many as a third had perceptual difficulties which could cause a considerable handicap in learning to read and write. Rutter, Graham and Yule (1970), in their comprehensive study in the Isle of Wight, found that reading skills were substantially impaired in almost one-fifth of the children with epilepsy. Stores and Hart (1976) investigated the *reading skills* of children with epilepsy attending normal schools. Their conclusions were as follows:

1. The reading skills of children with electrographically generalized epilepsy and subclinical seizure discharges appear to be no worse than those of nonepileptic matched controls
2. In contrast, children with persistent focal spike discharges tended to have lower reading levels than their nonepileptic matched controls

3. The inferior performance of the focal group was largely attributable to those children with left hemisphere focal spikes, and these were predominantly boys
4. The reading skills of epileptic boys, whatever their type of epilepsy, were inferior to those of epileptic girls
5. The long-term use of phenytoin was associated with lower levels of reading skills than were other forms of anticonvulsant medication.

Factors at home and at school

Quite apart from the effects of structural brain abnormality, seizure discharges and drugs on attention and learning ability in the child with epilepsy, it seems likely that unfavourable environmental factors at home and at school may adversely affect the development of the child's cognitive and social skills. Indeed, Hartlage and Green (1972) suggested that the academic achievement of the epileptic child may be more closely related to environmental factors than to any specific disability of neurological origin. In their study they found that the academic and social underachievement of children with epilepsy could be attributed, at least in part, to inappropriate dependency on their parents. They did not feel that this over-dependency was due to any single faulty attitude on the part of the parents (such as over-protectiveness), but rather to the direct impact of epilepsy and its treatment on the child's psychological development causing a delay in emotional growth.

Holdsworth and Whitmore (1974b), in a study of *the attitudes of teachers* towards children with epilepsy attending normal schools, found that these have been improving in recent years and that head teachers and class teachers were now more sympathetic towards these children and were anxious to treat them as normally as possible in school. They also found that many teachers showed an increased willingness to retain a child with epilepsy in school if his fits were not too severe or frequent. While they welcomed this improved tolerance on the part of the teachers, they felt that it may have misled the teachers into expecting a lower level of work from the children than they might have accepted had the children not been subject to epilepsy. This, in turn, led to underachievement by the children. However, they emphasized that it is not easy for teachers to maintain a balance between over-protection and under-protection where children with epilepsy are concerned.

It should be apparent from the foregoing discussion of this very complex problem that there may be many different factors concerned in the causation of learning difficulties in children with epilepsy. Furthermore, since it seems likely that cognitive defects may generate disturbed behaviour in these children, early recognition and treatment of these deficits may produce beneficial results both in the learning situation and in the personality development of the child.

THE ACQUIRED APHASIA SYNDROME

It seems appropriate at this point to mention an unusual disorder first described by Landau and Kleffner in 1957 which they called a 'syndrome of acquired aphasia with convulsive disorder in children'. It is now sometimes known as Landau's syndrome. They described six children who, after apparently normal acquisition of speech and language, developed aphasia for periods ranging from days to months or longer. Worster–Drought (1971) described a further 14 cases seen over a period of 10 years in which an acquired receptive aphasia was the outstanding symptom. Temporary aphasia is known to occur in association with certain types of epilepsy, particularly temporal lobe epilepsy, and usually follows a fit or a series of fits. In general, such aphasia recovers after a variable interval but may recur after further seizures. Temporary aphasia may also follow a head injury in childhood (so-called cerebral shock) or may be seen after an acute vascular accident such as an arterial thrombosis involving the dominant hemisphere, but slow recovery usually ensues in both instances. Speech may also be permanently lost in certain cerebral degenerative disorders, for example in Addison–Schilder's disease (Forsyth, Forbes and Cumings, 1971). However, in the syndrome of acquired aphasia previously normal children become aphasic, usually completely, without any evidence of other neurological abnormalities or a known focal brain pathology. At about the same time, or shortly afterwards, a proportion of the patients may have clinical epilepsy which may consist of generalized or partial seizures with predominantly motor components. The patients constantly display paroxysmal EEG abnormalities. Deonna et al. (1977) noted that spike foci were particularly located over the posterior territories of both hemispheres, i.e. mainly in the posterior temporal and parietal regions. The discharges were almost invariably bilateral and asynchronous over the two hemispheres and were nearly always with a left-sided predominance. In addition to the focal abnormalities, these authors noted multifocal slow spikes or bursts of slow spikes, usually bilateral but asynchronous, at one time or another in all of their patients.

The onset of the disorder has been reported as occurring from the age of three years up to nine years and it may be abrupt or gradual. The evolution of the condition is also variable. An onset may be followed by prompt recovery, and later recurrences and fluctuations may occur. At times, but again by no means invariably, the onset, recurrences and fluctuations may coincide with clinical epilepsy. However, in other cases the epilepsy may not occur or it may be very occasional, even though the typical EEG abnormality is present. Worster–Drought (1971) emphasized that the loss of comprehension of spoken language (receptive aphasia) was the crucial element of the disorder and that this was followed by loss of the ability to execute speech. A remarkable feature of this syndrome is that intelligence is usually unimpaired. The condition is frequently misinterpreted as the early stages of acquired peripheral deafness. Behavioural disturbances may coincide with the onset of the disorder and are usually due to an acute anxiety disorder in a child rendered incapable of understanding spoken language. Worster—Drought (1971) observed 14 cases over several years and concluded that the disorder was self limiting and did not progress beyond a certain point, although he commented that from the onset the course might run for several months before the disease process became quiescent. The long-term prognosis for full recovery is always doubtful. In Worster—Drought's series six children recovered more or less completely, three recovered partially and in the remaining five recovery was slight or very limited and the children were left with severe deficits in the comprehension and execution of spoken language. The author's experience with six cases of the disorder, seen over the past 12 years, has been similar to Worster—Drought's.

The aetiology of the syndrome is quite unknown. Landau and Kleffner (1957), in the original report of the condition, suggested that persistent epileptic discharges in parts of the brain concerned with linguistic communication result in a functional ablation of these areas as far as normal linguistic behaviour is concerned. Gordon (1964), writing of the concept of so-called central deafness, suggested that something similar to the 'deconnection syndromes' causing isolation of one part of the brain from another (which have been described in cases of adult dysphasia by Geschwind and Kaplan (1962)) might be present in children with severe specific language disorders who failed to develop normal understanding and execution of speech and language. He suggested that such a deconnection syndrome might arise as easily from a failure of normal connections to develop in the brain as from an acquired lesion. Perhaps new lesions of some kind may account for the strange syndrome of acquired aphasia. Gascon et al. (1973) thought that the EEG discharges might represent the cortical manifestation of a lower level subcortical deafferentiating process. However, as Foerster (1977) has pointed out, a dramatic improvement in language function does not necessarily occur when the EEG discharges disappear in these children and, in most cases, the improvement in language function lags behind EEG improvement.

Worster—Drought (1971) speculated that the underlying cause of the syndrome in some cases might be some form of low-grade selective encephalitis which particularly affects the temporal lobes, and Foerster (1977) was also in favour of a subacute inflammatory process with a self-limiting course. There is no definite evidence for this possibility, although one of the author's cases presented with aphasia developing in a setting of what might have been an encephalitic illness. Many authors, including the writer, have used anticonvulsant drugs in this syndrome. However, these drugs should only be used if clinical epilepsy is present. There is no evidence that they improve the paroxysmal abnormality in the EEG or that they affect the language disorder. Early diagnosis of this syndrome and its differentiation from deafness is important because these children do best in special schools dealing with aphasic children.

REFERENCES

Browne, T. R., Penry, J. K., Porter, R. J. and Dreifuss, F. E. (1974). 'Responsiveness before, during, and after spike-wave paroxysms.' *Neurology, Minneap.* **24**, 659–665

Deonna, Th., Beaumanoir, A., Gaillard, F. and Assal, G. (1977). 'Acquired aphasia in childhood with seizure disorder: A heterogenous syndrome.' *Neuropädiatrie*, **8**, 263–273

Fedio, P. and Mirsky, A. F. (1969). 'Selective intellectual deficits in children with temporal lobe or centrencephalic epilepsy.' *Neuropsychologia*, **7**, 287–300

Foerster, C. (1977). 'Aphasia and seizure disorders in childhood.' In *Epilepsy: The Eighth International Symposium*, pp. 305–306. Ed J. K. Penry. New York: Raven Press

Forsyth, C. C., Forbes, M. and Cumings, J. N. (1971). 'Adrenocortical atrophy and diffuse cerebral sclerosis.' *Archs Dis. Childh.* **46**, 273–284

Gascon, G., Victor, D., Lombroso, C. T. and Goodglass, H. (1973). 'Language disorders, convulsive disorders, and electroencephalographic abnormalities. Acquired syndrome in children.' *Archs Neurol., Chicago*, **28**, 156–162

Gastaut, H. (1965). 'Enquiry into the education of epileptic children.' In *Epilepsy and Education: Report on a seminar in Marseilles, April, 1964*, p. 3. British Epilepsy Association and International Bureau for Epilepsy

Geschwind, N. and Kaplan, E. (1962). 'A human deconnection syndrome.' *Neurology, Minneap.* **12**, 675

Gordon, N. S. (1964). 'The concept of central deafness.' *Clinics in Developmental Medicine, No. 13: The Child Who Does Not Talk*, pp. 62–64. London: Spastics Society and Heinemann

Hartlage, L. C. and Green, J. B. (1972). 'The relation of parental attitudes to academic and social achievement in epileptic children.' *Epilepsia*, **13**, 21–26

Holdsworth, L. and Whitmore, K. (1974a). 'A study of children with epilepsy attending normal schools, I: Their seizure patterns, progress and behaviour in school.' *Devl Med. child Neurol.* **16**, 746–758

Holdsworth, L. and Whitmore, K. (1974b). 'A study of children with epilepsy attending ordinary schools, II: Information and attitudes held by their teachers.' *Devl Med. child Neurol.* **16**, 759–765

Hutt, S. J. (1967). 'Epilepsy and education.' In *Proceedings of the 1st International Conference of the Association for Special Education*, p. 103. Stanmore, Middlesex: Association for Special Education

Hutt, S. J. and Jackson, P. M., Belsham, A. and Higgins, G. (1968). 'Perceptual-motor behaviour in relation to blood phenobarbitone level: A preliminary report.' *Devl Med. child Neurol.* **10**, 626–632

Landau, W. M. and Kleffner, F. R., (1957). 'Syndrome of acquired aphasia with convulsive disorder in children.' *Neurology, Minneap.* **7**, 523–530

Lennox, W. G., Gibbs, F. A. and Gibbs, E. L. (1936). 'The effect on the EEG of drugs and conditions which influence seizures.' *Archs Neurol. Psychiat., Chicago,* **36**, 1236–1245

Lynn, R. (1966). *Attention, Arousal and the Orientation Reaction.* Oxford: Pergamon Press

Mirsky, A. F. and van Buren, J. (1965). 'On the nature of the "absence" in centr-encephalic epilepsy: A study of some behavioural, electroencephalographic and autonomic factors.' *Electroenceph. clin. Neurophysiol.* **18**, 334–348

Ounsted, C. (1978). Personal communication

Ounsted, C. and Hutt, S. J. (1964). 'The effect of attentive factors upon bio-electric paroxysms in epileptic children.' *Proc. R. Soc. Med.* **57**, 1178

Ounsted, C., Lindsay, J. and Norman, R. (1966). *Clinics in Developmental Medicine, No. 22: Biological Factors in Temporal Lobe Epilepsy,* p. 110. London: Spastics International and Heinemann

Rutter, M., Graham, P. and Yule, W. (1970). *Clinics in Developmental Medicine, No. 35/36: A Neuropsychiatric Study in Childhood.* London: Spastics International and Heinemann

Stores, G. (1971). 'Cognitive function in children with epilepsy.' *Devl Med. child Neurol.* **13**, 390–393

Stores, G. (1973). 'Studies of attention and seizure disorders.' *Devl Med. child Neurol.* **15**, 376–382

Stores, G. (1975). 'Behavioural effects on anti-epileptic drugs.' *Devl Med. child Neurol.* **17**, 647–658

Stores, G. (1978). 'Sex-related differences in "attentiveness" in children with epilepsy attending ordinary school.' In *Advances in Epileptolgy, 1977,* pp. 54–57. Eds H. Meinardi and A. J. Rowan. Amsterdam and Lisse: Swets and B. V. Zeitlinger

Stores, G. and Hart, J. (1976). 'Reading skills of children with generalised or focal epilepsy attending ordinary school.' *Devl Med. child Neurol.* **18**, 705–716

Whitmore, K. and Holdsworth, L. (1971). *Some Observations from a Study of Children with Epilepsy who were Attending Ordinary Schools.* Durham, England: Spastics Society Study Group on Medical Aspects of Children with School Difficulties

Worster–Drought, C. (1971). 'An unusual form of acquired aphasia in children.' *Devl Med. child Neurol.* **13**, 563–571

CHAPTER 20

Diagnosis and Differential Diagnosis of Epilepsy

Paediatric neurology may be defined as the application of the neurological sciences to the developing, learning and growing child. As a discipline, it has contributed significantly to the ways in which the neurological problems of children, including epilepsy, are evaluated.

HISTORY TAKING

Careful and detailed history taking remains the essential cornerstone of accurate diagnosis. This will usually be obtained from the parents, and older patients may be able to contribute subjective information about their complaint. An eye-witness account of the attack by a parent, teacher or nurse, if the seizure occurs in hospital, is extremely useful in distinguishing the different types of epilepsy and in differentiating true epilepsy from other paroxysmal disorders. Attacks are often difficult to describe and asking the informant to mimic the attack is sometimes useful. A sequential account of the clinical feature should be obtained in an attempt to determine if there are focal or lateralizing features present.

It should be remembered, however, that the young patient may be quite unaware of the reasons for his visit to the doctor. A child with true petit mal, for example, may only be made aware that something unusual is happening by the reactions of those close to him. The child who has had a major tonic-clonic attack with have complete amnesia of the event and will remember only the circumstances in which he found himself on recovery. He will, however, realize that something very dramatic has taken place because of the concern shown by his family to him. It is important, therefore, to bear these matters in mind while taking the history from the parents if the child is present.

A full history should include any complaint of subjective sensations preceding the seizure (although an account of these is rarely obtained in young children), the characteristics and duration of the seizure itself and the occurrence of any postictal phenomena such as confusion, headache, drowsiness and sleep. Denis Williams (1968), writing about adults, has repeatedly emphasized the importance of asking about the circumstances in which the fit or fits occurred, remembering that anyone can have a fit under exceptional circumstances and that everyday events such as fatigue, fever, illness and emotional upset may precipitate an attack in those with an inherent susceptibility to convulse. Writers, from Hughlings Jackson onwards, have emphasized that epilepsy is a paroxysmal and recurring disorder in which there are disturbances of consciousness, sensation or behaviour of any sort which are caused primarily by cerebral disturbances (Williams, 1968). Since anyone can have a fit under exceptional circumstances, *the solitary seizure should not lead to a diagnosis of epilepsy* and all that that implies for the patient. The problem of the solitary fit is discussed more fully elsewhere in this book (*see* Chapter 8).

The history should, of couse, include a search for causes, and the family history, the mother's reproductive history, the circumstances of the pregnancy and birth, the events of the newborn period, the developmental milestones of the patient, and the history of any previous illnesses or injuries should all be taken into account. Paediatricians today have learned that early developmental aberrations are particularly relevant to the later progress of the child and disorders of growth, including intrauterine growth retardation, have a similar significance. Inquiries should be made with regard to the child's emotional development and current behaviour, and about his school progress and learning ability. In younger children aspects of play and the learning of skills should be discussed.

Clinical examination

Clinical examination of the child should include inspection for the external stigmas of diseases frequently associated with epilepsy, such as tuberose sclerosis and the Sturge—Weber syndrome. Posture, movements and adaptive behaviour are particularly important in infancy and later on, gait, speech and language development and the acquisition of simple skills should be observed and assessed. Evidence of crippling disorders

TABLE 20.1

'Soft' Neurological Symptoms and Signs

Overactivity
Impulsiveness
Distractibility
Irritability
Emotional immaturity
General clumsiness
Poor-visual motor function, e.g. in writing, drawing and catching a ball
Poor performance of skilled acts, e.g. in tieing shoelaces and fastening buttons
Abnormalities of gait, e.g. limp and failure to swing arms normally
Positive Fog test, i.e. the child is asked to walk on the outer sides of the feet,
    when associated movements of arms appear, particularly supination. May
    identify hemiplegia
Jumping, there is an inability to do so over the age of three years
Hopping, there is an inability to do so over the age of five years
Difficulties in picking up small objects – absence of pincer grip, athetoid move-
    ments, ataxia and tremor
Presence of abnormal movements or tremor on extending upper limbs anteriorly
    and spreading fingers
Difficulties in imitating gestures carried out by the examiner
Difficulties in performing rapid alternating movements, e.g. pronation/supination
Persistence of mirror or synkinetic movements in older children, e.g. when per-
    forming rapid pronation/supination, opposing thumb and individual fingers or
    performing rapid clenching movements of one hand
Crossed laterality
Speech problems and abnormal tongue movements

---

such as hemiplegia, in which the incidence of epilepsy may be as high as 50 per cent, should be looked for and even a mild degree of asymmetry in the face and limbs may be a clue to the presence of cortical atrophy on the side opposite to that on which somatic atrophy is present. Most paediatricians today are familiar with schemes of examination designed to detect the 'soft' neurological signs which may indicate the presence of neurological dysfunction (see Table 20.1). Information about these can be found in the monographs by Bax and MacKeith (1963), Paine and Oppé (1966) and Touwen and Prechtl (1970).

Formal neurological examination should include vital measurements (particularly of the head circumference); observation for any asymmetries in skull, face or limbs; auscultation for intracranial bruits; examination of the nervous system generally and, of course, examination of the fundi. A general physical examination should not be neglected; for example enlargement of the liver and the spleen may be associated with certain degenerative disorders of the central nervous system associated with seizures, and congenital heart disease may be complicated by cerebral thrombosis or cerebral abscess which may later be followed by the development of epilepsy. The assessment of the higher nervous activities probably comes under the heading of investigation, but the doctor experienced with children will usually be able to make a working estimate of the child's intellectual capacities without recourse to formal psychological testing which may, of course, be necessary later.

Syncopal attacks

Perhaps the commonest single error at all ages is to label *syncopal or fainting attacks* as epileptic. Syncope is exceedingly common and there are very few people who have not experienced this disturbance at some time during their lives. A typical faint usually has an apparent reason, such as standing still for a time (especially in school or in church), a warm and stuffy atmosphere, pain, emotional upset, the sight of blood or a lurid film or television presentation. Some people faint on exposure to cold which makes diving into the sea or swimming pools a risky business. A simple faint rarely happens without some warning and the onset is slower than in epilepsy. The usual premonitions are muscle weakness, tremor, nausea or a sinking feeling in the abdomen, sweating and light-headedness. These feelings may persist after a return to full consciousness in contrast to epilepsy where consciousness is clouded following the attack. Simple fainting usually occurs when the patient is standing or sitting and not when he is lying down. If the patient falls he tends to slump slowly to the ground or he may have time to reach a chair before falling, whereas falling in epilepsy is a sudden and dramatic event. An eye-witness account is invaluable because deathly pallor is the rule in fainting and the peripheral pulse is impalpable. If a deathly pallor does not occur and if unconsciousness lasts more than a few seconds then the attack is unlikely to be a simple faint.

The immediate cause of syncope is cerebral ischaemia and the attack may be aborted by lowering the head below the level of the heart or by lying down and, when that happens, consciousness is not lost. It is important to realize that patients in syncope may stiffen, jerk, be incontinent of urine or even bite their tongues by accident in falling during a simple faint. The jerky movements are always clonic and few in number and do not have the classic tonic-clonic sequence of epilepsy. Furthermore the clonic movements never precede a simple faint. In the author's experience, syncope can occur at any age in childhood from babyhood onwards, although it is probably most common in later childhood and early adolescence and in females.

Illingworth (1956) drew attention to an uncommon cause of syncope in early life due to abnormality and fusion of the cervical vertebrae in the Klippel—Feil syndrome. The usual story is that the child faints after any sudden movement of the neck. The attack is usually brief and leaves no sequelae. It was suggested that the cause of the syncope might be sudden compression of an abnormally placed medulla oblongata.

EEG examination is usually not necessary in the diagnosis of syncope unless atypical features are present. It is important to stress that even physicians experienced in the diagnosis of epilepsy can be misled by apparent syncopal attacks at times. The author's senior EEG technician has a series of such cases which she refers to caustically as examples of 'O'Donohoe's syncope'!

Parents should be reassured that syncopal attacks do no harm and, especially, that they do not damage the brain in any way. They should be advised that syncope may recur but that drug therapy is useless and pointless and even injurious to the patient. If the patient has already been put on a drug, usually phenobarbitone, then it should be stopped forthwith. One frequently obtains a family history of syncope in parents so presumably an unstable vasomotor centre can be inherited.

Breath-holding attacks

Another very common problem in early childhood, and one familiar to all paediatricians, is that of breath-holding attacks. These have been the subject of medical writing for centuries and the reader is referred particularly to the outstanding review by Lombroso and Lerman (1967) at the Children's Medical Center, Boston. The clinical story is that the child is, without warning, frightened, hurt, frustrated or angry; he cries vigorously for one or a few breaths and then holds his breath in the expiratory phase of respiration. After a few seconds he becomes more or less cyanotic, loses consciousness and falls limply. The limpness may be followed by a few jerks or even by a short period of stiffening. When such attacks occur frequently or are followed by longer periods of unconsciousness, or when apnoea and loss of consciousness supervene early after crying or even after a gasp only, or when marked stiffening or opisthotonus or even genuine convulsive movements develop then alarm and concern are aroused and it is not surprising that a diagnosis of epilepsy is suspected or misapplied to the patient. Although cyanosis is usual in breath-holding attacks, marked pallor may be present instead, and Lombroso and Lerman (1967) distinguished what they termed the cyanotic and pallid types of infantile syncope to cover these two types of attack.

The frequency of the attacks varies greatly, ranging from very occasional attacks to several times a day. Affected children soon outgrow their problem, and there is a sharp fall in frequency after the third birthday. In the Boston series (Lombroso and Lerman, 1967) 85 per cent of the children were free of attacks by five years of age. No significant relationship to either mental retardation or later epilepsy was found. The only reported fatality in a breath-holding attack probably followed the aspiration of gastric contents (Paulson, 1963). One striking observation by the Boston group was that 17 per cent of their cases went on to develop syncopal attacks later. Conversely, some adults suffering from syncope have a history of breath-holding attacks in early childhood.

Many different *mechanisms* for the attacks have been proposed. Emotional factors are certainly involved, and the attacks are most frequent during the normal developmental phase of negativism. Males predominate and many of those affected are described by their parents as being demanding and rather stubborn children. Heredity and familial factors are also important and, in the Boston series, a family history of breath holding was obtained twice as often among the patients compared with the controls (23 per cent against 11 per cent). The elements of surprise and unexpectedness in whatever triggers the attack have already been mentioned. Vulliamy (1956) suggested that the basic mechanism was an acute reduction in cerebral blood flow produced by a sharp rise in intrathoracic pressure or Valsalva-like manoeuvre caused by breath holding in the expiratory phase, similar to the mechanism of the 'fainting lark' to be described later (*see* page 198). The initial crying produced hypocapnia due to hyperventilation and this, it was suggested, caused cerebral vasoconstriction. Then, when the breath was held suddenly in expiration, the intrathoracic pressure rose suddenly producing a decrease in the effective perfusion pressure in the cerebral arterial vasculature by increasing jugular venous pressure and/or decreasing carotid arterial pressure. It has proved difficult to confirm this hypothesis experimentally in patients for obvious reasons.

Gastaut and Gastaut (1958) demonstrated that attacks similar to breath-holding attacks could be produced by ocular compression (the oculocardiac or oculovagal reflex) and they monitored ECG, EEG and respiration during these induced attacks. They demonstrated that the loss of consciousness in these reflexly induced episodes was due to acute cerebral hypoxia secondary to vagal cardiac arrest and respiratory arrest. They concluded that the basic pathological physiology of clinical breath-holding attacks was a 'familial hypervagotonia' which was reflexly triggered by emotional or external factors, such as a sudden blow on the head (particularly in the occipital region), and which resulted in cardiac and respiratory inhibition and sudden loss of consciousness due to cerebral hypoxia.

The Boston study (Lombroso and Lerman, 1967) also used the oculocardiac-reflex test on their patients (with resuscitation equipment on standby!) and used similar monitoring methods. They defined a positive result to the test as a period of cardiac asystole of two seconds duration or longer. They divided their cases into three groups, as follows:

1. The first and largest group (62 per cent) were children in whom the evolution of the attacks corresponded to the usually described pattern, i.e. a stimulus followed by vigorous crying, with apnoea and cyanosis preceding unconsciousness. Only one-quarter of this group had an asystole of two seconds duration or longer.
2. The second group (19 per cent) consisted of patients who lost consciousness much more quickly than the first group, with a minimum of crying and usually without cyanosis. Pallor was often described in this group and some went on to have stiffening or opisthotonus and convulsive movements. Nearly two-thirds of this group has a period of asystole lasting two seconds or more. Where periods of asystole of eight seconds or more were recorded, clinical convulsive seizures developed at the end of the attack.
3. In this group (19 per cent) clinical features of both types were present in the same individual.

Following this study Lombroso and Lerman (1967) proposed that two types of attacks could follow a noxious stimulus, i.e. cyanotic and pallid. They suggested that they were caused by different mechanisms, both leading to acute cerebral anoxia, and that both mechanisms could occasionally operate in the same child at different times. In the more common cyanotic type, they agreed that the mechanism suggested by Vulliamy (1956) was probably responsible, whereas in the pallid type they thought that the sudden circulatory failure secondary to asystole was clearly responsible. In both instances acute cerebral anoxia was the end-result and was responsible for the loss of consciousness. Lombroso and Lerman (1967) also demonstrated marked generalized slowing of activity in the EEG during the early hypoxic stage of the attack which was followed by flattening of the record (electrical silence) if the attack was prolonged and cerebral anoxia supervened. They suggested that the electrical silence in the EEG was probably due to cessation of cortical neuronal activity and that the stiffening, opisthotonus and tonic seizures occasionally seen in prolonged attacks were due to the release of brain-stem structures from control by cortico-reticular inhibitory fibres.

Lombroso and Lerman (1967) also found differences in the description of precipitating factors in the cyanotic group when compared with the pallid group. Emotional stimuli leading to frustration and anger were more commonly reported in the former, whereas minor injuries and sudden frights were more common in the latter. In the pallid group, unexpected blows on the head, especially in the occipital region, were also frequently provocative and were more likely to occur in toddlers learning to walk. This difference in triggering factors seems to tally with the alternative causative mechanisms proposed. They were surprised, as indeed most paediatricians have been, by the innocuous nature of the attacks as far as the child is concerned, considering their dramatic nature and rather terrifying pathological physiology. Stephenson (1978) reached similar conclusions in his splendid study and review of the problem.

In the Boston series (Lombroso and Lerman, 1967), 76 per cent of the patients commenced their attacks between six and 18 months of age, and most observers have reported them as being most frequent between the first and second birthdays. An onset in the early weeks of life was reported in a small number of patients in the Boston group, but Livingston (1972) felt that transient airway obstruction by aspirated milk or by mucus could simulate a breath-holding spasm. The author has seen undoubted breath-holding attacks in early infancy but has also seen episodes as described by Livingston and feels that the latter is the commoner cause of apnoeic spells in the young infant. Breath-holding attacks uncommonly begin after the age of two years.

As regards *treatment*, children with breath-holding attacks are often prescribed sedative or anticonvulsant drugs either because a mistaken diagnosis of epilepsy is made or because the attending doctor believes that these drugs prevent or reduce the frequency of the spells. There is absolutely no evidence to support this view and, as has been repeatedly stressed in this book, these drugs should be avoided in children unless they are genuinely indicated for conditions such as true epilepsy. However, Lombroso and Lerman (1967) suggested that the atropine derivatives might be tried in those patients who were having frequent and severe attacks of the pallid type because these medications might help by blocking the vagal arc of the reflex mechanism involved. The frequency of the attacks is often reduced after a correct diagnosis has been made and after advice and reassurance have been given, simply because parents worry less about the condition and the emotional temperature surrounding the problem is reduced.

Finally, parents have tried a large repertoire of counter stimuli to abort or terminate the attack with varying degrees of success. These include hearty slaps on the thighs or buttocks, the application of cold water or a wet flannel to the face, depressing the tongue and lower jaw with a blunt object and even throwing the child up in the air! Since recovery is invariable, the wise parent faced with a wrathful child might be better advised to avoid adding injury to insult and to simply do nothing.

Apparent fainting and sudden death

The syndrome of apparent fainting and sudden death in children is fortunately very rare but needs to be described briefly. Three different syndromes have been described as follows:

1. The syndrome of Jervell and Lange–Nielsen (1957) (also called the surdocardiac syndrome) is characterized by neurogenic deafness, attacks of ventricular arrhythmia and a prolonged Q–T interval in the ECG which is present between attacks
2. The syndrome described by my colleague Ward (1964) and also by Romano, Gemme and Pongiglione (1963), in which children have normal hearing but suffer from attacks of ventricular arrhythmia with a prolonged Q–T interval in the ECG (Ward–Romano syndrome)
3. A syndrome with multiple extrasystoles and attacks of ventricular arrhythmia, a prolonged Q–T interval and normal hearing.

The attacks are essentially similar to Stokes–Adams attacks in adults and in children they may occur after strenuous exercise. Ward's most recent case occurred in a girl who lost consciousness while swimming vigorously in a pool. Epilepsy, simple syncope and breath-holding attacks are often mistaken diagnoses. An ECG is mandatory in any child who has attacks of loss of consciousness after exercise. Prophylactic treatment with beta-blocking agents or with phenytoin (which shortens the Q–T interval) has met with limited success and, unfortunately, the life of a child with one of these syndromes hangs by a thread.

The fainting lark and mess trick

The 'fainting lark' and 'mess trick' are still occasionally practised by schoolboys. Usually. the method employed is to squat on the haunches and take several deep breaths. The individual then rises to his feet, closes his nostrils with his fingers and blows hard. Alternatively, the trick is played on a victim by others who persuade him to hyperventilate and then somebody standing behind him suddenly compresses his chest. Sudden brief loss of consciousness results in both instances. The first method is called the 'fainting lark' and the latter the 'mess trick'. In both the physiological mechanism is similar to that described for the cyanotic type of breath-holding attack; both are harmless but should be discouraged. Hysterical overbreathing in adolescents can produce a similar end-result.

Benign paroxysmal vertigo

The first mention of *benign paroxysmal vertigo*, like many other original observations in paediatrics, can be attributed to Still (1909). It was fully described by Basser in 1964. This condition is important because it is often confused with epilepsy, but a distinguishing feature is the absence of loss of consciousness. It occurs in children aged 1–5 years, who are bright and neurologically normal. There are multiple brief episodes of sudden onset and without warning and they may last for up to 30 seconds (but sometimes longer) during which the child is frightened, unsteady and may fall. He clings to his mother, may sweat or even vomit. If he is old enough to describe his symptoms, then he will refer to a sensation of rotation. He seeks something to support himself and, if this is not available he will sit down or crawl. Nystagmus may be observed. He has no amnesia for the attack or any postictal symptoms. The frequency of attacks varies from rare to several in a week and the EEGs are invariably normal, but caloric tests show abnormalities of vestibular function (Koenigsberger *et al.*, 1970). The evidence available points to a self-limiting peripheral lesion, but neither its precise location nor its nature are clear. The attacks wane with maturation and usually disappear by the age of four or five years.

Vestibular neuronitis is a condition which occurs in adults a few days after an upper respiratory tract infection. It can also occur in children but is not a paroxysmal disorder as is benign paroxysmal vertigo.

Vertigo can manifest itself as a symptom of temporal lobe epilepsy, usually with clouding or loss of consciousness, but this is very rare in the author's experience despite a recent report to the contrary (Eviatar and Eviatar, 1977). It must always be borne in mind that the list of *drugs* which can cause vertigo as a chronic side effect is endless, and acute accidental self-administered poisoning by drugs or alcohol producing vertigo is well known to those working in the admission departments of children's hospitals. In practice the main problem with recurrent vertigo in young children is to be aware of the existence of benign paroxysmal vertigo, to apply reassurance and avoid unnecessary medication.

Other disturbances

Young children, usually between 2½ and 3½ years of age, quite commonly engage in peculiar *ritualistic movements* when they are tired, particularly when they are put down to sleep. They may recur if the child wakens in the night. They may be seen while the child is sitting at table or in a highchair, particularly if he is bored. The usual pattern is one of slow squirming hand movements which are sometimes accompanied by lower limb movements. The eyes may appear blank or may turn up and the child may laugh or giggle in a rather inane fashion. The movements stop immediately when the child's name is called. The ritual is constantly being added to and may become quite prolonged. The remote withdrawn behaviour of the child alarms parents and it may be misdiagnosed as petit mal, in much the same way as day-dreaming at school in older children may be similarly mis-labelled. There can be no doubt that the child finds the movement patterns pleasant and relaxing and, at night, a means of dropping off to sleep.

At times, similar movements may be frankly *masturbatory*. Still (1909) wrote as follows: 'a girl of 5 years, was brought with a history that she would several times a day, when she thought herself not observed by her mother, rock herself backwards and forwards as she sat on her chair, at the same time turning red in the face, and perspiring, and then turning white as if exhausted. Inquiry showed that masturbation occurred at night also.' Masturbation in small children is more common in females. The parents should be told that it is a harmless habit, that the outcome will be favourable, that the condition has no connection with later adolescent or adult sexuality and that the child will suffer no ill-effects on his subsequent physical or mental development. The perineal area should be inspected for treatable causes of local irritation such as a rash and the possibility of threadworm infestation should be considered.

Night terrors (pavor nocturnus) afflict most children at some time, and adults are not immune from them either. They usually occur in the first few hours of sleep while the child is in deep non-REM sleep which is associated with high-voltage slow waves in the EEG. *Nightmares,* on the other hand, occur in the lighter REM sleep with which dreaming is associated and which is a feature later in the night or towards morning. A few strangled words or cries precede screaming and the child usually sits up staring and wide-eyed. He may stumble from his bed and appears terrified. He does not recognize his worried parents or respond to their comforting words. However, within minutes he settles down to sound sleep again and remembers little or nothing of the event next morning. It must be clearly understood that night terrors are not epileptic phenomena nor are they usually associated with any particular emotional disorder affecting the child at home or in school. Gastaut and Broughton (1965) polygraphically recorded episodes of night terror and, in every case, they demonstrated that the attack occurred during intense and sudden arousal from deep slow wave sleep. If the attacks are very frequent then diazepam, which significantly reduces the amount of non-REM sleep, may be prescribed at bedtime (2–4 mg orally). The doctor should firmly reassure the parents that the condition is common and benign and that the child will outgrow it.

Narcolepsy, in contrast to night terrors, is a disorder of sleep rather than a disorder of arousal. The characteristic symptom is recurrent daytime episodes of irresistible drowsiness and sleep. These may or may not be associated with the following:

1. Cataplexy, which is a sudden loss of muscle tone resulting in a fall to the ground while consciousness is maintained
2. Sleep paralysis, which is a sudden awareness, while falling asleep or during sleep, that one cannot move or cry out
3. Hypnagogic hallucinations which consist of vivid visual or auditory imagery occurring at the onset of sleep.

The irresistible sleep attacks are commonly the only symptom in childhood or they may be followed by any or all of the other symptoms after a variable period of time, often years. Cataplexy is the commonest associated phenomenon to develop. In those individuals with a history of cataplexy, sleep paralysis or hypnagogic hallucinations, investigations have shown that they are associated with the intrusion of REM sleep upon wakefulness. Loss of peripheral muscle tone is a normal physiological correlate of REM sleep, accounting for the cataplexy and sleep paralysis. The hypnagogic hallucinations resemble dreams recounted after awakening from normal REM sleep. In contrast to normal individuals who enter sleep through a prolonged non-REM period, people with cataplexy, sleep paralysis and hypnagogic hallucinations exhibit a prolonged initial REM period both in daytime attacks and in nocturnal sleep, and in this their sleep pattern resembles that of the neonate. Individuals who have only attacks of irresistible sleep without the other auxiliary features of the syndrome may not demonstrate this unusual transition to REM sleep but they show the normal descending pattern to non-REM sleep in both their daytime attacks and in nocturnal sleep. It has been suggested that the term narcolepsy should be restricted to those whose daytime attacks are characterized by the sudden transition from wakefulness to REM sleep and that, if this sequence is not present, some other condition is responsible for the attacks of involuntary sleep. Therefore, it seems wise to recommend careful EEG investigation in alleged cases of narcolepsy in order to determine the sequence of events.

The aetiology of narcolepsy remains obscure. Genetic factors are suggested by a positive family history in some instances. Emotional factors, particularly tension and anxiety, may precipitate attacks. In some children, the attacks may appear to be self-induced and associated with emotional problems in the family or school situation, but these cases should be investigated to determine whether they have true narcolepsy. Drugs such as the amphetamines, methylphenidate hydrochloride and the monamine oxidase inhibitors have been tried in treatment, and of these dextroamphetamine, which reduces REM sleep while minimally interfering with other sleep stages, seems very successful. A suitable dose would be 5 mg given in the morning, but smaller doses may be effective or larger doses may be required in some cases.

Narcolepsy is in no sense an epileptic disorder, but it may be misinterpreted as one. The 'sleep jerks', which occur in many normal children and adults while dropping off to sleep, may alarm parents and be misdiagnosed as epilepsy by some doctors, but they are normal phenomena (see Chapter 16). Even nocturnal enuresis and somnambulism may be labelled epileptic occasionally, particularly, or so it seems to the author, by psychiatrists. There is no evidence to connect these disorders with epilepsy although, of course, the child having a true nocturnal seizure may wet his bed. The reader interested in sleep disorders in infants and children is referred to the excellent reviews by Anders and Weinstein (1972) and Tassinari et al. (1977).

It is worth noting that delirium during acute febrile illnesses and even rigors may be mistaken for epileptic attacks. Children are prone to run much higher fevers with acute infections than are adults and rigors may be mistaken for febrile convulsions. Shivering and the lack of any real loss of consciousness will help to identify the rigor although the distinction can sometimes be difficult. However, it is a rather important clinical distinction in view of the current thinking about the importance of drug prophylaxis for children with febrile convulsions.

Hypoglycaemia may occasionally present a problem in differential diagnosis. Convulsions are one of the commonest presenting symptoms of hypoglycaemia at any age and have already been described in connection with neonatal hypoglycaemia. During infancy, rare metabolic disorders such as hypoglycaemia due to leucine intolerance and hereditary fructose intolerance may present with seizures. Over the age of one year the presenting problem may be the occurrence of fits or unusual drowsiness in the early morning only. Postictal stupor or confusion is usually prolonged after hypoglycaemic seizures. The symptoms at this age may be precipitated by vomiting, diarrhoea or deprivation of food and are likely to occur in a setting of intercurrent infection. The most likely cause of this symptom complex is the condition now usually called 'ketotic hypoglycaemia', defined by Colle and Ulstrom in 1964, which is considered to be responsible for perhaps half of the cases of hypoglycaemia occurring in early childhood. Attacks may continue to occur for some years unless prevented by treatment, but the long-term prognosis is excellent. The child is grossly ketotic during the attack and may occasionally exhibit marked hyperventilation. The condition may be familial and affect siblings. Acetonuria is an essential feature and the symptoms are rapidly relieved by giving glucose. Diagnosis requires observation in hospital and carefully controlled attempts at provoking hypoglycaemia by the administration of a ketogenic diet. Treatment consists of preventing ketosis by ensuring that regular meals are taken, especially during febrile illnesses, and by giving glucose supplements and alkalis when anorexia is present and the child is at risk of developing an attack (Ehrlich, 1971). In any hypoglycaemic child, whatever the cause, it is important to remember that hypoglycaemia and epilepsy may coexist, with the former precipitating the latter at intervals. The presence of persistent paroxysmal epileptic EEG abnormalities will usually clarify this situation and the child may need anticonvulsant medication in addition to the treatment for his hypoglycaemia. In view of its hyperglycaemic effect in some patients, mentioned in Chapter 24, phenytoin might be a suitable drug for treating such a combination of problems.

It has long been apparent to clinicians that there are striking points of similarity between epilepsy and *migraine*. Both are paroxysmal disorders and migraine is characterized by symptoms of central nervous system dysfunction, namely headache, vomiting, paraesthesiae, mental dulling and scotomas. Furthermore, migraine is often a familial disorder and epilepsy is linked in the public mind with heredity. Non-specific and non-epileptic EEG abnormalities have been reported in a moderate proportion of children with migraine and this has not helped matters in the medical mind. There is really no convincing evidence linking epilepsy and migraine, except that they are both paroxysmal disorders and both are common in childhood. However, the migraine attack is associated with vasoconstriction and a prolonged attack may occasionally lead to neuronal ischaemia and even infarction of the brain. Such an occurrence could be followed by atrophic changes and the later development of epilepsy, but such a sequence of events must be exceedingly rare (Editorial, *British Medical Journal*, 1977). The problem of migraine and migraine equivalents in children has been comprehensively reviewed by Brown (1977).

Migraine is often included in the group of recurrent disorders in childhood entitled '*periodic syndromes*'. Abdominal pain is a common periodic complaint in children and Apley and Naish (1958), in a survey of 1000 unselected schoolchildren, found that it occurred in one in every nine of the children studied. Emotional factors are usually responsible and an organic cause is rare (Apley, 1975). Epilepsy is also a common disorder in children, but whereas recurrent abdominal pain is most prevalent in the school child, convulsions occur more readily in the first five years of life. Does *abdominal epilepsy* exist as a clinical entity ? The fact that abdominal sensations can occur prior to epileptic seizures is widely accepted, and this sequence of events occurs quite frequently in temporal lobe epilepsy. Evidence exists for the central representation of abdominal sensation in the medial temporal area

(Penfield and Jasper, 1954). However, when people speak or write of abdominal epilepsy they mean something quite different from these prodromal syptoms of classic epilepsy. Douglas and White (1971) and O'Donohoe (1971) have reviewed the literature.

Douglas and White (1971) described 28 patients with recurrent abdominal pain in whom medical and surgical investigations were negative and who were then referred to a neurological consultation service for evaluation. Their ages ranged from four to 26 years and 16 were male; some of the older patients had had symptoms for many years. Their criteria for diagnosis of abdominal epilepsy were as follows:

1. The pain should be paroxysmal and of short duration, lasting a few minutes at most
2. There should be some coincidental transient disturbance of awareness or consciousness
3. There should be changes in the EEG acceptable as specifically epileptic in type
4. The patient should show a specific response to anticonvulsant medication.

By these criteria they accepted five cases as genuine and three others as probable. They explained their relatively high incidence of positive cases on the basis of selection.

No discussion concerning 'abdominal epilepsy' and its EEG correlates should omit a reference to the so-called 14 Hz and 6 Hz positive spikes or transients as first described by Gibbs and Gibbs (1951). This phenomenon consists of bursts of electrically positive sharp waves occurring in light sleep, which are of moderately low voltage and are maximal in the posterior temporal areas on one or both sides. The EEGs are obtained by using the standard bipolar method of recording. It was suggested by others that these waves could be correlated with the diverse symptoms of the periodic syndrome. Douglas and White (1971) discounted this idea and Eeg–Olofsson (1971), reviewing the normal development of the EEG in infancy and childhood, found that the phenomenon in question was infrequently present and appeared to be a normal developmental change reflecting the evolution of rhythm-generating systems in the brain. He found no connection with clinical symptoms.

In the author's experience, abdominal epilepsy is a very rare condition indeed and the causes of recurrent abdominal pain in children are usually those so well described by Apley (1975).

CONCLUSION

The differential diagnosis of epilepsy in children clearly involves a wide range of conditions. Making a correct diagnosis is of paramount importance to the patient and the key to this is careful history taking. The label of epilepsy is a passport to prejudice and, if wrongly applied, it can have a disastrous and even permanent effect on the patient's life. Jeavons (1975) has estimated that in most epilepsy clinics 20 per cent of the patients referred as having epilepsy do not have the condition, and this degree of misdiagnosis applies equally to children and adults. Furthermore, he emphasized that 20 per cent of patients in psychiatric hospitals diagnosed as having epilepsy do not have the condition. The same number of mistaken diagnoses has been found among patients referred to special centres for epilepsy (Parsonage, 1978). Doctors dealing with epilepsy should always look with suspicion at the phrase 'known epileptic' on the case-notes, and the word 'epileptiform' should be banished from the language of clinical medicine. These terms frequently indicate a reluctance on the part of the individual using them to take a detailed history of the patient's complaint and an additional lack of interest in or ignorance of the nature and clinical characteristics of epilepsy.

REFERENCES

Anders, T. F. and Weinstein, M. S. (1972). 'Sleep and its disorders in infants and children: A review.' *Pediatrics*, 50, 312–325

Apley, J. (1975). *The Child with Abdominal Pain*. Oxford: Blackwell Scientific

Apley, J. and Naish, N. (1958). 'Recurrent abdominal pains: A field survey of 1000 school-children.' *Archs Dis. Childh.* 33, 165–170

Basser, L. S. (1964). 'Benign paroxysmal vertigo of childhood. A variety of vestibular neuronitis.' *Brain*, 87, 141–152

Bax, M. and MacKeith, R. C. (1963). *Clinics in Developmental Medicine, No. 10: Minimal Cerebral Dysfunction*. pp. 82–84. London: National Spastics Society and Heinemann

Brown, J. K. (1977). 'Migraine and migraine equivalents in children.' *Devl Med. child Neurol.* 19, 683–692

Colle, E. and Ulstrom, R. A. (1964). 'Ketotic hypoglycaemia.' *J. Pediat.* 64, 632–651

Douglas, E. F. and White, P. T. (1971). 'Abdominal epilepsy: A reappraisal.' *J. Pediat.* 78, 59–67

Editorial (1977). 'Migrainous cerebral infarction.' *Br. med. J.* 1, 532–533

Eeg–Olofsson, O. (1971). 'The development of the electroencephalogram in normal children from the age of 1 through 15 years. 14 and 6 Hz positive spike phenomenon.' *Neuropädiatrie*, 2, 405–427

Ehrlich, R. M. (1971). 'Hypoglycaemia in infancy and childhood.' *Archs Dis. Childh.* 46, 716–719

Eviatar, L. and Eviatar, A. (1977). 'Vertigo in children: Differential diagnosis and management.' *Pediatrics*, **59**, 833–838

Gastaut, H. and Broughton, R. (1965). 'A clinical and polygraphic study of episodic phenomena during sleep.' In *Recent Advances in Biological Psychiatry*, Vol. 7, p. 197. Ed. J. Wortis. New York: Plenum

Gastaut, H. and Gastaut, Y. (1958). 'Electroencephalographic and clinical study of anoxic convulsions in children: Their place in the framework of infantile convulsions.' *Revue neurol.* **99**, 100–125

Gibbs, E. L. and Gibbs, F. A. (1951). 'Electroencephalographic evidence of thalamic and hypothalamic epilepsy.' *Neurology, Minneap.* **1**, 136–144

Illingworth, R. S. (1956). 'Attacks of unconsciousness in association with fused cervical vertebrae.' *Archs Dis. Childh.* **31**, 8–11

Jeavons, P. M. (1975). 'Misdiagnosis of epilepsy.' *Proceedings of the National Seminar on Epilepsy, Bangalore, India, 1975*, pp. 85–87. India: Indian Epilepsy Association

Jervell, A. and Lange–Nielsen, F. (1957). 'Congenital deafmutism and functional heart disease, with prolongation of the Q–T interval and sudden death.' *Am. Heart J.* **54**, 59–68

Koenigsberger, M. R., Chutorian, A. M., Gold, A. P. and Schvey, M. S. (1970). 'Benign paroxysmal vertigo of childhood.' *Neurology, Minneap.* **20**, 1108–1113

Livingston, S. (1972). *Comprehensive Management of Epilepsy in Infancy, Childhood and Adolescence*, p. 35. Springfield, Illinois: Charles C. Thomas

Lombroso, C. T. and Lerman, P. (1967). 'Breathholding spells (cyanotic and pallid infantile syncope).' *Pediatrics*, **39**, 563–581

O'Donohoe, N. V. (1971). 'Abdominal epilepsy.' *Devl Med. child Neurol.* **13**, 798–800

Paine, R. S. and Oppé, T. E. (1966). *Clinics in Developmental Medicine, Nos. 20/21: Neurological Examination of Children*. London: Spastics Society and Heinemann

Parsonage, M. J. (1978). Personal communication

Paulson, G. (1963). 'Breathholding spells: A fatal case.' *Devl med. child Neurol.* **5**, 246–251

Penfield, W. and Jasper, H. (1954). *Epilepsy and the Functional Anatomy of the Human Brain*, p. 422. Boston: Little, Brown and Company

Romano, C., Gemme, G. and Pongiglione, R. (1963). 'Aritmic cardiache rare dell' eta' pediatrica.' *Clinica pediat.* **45**, 656–683

Stephenson, J. B. P. (1978). 'Reflex anoxic seizures ('white breath-holding'): nonepileptic vagal attacks.' *Archs Dis. Childh.* **53**, 193–200

Still, G. F. (1909). *Common Disorders and Diseases of Childhood* Oxford: University Press. Also published as Still, G. F. (1938). *Common Happenings in Childhood*. London: Oxford Medical Publications

Tassinari, C. A., Terzano, G., Capocchi, G., Dalla Bernardina, B., Valladier, C., Vigevano, F., Daniele, O., Dravet, C. and Roger, J. (1977). 'Epileptic seizures during sleep in children.' In *Epilepsy: The Eighth International Symposium*, pp. 345–354. Ed. J. K. Penry. New York: Raven Press

Touwen, B. C. L. and Prechtl, H. F. R. (1970). *Clinics in Developmental Medicine, No. 38: The Neurological Examination of the Child with Minor Nervous Dysfunction*. Spastics International and Heinemann

Vulliamy, D. C. (1956). 'Breathholding attacks.' *Practitioner*, **177**, 517–519

Ward, O. C. (1964). 'A new familial cardiac syndrome in children.' *J. Ir. med. Ass.* **54**, 103–106

Williams, D. (1968). 'The management of epilepsy.' *Br. J. Hosp. Med.* **2**, 702–707

CHAPTER 21

The Investigation of Epilepsy in Childhood

In childhood epilepsy, as a general rule, investigations should be kept to the minimum necessary for making a firm diagnosis and for the exclusion of treatable causes. Linnett (1976) in an eloquent discussion on what he called 'the burden of epilepsy' as seen from the standpoint of a general practitioner, emphasized that, in the investigation of childhood epilepsy, a delicate balance had to be maintained between adding to parental anxiety by subjecting the child to a battery of interviews, tests and complex investigations, and the need to establish a firm diagnosis. He emphasized that the latter may make parental fears less dreadful and formless in the relief of knowing what it is they have to face. It is important to remember that the child may not be aware of his complaint or he may only be aware that something is wrong as a consequence of the reactions of his parents and siblings. Therefore, a full diagnostic onslaught in hospital may bewilder and frighten the small patient. If possible, investigations should be performed on an out-patient basis or, at the very least, the period of hospitalization should be minimized. A close liaison should be maintained at all times between the specialist, the parents and their family doctor, and the medical personnel involved should allow adequate time for explanation to the parents of what is taking place.

The extent of the investigations will, of course, be determined to a large extent by the type of epilepsy being studied and will be based on the 'working' diagnosis reached after full history taking and physical examination. At all times the physician should resist the modern mania for excessive investigation. This is always expensive and time consuming and frequently in the worst interests of the patient. There are no 'routine' investigations: there are only those that are indicated by the specific diagnostic problem presented by the patient.

LABORATORY INVESTIGATION

The investigation of epilepsy may, in certain cases, involve tests of renal function, serological tests (especially for viral infections), studies of the concentration of serum proteins and amino acids, chromosome analysis and even the highly elaborate studies involved in the differentiation of the various degenerative disorders of brain, nerve and muscle in childhood. The author usually advises measurement of the fasting true glucose, the serum calcium and the blood urea levels for all patients undergoing hospital investigation.

Specific neurological tests include diagnostic taps and plain skull radiography. Lumbar puncture should certainly not be regarded as a routine investigation. It is essential for the diagnosis of meningitis or encephalitis presenting with seizures or where seizures are associated with degenerative processes in the central nervous system such as metachromatic leucodystrophy or SSPE. In both conditions, a raised cerebrospinal fluid protein concentration may be found. Lumbar puncture should, of course, never be done where there is any suspicion of raised intracranial pressure.

RADIOGRAPHY

Plain radiography of the skull may be revealing in the secondary generalized epilepsies of early childhood where calcification consequent on tuberose sclerosis, intrauterine cytomegalovirus disease or congenital toxoplasmosis may be seen. Characteristic intracranial calcification may also develop later in the Sturge—Weber syndrome. Cerebral lesions occurring in early childhood frequently exert an influence on the growth of the skull bones. This was studied by Miribel, Vieto and Favel (1963). They demonstrated that where hemiplegia follows a hemiconvulsive episode in the first two years of life, hemiatrophy of the cranium on the affected side followed almost invariably and similar changes were frequent where the cerebral insult occurred between two and four years of age. From four years onwards the incidence of skull bone involvement decreased rapidly. They also felt that plain radiography might be useful where there was a history of obstetrical trauma since it might show localized abnormalities of skull growth in relation to sites of major cerebral damage.

In temporal lobe epilepsy due to mesial temporal sclerosis, there may be associated bony changes in the ipsilateral middle cranial fossa, including flattening of the vault, elevation of the base and enlargement of nearby air cavities in bone. The overlying skull may also be thickened. These X-ray changes may be useful additional evidence for lateralizing the brain lesion when surgery is being contemplated.

Epilepsy due to a condition such as a meningioma, so often associated with overlying hyperostosis of the skull or sometimes with bony erosion, is exceedingly rare in childhood.

Air encephalography (pneumoencephalography)

This is often of value in the investigation of intracranial lesions which are not obviously associated with raised intracranial pressure (*see* the section on CT scanning). It is used in investigation of the aetiology of partial epilepsies, in the study of post-traumatic intracranial complications and where space-occupying lesions are suspected. It should never be used for investigating the last without prior neurosurgical consultation and only after arranging for neurosurgical care. It should preferably be carried out by a radiologist familiar with neuroradiological techniques and their hazards. Direct ventriculography may have to be used where intracranial pressure is raised, but for this burr holes must be made in the skull and needles inserted through brain tissue.

Air encephalography studies are rarely necessary in the investigation of childhood epilepsy except, perhaps, in some of the partial epilepsies. The procedure carries a risk and severe headache may follow it.

Angiography

This may be of diagnostic value in three situations:

1. In the investigation of intracranial space-occupying lesions (haematomata, abscesses and neoplasms)
2. In the investigation of arteriovenous malformations and aneurysms
3. In the investigation of occlusion or stenosis of major vessels in the brain.

Again, it is important to remember that this procedure carries a risk and should preferably be done only by a competent neuroradiologist and only where specific indications are present. It may occasionally be useful in the investigation of a localized temporal lobe lesion.

TRANSILLUMINATION OF THE SKULL

It is worth remembering that simple *transillumination* of the skull in small children, using a torch fitted with a circular rubber extension applied to the skull, may be very informative in conditions such as hydrocephalus, porencephaly, hydranencephaly and localized brain atrophy. Fluid conducts light better than solid tissue and in a completely dark room one may clearly see the widespread diffusion of light through a fluid-filled area in the skull.

SCANNING TECHNIQUES

Gamma encephalography

This employs a gamma camera and the isotope technetium 99. It is a procedure which is of most value in the investigation of space-occupying lesions, including subdural haematomata (*see* section on CT scanning). It should be noted that occasionally abnormal uptake of the isotope may be found after repeated focal seizures in the absence of any demonstrable pathology. This is presumably due to alteration in the blood-brain barrier in the area and it soon returns to normal.

Computerized axial tomography

The imagination and ingenuity of two men, Hounsfield (an engineer) and Ambrose (a neuroradiologist) led to the introduction in 1973 of computerized axial tomographic scanning (CAT scan, CT scan, EMI scan; Ambrose and Hounsfield, 1973). This technique has led to a revolution in neuroradiological investigation and there seems to be no doubt that this revolution will be felt in all aspects of neurology. The CT scan is a method which gives quantitative readings of tissue density with a resolution sufficient to distinguish between the various intracranial soft tissues. This new technique has a special application in paediatric neurological investigation because it is painless and safe (the radiation exposure is considered to be relatively low), and because it is being adapted for children of all ages from infancy onwards (Gomez and Reese, 1976).

Schulte (1976), writing about CT scanning, commented that in recent decades diagnostic procedures had become more and more aggressive with sometimes quite remarkable complication rates including mortality. He went on to say that in this respect neurodiagnostic methods were in the forefront, and for that reason neuropaediatricians remained very conservative about these investigations when applied to children. He suggested that in paediatric investigation CT scanning should entirely replace radioisotope scanning with its exposure to inoculated radioactive material, and that pneumoencephalography and angiography should rarely be necessary now, the latter being reserved only for suspected abnormalities of the vasculature.

In an outstanding review of the present place of CT scanning in the neuroradiology of infants and children, Harwood–Nash and Fitz (1976) wrote as follows: 'In essence, CT has necessitated an altered emphasis of neuroradiological diagnostic techniques – an emphasis that is dependent on the clinical status of the patient, the suspected intracranial pathology, the degree of sophistication of modern neuroradiological equipment, and the expertise possessed by the paediatric neurologist. Increasing experience with and sophistication of CT will also improve its diagnostic significance. Due to the impact of CT, our present experience is that the use of so-called screening pneumoencephalograms and angiograms for such conditions as epilepsy or possible cerebral atrophy has markedly decreased. We still perform angiography and/or contrast air studies to study congenital anomalies of the brain and certain tumours (e.g. brain stem tumours, masses in or around the third ventricle), for we believe the geography and character of mass lesions must still be precisely defined to obtain a successful surgical result. In our hands, therefore, CT has become a valuable initial and additional investigative tool rather than a replacement technique.' They later go on to say that: '. . . we do not believe that CT will replace angiography and pneumoencephalography to any great extent in the near future. They will better show the trees within the wood so to speak, the site of the latter having been determined by CT. For demonstrating the content of mass lesions, however, CT will remain paramount. The routine screening functions of standard neuroradiological procedures will disappear.' They later emphasized, however, that their predictions for the future place of CT scanning might prove quite wrong since, as they put it, month by month, 'new computer machines and more sophisticated computer programs are budding like the veritable maple tree in the spring', and as a consequence present machinery might soon be obsolete.

Gastaut and Gastaut (1977), in an extensive review of their experience with CT scanning in epilepsy generally, reported that in patients with various types of epilepsy the method gave accurate information about frequency, topography and severity of morphological lesions and markedly increased the ability to establish the aetiology (*Figure 21.1*). However, in patients with presumed primary generalized epilepsies the yield of cerebral lesions with CT scanning has ranged from 0–10 per cent (Gastaut, 1976). Zimmerman, Niedermeyer and Hodges (1977) have applied the technique to the severe secondary generalized epilepsies of the so-called Lennox–Gastaut syndrome. In a study of 38 patients they showed normal findings in 20 and abnormalities in 18, and diffuse cerebral atrophy was found to be the most common abnormality.

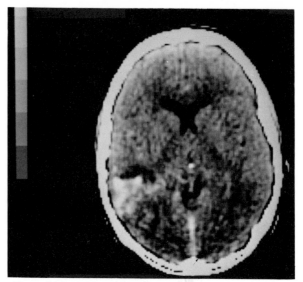

Figure 21.1. CT scan showing large left posterior temporal angioma, following the injection of contrast medium

Diffuse cerebral abnormalities were found in greater numbers with advancing age of the patients.

It is clearly still too early to know just what new knowledge about childhood epilepsy this revolutionary technique will provide, but there is no doubt that it will be considerable. It offers exciting prospects over the next decade for all those interested in the welfare of children with epilepsy.

Echoencephalography

Echoencephalography, and particularly methods designed to detect ventricular landmarks by two dimensional ultrasonography (Erba and Lombroso, 1968), has been used in neurological investigation in children and is safe and painless. It will probably be superseded by CT scanning and it plays little part in the investigation of epilepsy in the paediatric age-group.

ELECTROENCEPHALOGRAPHY

The investigation par excellence for epilepsy is, of course, the EEG. It has been said that the EEG was the glass slipper for the Cinderella disease of epilepsy. The story of Hans Berger's discovery of the human EEG in 1924 has never been better told than by Gloor (1974) at the Hans Berger Symposium which was held in Edinburgh in 1973 to celebrate the centenary of his birth.

Berger was the first to prove the correctness of Hughlings Jackson's hypothesis that an epileptic seizure was a manifestation of exaggerated discharges of grey matter taking place in an area of brain functionally related to the clinical symptomatology of the seizure although, as Gloor points out, he was completely unaware of having done so, probably because his knowledge of English was poor and he was not familiar with Hughlings Jackson's writings. Berger was also the first person to record an absence attack in which he demonstrated the occurrence of regular rhythmic high voltage slow waves at the rate of 3/second. He failed to demonstrate the associated spikes and felt that he had recorded an artefact. The validity of his pioneering work was later confirmed in Great Britain by Adrian and Matthews (1934) and by workers in other countries.

The EEG measures differences in electrical potential arising between different parts of the head resulting from the spontaneous activity of the underlying brain. The growth of electroencephalography as a science since the twenties has really paralleled that of its instrumentation, for when measured through the skull from electrodes placed on the unshaven scalp these potentials commonly show a voltage difference between the leads of only about 50 μV and only rarely in man do they exceed 200 μV. They are usually, therefore, about one-tenth or less of the magnitude of ECG potentials. Consequently they need considerable amplification before they can be recorded. The development of the modern thermionic valve made such amplification possible but the EEG machines using valves were large and cumbersome. The invention of the transistor in 1948 has led to the development of the modern compact and often portable machines.

In the usual method of recording, potentials from several pairs of electrodes are led in through differential input stages and registered simultaneously, each pair of electrodes having its independent amplifying system and recording unit. Recordings between members of a pair of electrodes may be bipolar (i.e. from two electrodes which are over active brain) or unipolar (i.e. where one electrode is over active tissue and the other is over a distant and relatively inactive point; usually the mastoid process is used although there is no truly inactive point anywhere on the head). The bipolar method of recording is in universal use today.

Those seeking further information concerning the electrical activity of the nervous system should consult Brazier (1968). The EEG has *limitations as an investigative tool*. It is a fussy technique requiring much attention to detail, particularly in the electrode placement and maintenance of apparatus in order to obtain good artefact-free recordings. It can pick up electrical signals from a limited area of the brain only, mainly from the convexity of the cerebral hemispheres. The small size of the potentials has already been mentioned and they are further attenuated by the distance of the electrode from the actual source of the activity. Perhaps most important of all, the abnormal patterns of electrical activity recorded are, except in very rare instances, nonspecific with regard to pathology. This point will be discussed further. Also, it is important to remember that dead brain tissue does not produce abnormal electrical potentials. It is the surrounding and altered living cerebral tissue which undergoes changes of normal electrical activity which are then registered in the EEG recording.

The *advantages of the EEG examination* are that it is painless, fairly brief and relatively inexpensive. It is non-invasive when compared with some neuroradiological investigations, and even the invasive modifications employed in some adult examinations, such as the use of sphenoidal electrodes, are seldom used in childhood. Permanent records of the electrical activity of the brain are immediately obtained and easily stored for comparison, if necessary, with later recordings. The EEG can be studied during attention or at rest and also during sleep and the degree of abnormality may vary from one state to another, particularly in the case of epilepsy.

EEG techniques in childhood

As has been emphasized in other sections of this book, epilepsy is most common in the early years of life and it is in taking recordings from babies and young children that most technical difficulty is experienced. The author is convinced that such recordings are best done in an EEG department specializing in paediatric EEG, and having the services of technicians with special experience in this particular field of electroencephalography. The technician should be able to allow time to play with the child and gain his or her confidence and co-operation. The recording room should be quiet and look as unclinical as possible. Soft furnishings, cheerful colours and plenty of toys, especially small toys for use during the recording, are essential. Sedation should rarely be necessary except for very disturbed children. In the author's department, the product most commonly employed to placate rather than sedate is chocolate drops! The child should be given every opportunity to drop into a natural sleep if possible, since sleep is perhaps the most potent of all activating procedures in childhood epilepsy. Routine recordings are made either with the subject sitting or recumbent, or frequently the former followed by the latter, and activation by hyperventilation and intermittent photic stimulation, using a rapidly flickering light, is used where appropriate. The use of stick-on rather than pad electrodes is essential in babies and young children if artefact-free records are to be obtained and, in many paediatric EEG departments, stick-on electrodes are used exclusively.

Interpretation of EEGs in childhood

The interpretation of EEG recordings from children, particularly infants and small children, requires special knowledge and experience on the part of the examiner and should preferably be done by an individual versed in the problems of neuropaediatrics. There are considerable differences from adults and changes in the EEG, both in the waking state and during sleep, occur from infancy through early childhood and up to late childhood (Petersen and Eeg–Olofsson, 1971). In fact, the EEG may not reach a state indistinguishable from an adult record until the midteens.

Throughout the neonatal period, infancy and childhood the EEG pattern is much more easily disturbed by intercurrent metabolic and toxic changes than is an adult EEG recording. The normal response of the child's EEG to hyperventilation is an example of this. Cerebral lesions cause more widespread and marked abnormalities than would a comparable lesion in an adult. The EEG abnormalities seen in children suffering from epilepsy, whatever its type, are similar to those found in adults, but they are usually of larger amplitude, more widespread and are associated with a more generalized disturbance of brain rhythm than would be the case in an adult. There are also certain specific EEG patterns in children with diseases such as SSPE, neuronal ceroid lipofuscinosis (Batten–Vogt disease) and, of course, infantile spasms. As with paediatric neurology in general and childhood epilepsy in particular, the EEG of an infant or child is the result of a complex interplay of pathological, metabolic and maturational factors in the individual being studied.

Electroencephalography has precise but limited applications, and the study of the electrical activity of the brain should not be regarded with greater veneration than the study of any other function of the body, nor should an abnormal EEG be regarded as more significant than any other abnormal physical sign. Any neurological problem in a child or an adult should be assessed as a whole. An EEG may be able to tell us how the patient's brain appears to be working and whether the patterns present are within the normal range of maturity of his age. The responses to various stimuli can be assessed and differences in the function of the two hemispheres and between homologous areas of the brain can be studied.

In general, clinicians unfamiliar with the EEG ask too much of the investigation, both in adults and children, and are often disappointed by the results. It is appropriate to quote Denis Hill (1958) on this point. He wrote: 'The EEG is often used as a means of helping to decide whether a given patient's symptoms are epileptic or psychogenic or are due to some noncerebral cause, such as syncope. I believe this is an improper use of the technique and that in fact the results of doing this can be misleading. A single routine normal EEG is not evidence against epilepsy, nor indeed is the finding of epileptic discharges in the EEG evidence that the patient's symptoms are necessarily epileptic in nature. Such discharges occur in the EEGs of some nonepileptic persons, in many with degenerative brain disorders, in some psychotics, and in cases of behaviour disorder. The prescription of anticonvulsants on the finding of such discharges in the EEG is unjustifiable and often illogical, and may lead the clinician to overlook more important issues for his patient. The recognition of the epileptic nature of any symptom or group of symptoms is, I believe, a clinical task and must remain so. When the clinician requests an EEG to confirm the diagnosis he is not so much interested in the question of whether the EEG demonstrates focal discharges in the expected area — he is merely disappointed but does not alter his diagnosis if it does not — as in the question of whether the EEG demonstrates the presence of a pathological process, either a local lesion or a diffuse one, which is of such importance for the prognosis.' Although these remarks concern adults, they are also largely applicable to children.

One happy circumstance for the paediatric electroencephalographer is that the interictal records of children with epilepsy are more likely to show abnormalities than those of epileptic adults, and these may include spikes, spike and wave complexes and other paroxysmal abnormalities. These EEG findings are not specific for epilepsy but they are vastly more common in those who have had fits than in those who have not. The EEG will not usually tell us why the young patient has epilepsy although it is established that certain EEG patterns are associated with a predominantly inherited or genetic origin for the seizures while other EEG abnormalities are more likely to be caused by acquired brain damage. The EEG can be helpful in categorizing the type of epilepsy from which the child is suffering and this aspect of things has been described in more detail in the chapters dealing with the particular varieties of epilepsy.

A widespread misconception about the EEG is that it will always or even usually tell the clinician if the patient's epilepsy is improving and, therefore, that it can be used to decide whether or not it is safe to stop treatment or even, at a later date, if it is safe for the patient to drive a car — this is not so. Epilepsy is a clinical state and consists of having fits and not simply of having abnormal brain-waves, and assessment of improvement should be predominantly a clinical exercise.

The EEG has much to contribute in deciding whether or not the patient is a suitable case for temporal lobectomy, but the techniques now employed in centres where the operation is done are much more elaborate than those of an ordinary EEG department. However, the consistent finding in routine recording of a unilateral temporal lobe focus in a patient with intractable epilepsy is a useful starting point.

Non-specific nature of EEG abnormalities

The question of whether seizures are due to a space-occupying lesion is one that agitates the minds of parents and their doctors but, as discussed elsewhere, supratentorial tumours are very uncommon in childhood. It is important to emphasize, in this context, that the EEG never directly indicates a pathological process. A delta wave abnormality in the EEG may be caused by tumour or abscess, by infarct or haemorrhage, by a local area of demyelination or by many other lesions. A change in the abnormality, for better or worse, in serial recordings may be useful in differentiating the various diagnostic possibilities. It should be re-membered, as mentioned previously, that the abnormal waves are not produced by the tumour or abscess or whatever, but by damaged brain cells in the vicinity. One further pitfall is that, since the brain appears to function by conveying electrical impulses from one area to another, abnormal activity can sometimes be recorded from areas which are relatively remote from their site of origin and 'mirror foci' may occur on the contralateral side from the area of primary abnormality.

In the early days of the EEG a great deal of emphasis was laid on the need for accurate electrical localization. Fortunately, the great advances in neuroradiology have rendered such accuracy unnecessary and the EEG should now be able to find its proper place in the scheme of neurological investigation. As Matthews (1964) has written: 'There is a serious need to find a middle course between blind acceptance of the EEG as a routine investigation and the attitude summarized by dismissing an EEG department as "another waste-paper store". Change will be difficult while every doctor expects his epileptic patients' problems to be solved by the EEG, and every patient demands it. Under such demands few electroencephalographers can claim never to have written such futilities as "the record is compatible with epilepsy", well knowing that this applies to every record ever taken.'

EEG AND CLASSIFICATION OF CHILDHOOD EPILEPSY

Attempts to classify epilepsy in childhood in relation to EEG criteria have not been successful, mainly because the younger the child the more diverse the EEG abnormalities which correspond with the variable clinical manifestations of epilepsy in the young.

The role of EEG investigation in the neonate with seizures is discussed in Chapter 3. The grossly disorganized EEG pattern called *hypsarrhythmia* is seen in infants with infantile spasms but is a nonspecific reaction on the part of the brain to a variety of insults. Hypsarrhythmia can also occur in severely mentally handicapped children who may not have clinical epilepsy. Friedman and Pampiglione (1971) studied 105 children who had shown the EEG features of hypsarrhythmia in the first year of life and who were followed-up for a minimum of seven years. Irrespective of the presenting symptomatology, and to some extent regardless of therapy, mortality in the group was of the order of 25 per cent and occurred mainly before the age of three years, and the incidence of mental subnormality in the survivors was 77 per cent. Only 18 children attained fairly normal standards of mental development and could attend ordinary schools. They concluded that hypsarrhythmia was a physical sign of grave prognostic significance, whatever the clinical picture at the time. It is important to realize that the EEG in many of these patients may eventually show no abnormality at all, in spite of serious and permanent mental handicap. In those who continue to have epilepsy, the hypsarrhythmic pattern may change into generalized repetitive slow spike-wave complexes.

Aicardi (1973) has written comprehensively about the slow spike-wave patterns which are frequently but by no means invariably seen in the myoclonic epilepsies. The main features are triphasic slow spikes or sharp waves followed by a slow component of variable shape occurring in runs of several seconds or minutes bilaterally. The rhythm is between 1.5 and 2.5 complexes/second and is often irregular, as are the spacing, configuration and distribution of the complexes in various leads. There is a tendency for the slow spike waves to be better defined in the frontal regions. This slow spike-wave pattern is usually interictal, usually insensitive to stimulation (hyperventilation, flicker stimulation) and is activated by sleep, during which it tends to reinforce and become continuous. There is a tendency to equate this particular type of EEG pattern with the most severe type of myoclonic epilepsy (the so-called Lennox—Gastaut syndrome) but, as Aicardi points out, diffuse slow spike waves may be seen not only in the Lennox—Gastaut syndrome but also in a wide array of epileptic phenomena including other myoclonic epilepsies, minor status epilepticus and in association with some of the clinical manifestations of temporal lobe or psychomotor epilepsy. The slow spike-wave pattern, when seen in association with severe myoclonic epilepsy of the Lennox–Gastaut type, is an indication of a poor prognosis for later intellectual development.

Aicardi and Chevrie (1973) studied a large group of children under three years of age who had *seizures and paroxysmal EEG abnormalities*, other than hypsarrhythmia and slow spike waves, and they compared them with a control group in the same age range who had seizures but no paroxysmal EEG abnormalities. All types of seizure, including febrile convulsions, were considered. They showed that seizures in young children associated with paroxysmal EEG abnormalities belonged preferentially to certain types of epilepsy with a bad mental outcome and vice versa. Febrile convulsions, which have a favourable prognosis, were seldom associated with a paroxysmal EEG abnormality (at least not under three years of age). Conversely, seizures due to organic brain damage were characterized both by poor mental outlook and by the frequent occurrence of EEG paroxysms. However, they showed that patients with generalized spike waves occurring at a rate of 3 complexes/second had a more favourable intellectual outcome than patients with paroxysmal patterns such as generalized or lateralized spikes. Patients with these regular spike-wave patterns were, on the whole, older when their epilepsy started, fewer had gross brain pathology and more had a positive family history of epilepsy. They pointed out, however, that under two years of age the spike-wave patterns at 3 complexes/second were usually associated with or heralded the epilepsies with myoclonic features, whereas in older children they were associated with primary generalized epilepsy of the petit mal type. They concluded that children with paroxysmal abnormalities in their EEGs, especially when these were discovered in the first two years of life, belonged to the more severe group of childhood epilepsy, while children without paroxysmal abnormalities under the age of three years tended to have a better prognosis for their seizures.

As discussed elsewhere, the *interictal EEG* in children who have had *febrile convulsions* is usually normal. However, if records are taken within a day of the attack over three-quarters of the children will show slow wave disturbances which are often more marked over one hemisphere. These abnormalities persist in a third of cases for about 3–5 days. Focal slow wave disturbances following a febrile seizure increase the chance of subsequent spike foci developing later in the EEG, but such foci are less common than generalized bursts of slow spike and wave discharge of short duration which should not be confused with the EEG abnormality of the true petit mal absence, the classic spike-wave complexes occurring at the rate of 3/second. Lennox–Buchthal (1973) found that neither of these findings had any predictive value with respect to the risk of developing epilepsy later, although all the children in her series who did develop epilepsy later had shown spikes or spike and slow wave complexes in earlier records. *Focal spike discharges* have a limited value in localizing brain lesions in children. As already mentioned, they are usually accompanied by more widespread disturbances of electrical activity around the main epileptogenic area and by more general disturbance in the record than in adults. Trojaborg (1968) carried out follow-up studies over periods ranging from 3–15 years in 242 children who had spike foci in their EEGs. Of these children 85 per cent showed a change in spike location during the study, and in half the change was from one hemisphere to another. All who report on children's EEGs will be familiar with this common and sometimes embarrassing phenomenon. Trojaborg concluded that spike discharges alone are of limited value as an indication of focal cortical damage in children, and that electroclinical correlations are not reliable unless serial examinations over several years show consistent focal abnormalities. It is interesting to consider this feature in the light of what has already been said in Chapter 9 about 'benign focal epilepsy of childhood', where the spike discharges are considered to represent a functional disturbance of a part of the brain rather than actual localized damage.

The persistence of focal spikes for many years after a child has been free of seizures is also well known. Trojaborg found persistent spikes in 52 per cent of his patients who had been free of seizures for more than two years, and some were followed-up for as long as 10 years. This common observation again highlights the limitations of the EEG with regard to the clinical management of epilepsy. Seizures are clinical events to which the frequency and incidence of EEG spikes are sometimes poorly related. The EEG must be used in the problems of childhood epilepsy with discrimination. Excessive reliance on the so-called routine EEG as a diagnostic tool should be avoided and findings should be evaluated in the context of the patient's individual situation. It is important to realize that seizure discharges (whether generalized or focal, spontaneous or evoked) may be found in the EEGs of a proportion of normal children, i.e. children with no history of clinical epilepsy.

There is increasing interest in the accurate diagnosis of *temporal lobe epilepsy* in childhood. The difficulties of recording EEGs from the mesiobasal parts of the temporal lobes have been well known since Gibbs and Gibbs (1952) observed that in psychomotor epilepsy a standard EEG recording had only a 30 per cent chance of demonstrating an abnormality whereas a record taken from a sleeping patient was about three times as likely to do so. A sleep EEG is now regarded as the standard minimum procedure in the investigation of any case of temporal lobe epilepsy. Indeed, it should be standard practice in any paediatric EEG department to encourage as many patients as possible to drift into sleep during the recording. The experienced technician, working in the right surroundings and with time to devote to the individual patient, will achieve this goal in a surprisingly large proportion of patients. Occasionally, in restless difficult patients, sleep records may be obtained following mild sedation with a barbiturate and/or a phenothiazine drug. Using sleep records in this way, 80–90 per cent of the patients with temporal lobe epilepsy will show one or more temporal lobe foci and possibly other abnormalities. The use of sphenoidal electrodes, i.e. electrodes inserted to record from the under surfaces of the temporal lobes anteriorly, should only be considered for use in children who are being investigated for possible neurosurgery. Nasopharyngeal electrodes, which are passed in through the nose, have been used in adults to record from the mesiobasal parts of the temporal lobes, and smaller modifications of these are available from Grass Instruments of Quincy, Massachusetts, USA, for use in babies and young children. It must always be remembered that an EEG abnormality over the temporal lobe does not make a diagnosis of temporal lobe epilepsy. The historical and behavioural data and the EEG and radiological data must all add up to a diagnosis of this type of epilepsy before such a diagnosis is accepted, and this is particularly important in differentiating various psychic aberrations which may be mistaken for the behavioural changes of temporal lobe or psychomotor epilepsy.

EEG FINDINGS AND FREQUENCY OF SEIZURES

One particular problem with the EEG diagnosis of temporal lobe epilepsy, and indeed with other types of focal epilepsy, is that there does not seem to be any close relationship between the occurrence of focal spikes and seizure frequency. In fact, recordings of actual temporal lobe seizures have shown that the EEG spike and the epileptic seizure are not very closely related to each other, although they are both related in some way to the epileptic properties of the cerebral lesion. This is one reason why the frequency of spike discharges in the partial or focal epilepsies should not be used to assess the efficacy or otherwise of a particular anticonvulsant drug. On the other hand, the frequency of occurrence of short bursts of spikes and of spike-wave complexes in children with generalized convulsive seizures and true petit mal is very definitely related to the frequency of actual attacks, and can provide a good index of possible therapeutic benefit from a particular drug. The medication may be given parenterally during an actual EEG recording and its effects, when given on a regular daily basis, may be monitored by serial EEG recordings at intervals.

Apart from their possible effects on seizure discharges, *drugs* can have their effect on the EEG in other ways. The barbiturates and benzodiazepines induce fast activity in the record under normal circumstances and a lateralized or focal deficit of fast activity may be indicative of localized cortical abnormality, e.g. atrophy (Pampiglione, 1952).

NEWER TECHNIQUES IN ELECTROENCEPHALOGRAPHY

Telemetry, which is essentially the provision of a radio link between the patient's head and a recording apparatus, has been used in special centres for the investigation and treatment of epilepsy for many years, such as at the Park Hospital for Children in Oxford. The opportunity to record the EEG during an attack rarely presents itself during routine investigation. Recording of an attack is, of course, overwhelming evidence in favour of a diagnosis of epilepsy. On the other hand, as had already been emphasized, epileptic changes in the interictal EEG do not prove that all of the patient's symptoms are due to epilepsy. For these and other reasons it is often desirable to monitor a patient's EEG for a prolonged period in order to obtain a recording during an attack. Many systems have been devised for this purpose. Radiotelemetry has been used for the transmission of the EEG over short distances to a receiver which transfers the data to either a magnetic tape or an EEG machine or both. Such a method eliminates the restriction of movement imposed by the wires used in routine EEG recordings, but the patient must still be confined within the radius of the range of the transmitter, usually not more than 20 metres from the receiver.

Recently this problem has been overcome by the use of a cassette recorder (Ives and Woods, 1975). The method was originally devised for prolonged ECG recordings and the cassette recorder is available from Oxford Medical Systems Ltd*, England. It will record for just over 24 hours from four channels using a standard C120 cassette. Problems with 'noise level' in the recording are overcome by using the recorder connected to a small preamplifier. Standard silver electrodes are attached to the scalp using gauze and collodion. The cassettes are later played back on a high-speed playback unit and the EEG write-out is made by an EEG machine using a special ink-jet technique which permits a very high frequency recording to be made. In this way a 24-hour recording can be written out in just over one hour. One great advantage of this new technique is that the patient can wear the unobtrusive equipment for a prolonged period and can even wear it at home for a few days, renewing the electrode jelly and replacing the cassettes as required. In

* Oxford Medical Systems Ltd, Nuffield Way, Abingdon, Oxford, OX14 1B2.

patients with known epilepsy the method can give a clear picture of the influence of environmental and other factors, particularly sleep, on the frequency of seizure discharges, and, in patients with transient symptoms of unknown origin, it can sometimes be of great value in excluding epilepsy as a cause. At present, the experience with this new method of investigation is limited, but increasing experience and improved technology will probably widen its application to the study of epilepsy in the future.

REFERENCES

Adrian, E. D. and Matthews, B. H. C. (1934). 'Berger rhythm: Potential changes from occipital lobes in man.' *Brain*, 57, 355–385

Aicardi, J. (1973). 'The problem of the Lennox Syndrome.' *Devl Med. child Neurol.* 15, 77–81

Aicardi, J. and Chevrie, J. J. (1973). 'The significance of electroencephalographic paroxysms in children less than 3 years of age.' *Epilepsia*, 14, 47–55

Ambrose, J. and Hounsfield, G. (1973). 'Computerized transverse axial tomography.' *Br. J. Radiol.* 46, 148

Brazier, M. A. B. (1968). *The Electrical Activity of the Nervous System*, 3rd Edn. London: Pitman Medical

Erba, G. and Lombroso, C. T. (1968). 'Detection of ventricular landmarks by two dimensional ultrasonography.' *J. Neurol. Neurosurg. Psychiat.* 31, 232–244

Friedman, E. and Pampiglione (1971). 'Prognostic implications of electroencephalographic findings of hypsarrhythmia in first year of life.' *Br, med. J.* 4, 323–325

Gastaut, H. (1976). 'Conclusions: Computerised transverse axial tomography in epilepsy.' *Epilepsia*, 17, 337–338

Gastaut, H. and Gastaut, J. L. (1977). 'Computerized axial tomography in epilepsy.' In *Epilepsy: The Eighth International Symposium*, pp. 5–15. Ed. J. K. Penry. New York: Raven Press

Gibbs, F. A. and Gibbs, E. L. (1952). *Atlas of Electroencephalography, Vol. 2: Epilepsy.* Cambridge, Massachesetts: Addison–Wesley

Gloor, P. (1974). 'Hans Berger – psychophysiology and the discovery of the human electroencephalogram.' In *Epilepsy: Proceedings of the Hans Berger Centenary Symposium*, pp. 353–373. Eds P. Harris and C. Mawdsley. London, New York and Edinburgh: Churchill Livingstone

Gomez, M. R. and Reese, D. F. (1976). 'Computed tomography of the head in infants and children.' *Pediat. Clins N. Am.* 23, 473–498

Harwood–Nash, D. C. and Fitz, C. R. (1976). 'Computed tomography.' In *Neuroradiology in Infants and Children*, Vol. 2, pp. 461–504. Saint Louis, USA: C. V. Mosby and Company

Hill, D. (1958). 'Value of the EEG in diagnosis of epilepsy.' *Br. med. J.* 1, 663–666

Ives, J. R. and Woods, J. F. (1975). '4-channel 24 hour cassette recorder on long-term EEG monitoring of ambulatory patients.' *Electroenceph. clin. Neurophysiol.* 39, 88–92

Lennox–Buchthal, M. A. (1973). 'Febrile Convulsions: A Reappraisal.' *Electroenceph. clin. Neurophysiol.* Suppl. 32

Linnett, M. J. (1976). 'People with epilepsy – the burden of epilepsy.' In *A Textbook of Epilepsy*, pp. 1–14. Eds J. Laidlaw and A. Richens. Edinburgh, London, New York: Churchill, Livingstone

Matthews, W. B. (1964). 'The use and abuse of electroencephalography.' *Lancet*, 2, 577–579

Miribel, J., Vieto, N. and Favel, P. (1963). 'Value of simple radiography of the skull in epilepsy.' *Epilepsia*, 4, 261–284

Pampiglione, G. (1952). 'Induced fast activity in the EEG as an aid in the location of cerebral lesions.' *Electroenceph. clin. Neurophysiol.* 1, 79

Petersen, I. and Eeg-Olofsson, O. (1971). 'The development of the electroencephalogram in normal children from the age of 1 through 15 years. Nonparoxysmal activity.' *Neuropädiatrie*, 2, 247–304

Schulte, F. J. (1976). 'The CCT revolution.' *Neuropädiatrie*, 7, 135

Trojaborg, W. (1968). 'Changes of spike foci in children.' In *Clinical Electroencephalography of Children*, pp. 213–225. Eds P. Kellaway and I. Petersen. Stockholm: Almqvist and Wiksell

Zimmerman, A. W., Niedermeyer, E. and Hodges, F. J. (1977). 'Lennox–Gastaut syndrome and computerised axial tomography findings.' *Epilepsia*, 18, 463–464

CHAPTER 22

The General Management of Childhood Epilepsy

To have a correct outlook on the general management of epilepsy and its problems, one must constantly remember that seizures are symptoms in their own right and not disorders. Caring for the patient with epilepsy means much more than prescribing anticonvulsant drugs in an attempt to control the attacks. In the broad context of childhood epilepsy, probably the minority of the patients will suffer from epilepsy alone; the rest will have, in addition, intellectual difficulties and defects of cognitive function, behavioural problems or perhaps some other neurological deficit. Surveys in various countries support these observations (Green and Hartlage, 1971; Pazzaglia and Frank—Pazzaglia, 1976; Stores, 1978), and they are discussed in detail in Chapters 18 and 19.

Correct diagnosis essential

The management of epilepsy cannot be started until a correct diagnosis has been made. It is difficult to over-emphasize this point, and for this reason a great deal of attention was devoted to diagnosis and differential diagnosis in a preceding chapter. Modern drug therapy is semispecific in its effects and therefore an accurate diagnosis of the type of epilepsy from which the patient is suffering is mandatory. Similarly, since the circumstances of each patient's epilepsy tend to be highly individual and are important for the establishment of a comprehensive plan of management, diagnostic study implies not only an investigation of the type of seizure, its frequency and severity, but also a determination of any conditioning or precipitating factors which may be present. The identification of any localizing factors is of importance and may be suggested by the case history, by the neurological examination or by special investigations.

The author has arbitrarily chosen to adopt the *International Classification* (Gastaut, 1970) for the purpose of categorizing the various types of childhood epilepsy described in this book. As already mentioned, this new classification has the virtues of being acceptable on an international level and of facilitating the exchange of information about epilepsy. However, Taylor (1977) has emphasized the dangers of classifying illnesses as opposed to diseases. One danger is that the categories, being arbitrary, can develop a valid existence which is nevertheless independent of physical reality. As he points out, symptoms such as fever, cough, pain or epilepsy can all be studied at a phenomenological level but simply cannot be contained within independent categories.

DISEASE, ILLNESS AND PREDICAMENTS

If we accept the advantages and limitations of classification as applied to epilepsy, we can then consider epilepsy, as Taylor (1977) has suggested, under the separate headings of disease, illness and predicaments.

Disease

In epilepsy, as with other symptoms, the physician seeks *diseases* which are known to be relevant to the presenting symptom. These will include congenital abnormality, acquired brain injury, infections of the central nervous system and new growths of various kinds. Possible genetic influences will also be considered. Disease diagnosis includes both specifying structural and functional changes and providing a description of the causal mechanisms involved.

Knowledge about diseases grows with research and in the case of epilepsy it is likely to grow still more in the future with the advent of revolutionary new methods of investigation such as CT scanning. This may be of crucial importance for the illness of epilepsy because diseases allow scope for specific remediation by attacking and possibly eliminating or arresting the disease process involved. However, in the case of many of the known diseases of which epilepsy is a symptom nothing can be done or, alternatively, needs to be done, and the treatment of the symptoms alone is adequate therapy.

Illness

'This is the process of declaration of disease in its symptomatic form.' 'Unless it is predicated that all is already known about all diseases it has to be accepted that the concept of illness is valid without discoverable disease' (Taylor, 1977). This leads to an acceptance of a classification of epilepsy based on clinical symptomatology. Knowledge of disease is enhanced by classification, provided that we never allow ourselves to become hidebound and the captives of our own classifications. Diagnosis of illness consists of description and, as has been seen, this is particularly true of epilepsy. Taylor reminds us that in the absence of disease definition all therapy is empirical, which again has been true of the drug therapy of epilepsy from the introduction of bromides onwards.

Predicaments

Taylor (1977) uses the word 'predicaments' meaning the complex of psychological and social difficulties which bear on the individual as a result of having a chronic illness. He further emphasizes that people are expected to 'get well soon' and if they fail to do so they lose the status of being ill. People who are normally well and who develop acute illnesses tend to get more sympathy than those who have a chronic disorder. Illness which persists is not so supportable socially as is acute illness, particularly if, as happens with epilepsy, there is no definite underlying disease.

The predicament of an individual is more personal than environmental – it is how the individual is placed in his particular environment. As Taylor so beautifully puts it, the predicament of an individual with a chronic illness is much less that of a textbook description of the illness and much more of an up-to-date chapter in his personal autobiography. Predicaments are influenced by social *mores* and by the expectations of affected individuals and their families and friends. The diagnosis of a predicament requires time and discernment and knowledge of the predicament grows with understanding (Taylor, 1977). Anyone who has looked after children with epilepsy over many years will be very familiar with this fact. It is one of the reasons why an affected child who sees the same physician over a period of years is likely to do far better than one who sees a succession of interns, residents or registrars at a hospital. The single physician, while he may produce little change in the disease or even the illness, may be able to influence the patient's predicament in all sorts of ways, i.e. psychological, social or otherwise.

In summary, if diagnosis is crucial for the proper management of epilepsy, then the diagnostic task should be to discover the disease (if possible), describe the illness and discern the predicament. This diagnostic triad is dependent on different philosophies, has different purposes and demands the development of separate skills. The attending physician will certainly have to call on people from other disciplines to help him complete the task. As with so many chronic diseases in childhood, a multidisciplinary approach is used. Successful therapy depends on having a broad approach to the physical, neurological and psychological aspects of each patient's problem. These points will be mentioned again when special centres for epilepsy are discussed.

ACCEPTANCE AND THE TERM EPILEPSY

The acceptance of any chronic disorder and its limitations is difficult. It depends not only on factors such as the severity of the illness and the degree to which it handicaps the patient, but also on the inherent personality of the affected individual and on the understanding of the illness itself by the patient and/or his family. In the case of epilepsy, acceptance is particularly difficult because the afflicted individual and his family must acclimatize themselves not only to his illness and its associated hazards and complications, but also to the unfortunate adverse attitudes of society towards the entire epileptic population. Because of this dual difficulty, epilepsy is especially a disorder in which understanding and insight are exceedingly important factors in helping the patient and his family to learn acceptance. It should always be remembered that few experiences can be more frightening for parents than to see their child in a convulsion, and the basis of management must be sympathetic and knowledgeable advice, bearing in mind that epilepsy is still a word which causes misunderstanding and fear. Some physicians and clinics have adopted the policy of concealing the word 'epilepsy' from the patient and his parents and a variety of other more euphemistic terms have proliferated. The author agrees with Livingston (1972) that it is better not to withhold the term 'epilepsy' from the parents and the older patients. He points out that it is impossible to hide the word 'epilepsy' because it is used in medical textbooks, is seen in newspapers and magazines and is heard on radio and television. He believes that alternative terms are likely to create confusion and puzzlement for the patient and his parents, and that it is better to face the problem honestly and to explain that the word 'epilepsy' is derived from a Greek word 'epilepsia' meaning to be seized.

Parents' reactions

Livingston (1972), in an excellent account of the general management of the epileptic child, describes the first reaction of many parents to a diagnosis of epilepsy as being one of horror and frequently of disbelief. Many parents have a feeling of guilt stemming from the belief that they have brought a child into the world with a 'horrible disease'. He emphasizes that there is a general belief that epilepsy is a shameful disease, and that the physician should, with tact and understanding, make the following points to them:

1. There is no definite proof that epilepsy is unquestionably an inherited disease
2. There is no reason why epilepsy should carry a stigma
3. They should look upon epilepsy as a disease differing in no way in its social implications from other diseases such a rheumatic fever, tuberculosis or diabetes.

Livingston also points out that the parents must be made to realize that nothing they have done or not done has contributed to the development of epilepsy in their child. Parents may believe that the condition has resulted from some error of omission or commission on their part, or even that the development of epilepsy is a 'punishment for their sins'. Such feelings may affect their attitude towards the child leading to either over-protection or rejection. Ward and Bower (1978) deal with these problems in detail in their excellent study.

Parents will want to know how much to tell the child. Obviously this will vary between patients, depending on the severity of the illness, the age of the child and the likelihood of his understanding the situation. Livingston (1972) believes that explanations of the illness are probably best given to the child by the parents after they themselves adequately understand the disorder, and that the doctor should indicate to the child that he understands how the child feels as a seizure comes on and after it is over. He emphasizes that the term 'epilepsy' should not be concealed from the child as he gets older, and he believes that generally the time when the child can best accept and understand the full implications of epilepsy is when he reaches his early teens. A child who is not kept informed in this way may end up by being enlightened by outsiders and may then feel resentment against his parents because they concealed the information. The handicapping nature of epilepsy should not be minimized and, for the epileptic child or adolescent, this is usually related to what he can or cannot do.

In general, patients who are having seizures or who have been free from them for only a short time should be prohibited from climbing to any dangerous height and from participating in unsupervised swimming. Activities such as team sports and gymnastics are to be encouraged, if feasible, because they tend to encourage feelings of normality, independence and well being in the child. The question of bicycling may present difficulties and may have to be prohibited for a short time until the frequency of the attacks and the response to treatment are better defined. In adolescence, the patient will want to know about the likelihood of driving a car and about possible employment. In general, it is best for the patient to accept certain limitations in living imposed by the epileptic disorder while at the same time maintaining the highest degree of normal activity as possible. He should be taught 'to live with his epilepsy' and to disregard, as far as possible, society's prejudice and ignorance about the condition.

Teachers and schooling

The question of telling teachers and school authorities about the child's epilepsy usually arises. While attitudes about this point will vary from case to case, it is best to inform teachers, particularly if the child's attacks are likely to occur at school.

It is essential that student teachers be informed about the nature of epilepsy and encouraged to have an enlightened and optimistic attitude towards the condition. They should be taught about the emergency treatment of a child having a major seizure in the classroom.

The teacher is the key to the school situation in much the same way as the parents are the key to the family situation. A capable teacher who can handle a seizure in the classroom with composure and who can then calmly explain the situation to the other children will contribute enormously towards improving attitudes about the disorder. This is a positive contribution not only to the afflicted child but also to the social education and development of desirable attitudes of the class as a whole. Furthermore, the teacher is often in the best position to evaluate the educational needs of the children with epilepsy with whom he deals and should be consulted on this matter.

Nowadays, it should be possible in cases of uncomplicated epilepsy to control fits sufficiently for them not to disrupt a child's schooling unduly. In fact, many epileptic children never have fits at school (Henderson, 1953), probably because their attention is engaged in class.

It is generally agreed that the child with epilepsy should be raised in circumstances, both at home and at school, which approximate to normal as nearly as possible. Extremes of neglect and over-protection should be avoided. Children with epilepsy are no less children because of their epilepsy, but they are children at a disadvantage and this is a fact which must be grasped if they are to develop their capabilities fully.

The question of the need for *special schools* with epilepsy needs consideration here. There are six such schools in England and one in Scotland. It is important to realize that while special educational methods are required for the blind, deaf and mentally handicapped, no such methods are required for the children with epilepsy and there is no reason why they should not attend ordinary schools. The child with severe intractable epilepsy who is mentally handicapped as well should be looked after by the mental handicap service. Probably only about 1 per cent of epileptic children require special schooling because of epilepsy alone.

Grant (1976), who has great experience of this particular aspect of the care for children with epilepsy, feels that although it is a general policy to keep all children with epilepsy in normal schools, it is likely that many have potential which is under utilized. He considers that the child with frequent seizures, emotional problems, maladjustment and social rejection by his peers can often obtain considerable benefit from a period of residential treatment in a school for children with epilepsy, if a suitable one is available. He points out that in such a school the seizure is only a passing incident which causes a minimum of disturbance and allows the child time to come to terms with his disability. He thinks that the period of transition from primary to secondary education is particularly difficult and that temporary residential schooling can often prevent the development of serious emotional and social complications. Such temporary residential schooling may be particularly important for the child who, apart from having epilepsy, is under privileged through social class, intelligence, previous erratic schooling or disturbed family background.

Intelligence levels and testing

The parents of children with seizure disorders and their doctors are always concerned with the prognosis for intellectual development and academic attainment, and the child with epilepsy should, ideally, have a full psychometric assessment. If possible, this should be carried out by an experienced and skilled psychologist who is familiar with and sympathetic to the problems of epileptic children. It appears that too often, in the author's experience, psychologists seem to harbour the same preconceived ideas and prejudices about epilepsy as society in general. It is not adequate simply to perform a battery of IQ tests. The possible effects of drugs and of subclinical discharges mean that a single IQ estimation, particularly if low, should be interpreted with caution. Ounsted (1971), in his review of some aspects of seizure disorders, emphasizes that the responses to intelligence tests fluctuate unpredictably in children with seizures. This fact was established as early as 1924 by Fox who showed that there were remarkable fluctuations, both upwards and downwards, in the levels of intelligence attained by these children. Furthermore, these fluctuations are often independent of the factors of medication and frequency of seizures although these factors may influence the results of testing at times, particularly in those children subject to episodes of minor epileptic status (Brett, 1966).

Another point which emerges from a study of the literature on intelligence in children with epilepsy is that opinions vary enormously, presumably depending on the particular sample of epileptic children the author has studied. Indeed, Rodin (1968) felt that the problem of intelligence in children with epilepsy was far from settled and that the answer must await 'more long-term interdisciplinary work between neurologists, psychiatrists, psychologists, and electroencephalographers'. It is probably fair to generalize to the extent that the mean IQ is likely to be average in children whose epilepsy is uncomplicated by organic brain disorders such as mental subnormality and cerebral palsy.

Rutter, Graham and Yule (1970) produced an IQ figure of 102 on the Wechsler's Intelligence scale in children with epilepsy which was uncomplicated by organic brain disorders. Their very careful study of children in the Isle of Wight showed clearly the dangers of using unrefined averages when studying the intelligence levels of children with epilepsy. Many previous studies which had included children who derived their epilepsy from organic brain disorders, such as mental subnormality and cerebral palsy, had suggested that the IQ distribution in epilepsy generally was skewed towards the lower end of the scale. Taking cognisance of this fact, Rutter, Graham and Yule (1970) showed that the intelligence of children with such organic brain disorders arising above the brain stem and associated with epilepsy was well below average. When the 28 per cent of children with these disorders were considered together with the 72 per cent of children with epilepsy uncomplicated in this way, the IQ level of their whole epileptic child population was also well below average. Considered separately, however, the remaining children with uncomplicated epilepsy were found to have the same IQ distribution as the general population of children and many children were of above average and even superior intelligence. Thus, while one of the underlying causes of epilepsy may also be a cause of low intelligence, the fact of having fits is not in itself an indicator of low intelligence. It is probably reassuring for parents to hear the long list of famous epileptics in history, which includes Socrates, Julius Caesar, Alexander the Great, Dante, Byron and Dostoevski.

One may also look at this problem in another way, i.e. by considering the intelligence level in different types of childhood epilepsy. Normal intelligence is usually found in patients with primary generalized epilepsy of the petit mal or grand mal type and in the partial epilepsies with elementary or simple symptomatology as for example in benign focal epilepsy of childhood. Ounsted, Lindsay and Norman (1966), in their study of temporal lobe epilepsy in childhood, found that 68 of their series of 100 children had intelligence test results within the range required for normal schooling, but they also found that many of these children had learning difficulties. Fedio and Mirsky (1969) found specific patterns of intellectual impairment in children with unilateral temporal lobe abnormalities and epilepsy. Within the first decade of life, they found that involvement of the left temporal lobe imposed limitations on the development of verbal intelligence and on the learning and/or memory capacity for verbal material. Nonverbal functions were spared. The converse was true for children with right temporal lobe epilepsy; these were more likely to have perceptual difficulties related to visuospatial learning. The authors pointed out that the results were similar to those obtained in adults with comparable cerebral dysfunction, and that they supported the view that cerebral differentiation of intellectual processes was established in childhood and that early and late cerebral injury produced comparable results in childhood and adult life. As was emphasized in early chapters of this book, the serious types of epilepsy which commence in infancy and early childhood, such as infantile spasms and the severe varieties of myoclonic epilepsy, are very frequently associated with mental handicap which is often profound. Finally, it is important to stress to parents that seizures themselves, even when frequent, are seldom responsible for a gross decline in intelligence unless the attacks are of long duration or unless the clinical story is punctuated by episodes of major status epilepticus (see Chapter 14).

It is widely accepted that there is a connection between complicated epilepsy and lower social class, although this is by no means a clear-cut association. It may be that lower standards of medical care together with an adverse environment could lead to a higher incidence of disorders which result in epilepsy. The theory of what is called social drift may also be relevant. According to this theory persons with some form of handicap are unable to maintain their position in the social hierarchy and drift downwards to the lower social class occupations. In the case of epilepsy, however, incidence of new cases is highest in the formative years before employment is sought, so it may be more characteristic for people with epilepsy to tend to find jobs with a lower social status than their parents early in life.

Precipitating factors

The identification of possible precipitating or conditioning factors in the causation of seizures in the individual patient is important in the management of epilepsy. Some people with epilepsy, for example, have all or most of their attacks during *sleep*. The association between sleep and epilepsy is dealt with in another chapter (*see* Chapter 16). The relationship of epilepsy to *menstruation* is also well known and refers to the fact that in some females seizures are observed to occur immediately before or shortly after the beginning of the monthly period, or they are more frequent and severe at that time.

Hyperventilation may precipitate epileptic attacks and this is probably a specific effect in true petit mal. Curiously enough, however, the over-breathing associated with normal physical exertion rarely, if ever, causes absence attacks. *Photic stimulation* as a trigger mechanism of seizures is discussed with other causes of reflex epilepsy in Chapter 11.

Emotional disturbances such as excitement, fear, frustration, tension and anxiety may act as precipitants of attacks in some patients, particularly in older children and teenagers (Gastaut and Tassinari, 1966). However, as Livingston (1972) points out, the physician should be wary of over-emphasizing this point to parents in case they respond by over-protecting the child and shielding him from the normal and often emotionally exciting circumstances of everyday life. This in turn may lead to a neurosis connected with his epilepsy and a deep sense of being different from his peers. Livingston (1972) also believes that a change of environment may favourably affect the course of epileptic seizures, particularly in children, and he cites some interesting case histories to prove his point. He quotes Hippocrates who in the fifth century B.C. stated: 'Epilepsy in young persons is most frequently removed by changes of air, of country and of modes of life.'

Fever is, of course, an important cause of convulsions in early childhood but illness and high temperature may also cause a convulsion in an older child with epilepsy. *Lack of sleep, chronic fatigue and alcohol* may act as precipitants, particularly in adolescence. Sometimes a combination of factors may operate; for example one of the author's adolescent patients, at a time of great emotional stress in the family, developed partial seizures of complex symptomatology with the EEG showing a temporal lobe focus. He was described by his mother as 'sitting up most of the night talking to his friends, smoking French cigarettes and drinking black coffee'. Advice about a more orderly way of life, an improvement in the emotional climate and the prescription of carbamazepine for some months led to a complete and permanent cessation of his epilepsy and the EEG returned to normal.

The sudden *withdrawal of anticonvulsant drugs* is a common cause of an increase in the frequency of seizures or even of status epilepticus. The barbiturates and, to a lesser extent phenytoin, are particularly important in this respect. There is no justification for withdrawing anticonvulsant medication suddenly prior to an EEG examination, and happily this deplorable and dangerous practice seems to be dying out. Occasionally, where there is doubt about the diagnosis of true petit mal and the patient is already taking ethosuximide, it is reasonable to withdraw the drug slowly prior to an EEG examination. Sometimes, drug therapy has to be discontinued abruptly because of untoward reactions caused by the drug. In some instances it may be wise to protect the patient by the administration of a different anticonvulsant.

DYSTONIC REACTIONS TO DRUGS

Many of the commonly used anticonvulsants may act as convulsants when taken in toxic doses. A rather different problem, now familiar to most paediatricians, is the occurrence of neurotoxic reactions with the phenothiazine drugs and with metoclopromide, causing extrapyramidal movement disorders (Mowat, 1973). The toxic effects develop acutely at both excessive and therapeutic doses. The most common movements are sudden episodes of opisthotonus accompanied by marked deviation of the eyes and torticollis, but without loss of consciousness. Dystonic movements of the tongue, face and neck muscles, drooling, trismus, ataxia, tremor, episodic rigidity and oculogyric crises are also seen. The violent dystonic movements may mimic clonic seizures but, although the patient may be drowsy from the drug, he remains conscious. Diagnosis rests on the history of drug ingestion. There appears to be an element of idiosyncrasy in those patients who develop the syndrome on therapeutic doses of the drug. Benztropine mesylate intravenously or diphenhydamine intravenously, and later orally, act swiftly as effective antidotes.

DRUG THERAPY AND THE PATIENT

The following chapters will be devoted to the drug therapy of epilepsy and the adverse effects of such treatment. Treatment with anticonvulsant drugs is likely to remain the cornerstone of therapy in the foreseeable future. It is salutary, therefore, to consider that among adults with epilepsy it has been estimated that 30 per cent of those suffering from repeated seizures never consult a doctor at all (Janz, 1976). A recent field survey among adults in Warsaw by Zielinsky (1974) disclosed that 37 per cent of all patients who had had more than two epileptic attacks had never taken an anticonvulsant drug and that, at the time of the survey, only 35 per cent were being given drug treatment. Admittedly, of the patients in the Warsaw study who had never been treated, most were suffering from mild forms of epilepsy; only a quarter of them had consulted a doctor and one-third had been free of seizures for more than five years. Among the untreated patients, many were subject to focal attacks or absences which they did not regard as requiring treatment, and major seizures were infrequent. Other patients, including those with major attacks, simply did not want to be treated, or thought that epilepsy was untreatable or refrained from consulting a doctor because they were afraid of being admitted to hospital and subjected to diagnostic procedures. Others had been treated and discontinued their medication because of side-effects or had discontinued their drugs because they considered them ineffective or they had become free of attacks.

While these observations are not directly applicable to children with epilepsy, they do, nevertheless, provide food for thought where the efficacy or otherwise of drug therapy is concerned. The reasons why these observations are less likely to apply to children are apparent from a commentary by Janz (1976) on his own work and on Zielinsky's findings. He points out that epilepsy differs from most other illnesses in that it is not the epileptic attacks which entail suffering for the patient, but rather their repercussions *vis-à-vis* society. The manifestations of epilepsy which make the strongest impression upon the onlooker − the sudden cry, the fall and the muscle contractions of the clonic stage − are suffered by the patient but are not really experienced by him. What actually impinges upon the patient's consciousness during an attack is in no way comparable with the shock experienced by the onlooker − usually parents, guardians or teacher in the case of a child. As Janz (1976) says: 'patients with epilepsy experience their illness chiefly as mirrored in the reactions of their fellow men.' Where children are concerned, the latter are likely to seek medical help in order to try to prevent a recurrence of the shocking event they have witnessed. Therefore, we can conclude that the motivation to seek treatment for epilepsy occurring in children is far greater than it is among adults with epilepsy.

Patient compliance

The only absolute indication for drug therapy is chronic epilepsy, i.e. the repeated occurrence of seizures at fairly frequent intervals. The problems of the individual with the single seizure are dealt with elsewhere (*see* Chapter 8). The use of prophylactic anticonvulsant medication is discussed in connection with the dangers arising from repeated febrile convulsions (*see* Chapter 6) and also where the prevention of post-traumatic epilepsy is concerned (*see* Chapter 13). When anticonvulsant medication is prescribed in any situation, it is only likely to be successful if the patients take their drugs conscientiously, regularly and in adequate doses over prolonged periods of time. Such a degree of patient compliance is essential if an unsatisfactory response to therapy is to be avoided. The patients should be carefully instructed concerning the importance of regular medication and should be familiar with the names of the drugs being used and their dosage schedules. In some countries, small containers subdivided to hold the daily doses for a week are used. It is the author's practice to write out the patient's dosage schedules for the parents, since solely verbal instructions may easily be forgotten or confused.

Changing drugs

Changing from one drug to another should be done carefully, gradually withdrawing one drug and simultaneously introducing another in a stepwise fashion. Another method used for effecting a changeover of medication is to add the new drug to the old regimen, await the effects of the combined medication and then, if necessary, withdraw the original drug slowly. In this way one can assess the effect of the combined medication compared with monotherapy with either the old or the new drug. It is the author's practice to aim at twice daily medication if possible. Because the half-lives (i.e. the time taken for one-half of a given dose to be eliminated from the body) of most anticonvulsants are long, there is not much point in trying to adapt the daily dosage schedule to the time of day at which attacks are most likely to occur, although in certain mild types of epilepsy, such as benign focal epilepsy of childhood, the administration of medication at bedtime only may often be sufficient. Some parents become quite obsessional about giving the drugs at unsuitable times, such as 6.00 am or 12.00 midnight, in the mistaken belief that this will prevent seizures occurring predominantly in the early morning or during sleep. However, this should be discouraged since it disrupts the child's normal day and is likely to be ineffective.

Quite apart from the precipitating or conditioning factors described earlier, children with epilepsy may inexplicably have good periods and bad periods, and parents should be discouraged from arbitrarily increasing the dosage of drugs in the bad periods because this may easily lead to overtreatment and its consequences. Similarly, with certain types of epilepsy associated with structural brain disease and mental and neurological handicap, parents should be instructed that seizures are unlikely to be controlled fully and that they should accept a certain 'inevitability of epilepsy' and learn to live with it, again without constant changes and increases in drug therapy.

SPECIAL CENTRES: THE MULTIDISCIPLINARY APPROACH

Because of the complexities of diagnosis and management of epilepsy, the question of the need for special centres and clinics for epilepsy needs consideration and has been reviewed in detail by Brown (1976). As he points out, there has been a veritable explosion of knowledge about the genetics, electrophysiology, neurochemistry and pharmacology of epilepsy in recent years making it difficult for anyone but the specialist to keep abreast of the changing epileptic scene. There has been a remarkable increase in knowledge of the adverse effects of anticonvulsant drugs (to be described later), including the recognition of various clinical syndromes, making it imperative that the physician dealing with epilepsy should have access to facilities for monitoring the levels of these drugs in the blood plasma. Something approaching a third of all epileptic children are mentally retarded to a greater or lesser degree (*see* Chapter 14) and many have behavioural difficulties. These include the hyperkinetic behaviour and other difficulties of the child with temporal lobe epilepsy, and the withdrawn autistic behaviour of the child who has had infantile spasms or severe myoclonic epilepsy and also a host of less severe reactions including enuresis, encopresis, phobias and anxieties. The educational and learning difficulties of the child of normal intelligence with epilepsy have already been discussed (*see* Chapter 19). Medicosocial problems are also common in the family with an epileptic child — the predicaments of the patient and his family.

It is clear that the child with epilepsy needs a multidisciplinary approach but, because of the way in which the growth and development of the child are so intimately linked with the type of epilepsy which may afflict him, in contrast to the relatively unchanging state of the adult, it seems unlikely that special centres for epilepsy are the answer as far as paediatric epileptology is concerned. The multidisciplinary approach to epilepsy in childhood should involve the participation of people with many different skills and interests, but not necessarily working under the same roof. The family doctor will have the closest contact with the family in their predicament, and the paediatrician will be involved when the child is first referred with epilepsy. The paediatrician is in the front line as far as the prevention of epilepsy is concerned and this will be discussed in another chapter (*see* Chapter 27). The community physician, the teacher, the child psychiatrist and the psychologist may all be involved. A special out-patient clinic for children with epilepsy, based in a children's hospital or in the children's department of a general hospital and under the supervision of a paediatrician with a special interest in epilepsy or of a paediatric neurologist, is particularly valuable because it allows time to be alloted to the parents for discussion of their problems and also because it ensures continuing care by one concerned physician. The place of special schools for children with epilepsy has already been mentioned.

Finally, there is a need for a few highly specialized 'centres of excellence' where intractable and difficult cases can be studied in detail using all available modern techniques, and where the psychotherapeutic management of the whole family in their predicament can be undertaken. An outstanding example of such a centre is the Park Hospital in Oxford where a distinguished group of specialists representing several disciplines has made many outstanding contributions to the understanding and management of childhood epilepsy (Ounsted, 1974).

REFERENCES

Brett, E. M. (1966). 'Minor epileptic status.' *J. neurol. Sci.* **3**, 52–75
Brown, J. K. (1976). 'Special clinics for epilepsy.' *Devl Med. child Neurol.* **18**, 809–811
Fedio, P. and Mirsky, A. F. (1969). 'Selective intellectual deficits with temporal lobe or centrencephalic epilepsy.' *Neuropsychologia*, **7**, 287–300
Fox, J. T. (1924). 'The response of epileptic children to mental and educational tests.' *Br. J. med. Psychol.* **4**, 235–248
Gastaut, H. (1970). 'Clinical and electroencephalographical classification of epileptic seizures.' *Epilepsia*, **11**, 102–113
Gastaut, H. and Tassinari, C. A. (1966). 'Triggering mechanisms in epilepsy: The electroclinical point of view.' *Epilepsia*, **7**, 85–138
Grant, R. H. E. (1976). 'The Management of epilepsy.' *Scott. med. J.* **21**, 11–22
Green, J. B. and Hartlage, L. C. (1971). 'Comparative performance of epileptic and non-epileptic children and adolescents on tests of academic, communicative and social skills.' *Dis. nerv. Syst.* **32**, 418–421
Henderson, P. (1953). 'Epilepsy in school children.' *Br. J. prev. soc. Med.* **7**, 9
Janz, D. (1976). 'Problems encountered in the treatment of epilepsy.' In *Epileptic Seizures – Behaviour – Pain*, pp. 65–75. Ed. W. Birkmayer. Bern, Stuttgart, Vienna: Hans Huber
Livingston, S. (1972). *Comprehensive Management of Epilepsy in Infancy, Childhood, and Adolescence*, pp. 123–166. Springfield, Illinois: Charles C. Thomas
Mowat, A. P. (1973). 'Dystonic reactions to drugs.' *Devl Med. child Neurol.* **15**, 654–655
Ounsted, C. (1971). 'Some aspects of seizure disorders.' In *Recent Advances in Paediatrics,* pp. 363–400. Eds D. Gairdner and D. Hull. London: J. and A. Churchill
Ounsted, C. (1974). 'A special care centre for children with seizures.' *Health Trends*, **6**, 69–71
Ounsted. C., Lindsay, J. and Norman, R. (1966). *Clinics in Developmental Medicine, No. 22: Biological Factors in Temporal Lobe Epilepsy.* London: Spastics Society and Heinemann
Pazzaglia, P. and Frank–Pazzaglia, L. (1976). 'Record in grade school of pupils with epilepsy: an epidemiological study.' *Epilepsia*, **17**, 361–366
Rodin, E. A. (1968). *The Prognosis of Patients with Epilepsy*, p. 154. Springfield, Illinois: Charles C. Thomas

Rutter, M., Graham, P. and Yule, W. (1970). *Clinics in Developmental Medicine, Nos. 35/36: A Neuropsychiatric Study in Childhood*, pp. 133–150. London: Spastics International and Heinemann

Stores, G. (1978). 'School-children with epilepsy at risk for learning and behaviour problems.' *Devl Med. child Neurol.* **20**, 502–508

Taylor, D. C. (1977). *Epilepsy: Disease, Illness and Predicament.* A paper presented at the Colby Epilepsy Course in Maine, USA, July 1977, and made available to the author. (Also reproduced on audiocassette by Medisette)

Ward, F. and Bower, B. D. (1978). 'A Study of Certain Social Aspects of Epilepsy in Childhood.' *Devl Med. child Neurol.* **20**, Suppl. 39

Zielinsky, J. J. (1974). 'Epileptics not in treatment.' *Epilepsia*, **15**, 203–210

CHAPTER 23

Anticonvulsant Therapy

The control of seizures is the essential and most important problem for all patients with epilepsy. Treatment with anticonvulsant drugs is the standard form of therapy today and this situation is unlikely to change in the foreseeable future. The use of such drugs began with the discovery of the effectiveness of bromides in 1857, followed by the introduction of phenobarbitone in 1912 and phenytoin in 1938. Since then, there has been a steady expansion in the therapeutic armamentarium.

However, the most important advance in the drug therapy of epilepsy in recent years has been the emergence of the clinical discipline called *pharmacokinetics*. This is the science which studies the absorption, distribution and elimination of drugs and the factors, both genetic and environmental, which influence these processes. In this context, elimination means the combined processes of excretion and inactivation of drugs. The development of techniques for measuring serum levels of anticonvulsants in low concentration has made it possible to study their pharmacokinetics accurately and scientifically and, in particular, to study the relationship between drug dosage and serum levels. As a result the era of the empirical management of epilepsy by drugs is passing and, furthermore, a great deal of new knowledge has been gained about the ill-effects of these drugs on patients. Often, in the past, the ill-effects have outweighed the benefits conferred by seizure control.

Another consequence of this new knowledge is that the days of polypharmacy for epilepsy are over and *monotherapy* is becoming the rule rather than the exception. Gordon (1976) contends that there are strong arguments today for trying to find out whether a child's seizures can be controlled by one drug alone before considering the use of two drugs simultaneously. In order to do this successfully, he thought

241

that the clinician needed facilities for accurate estimation of drug levels in the blood. He recommended that treatment should be carefully planned and controlled, and that it was no longer excusable to leave dosage to chance and indulge in polypharmacy just because fits continued despite treatment. Many would feel that it is as illogical today to treat epilepsy without the availability of estimations of anticonvulsant blood levels as it would be to use anticoagulants without prothrombin times or antidiabetic agents without determining blood glucose levels.

The careful selection of anticonvulsants designed to control a particular kind of epilepsy and the control of therapy by monitoring serum levels have been the really significant advances in the management of epilepsy in recent years. At the same time, however, it should be remembered that the clinical response of the patient is still of paramount importance and that there is more to the treatment of epilepsy than the dispensing of pills. Indeed, there are disadvantages in the routine use of drug assays which will be considered later.

METABOLISM OF ANTICONVULSANTS

Anticonvulsant drugs are usually administered orally and most are absorbed rapidly, phenytoin rather more slowly than the others. Once absorbed they enter the circulation and are distributed to all parts of the body. The various drugs are bound reversibly to plasma proteins to a greater or lesser degree: phenytoin and carbamazepine to the greatest extent, phenobarbitone partially and primidone and ethosuximide hardly at all. The protein-bound drug serves as a reservoir to maintain the level of free drug in the plasma at a constant level and also to prolong the effect of the drug. The rates at which a drug diffuses across the blood-brain barrier depends on the availability of unbound or free drug in the plasma. The concentration of the drug in plasma creates a gradient across the blood-brain barrier. Most anticonvulsants are lipid soluble and distribute rapidly in brain tissue after crossing over from the plasma. The action of an individual drug on the brain is determined by its concentration in brain tissue, and it is generally accepted now, as a result of experimentation, that the estimated serum concentrations of the various drugs are representative of their concentrations in the brain.

The duration of activity of anticonvulsant drugs is dependent on their rate of *biotransformation* in the body. Generally, this produces inactive metabolites, but occasionally, as for example with primidone, active metabolites may result, but the latter are usually of lower potency than the parent compound. Most biotransformations of anticonvulsants take place in the liver by enzymes located in the endoplasmic reticulum

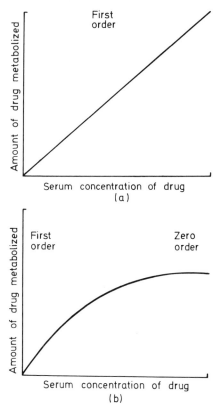

Figure 23.1. Kinetics of drug metabolism. With first order kinetics (a) the amount of drug metabolized is proportional to the serum concentration, whereas with saturation kinetics (b) there is a ceiling to the amount of drug metabolized. (From Dr A. Richens, Drug Treatment of Epilepsy, 1976, by courtesy of Henry Kimpton, Publishers, London)

(microsomes). A frequent metabolic step is hydroxylation followed by conjugation with glucuronic acid or sulphate. This results in the inactivation of the compound and in its increased water solubility which is necessary for excretion via the kidneys. The rate at which these drugs are metabolized is governed by the activity of the microsomal enzymes, and this activity is under genetic control and tends to vary from individual to individual. It is also affected by age, sex, diet and by other drugs. Children, for example, generally metabolize drugs more rapidly than adults. More will be said about the effects of other drugs later, but in general it may be stated that some drugs increase the activity of these enzymes (enzyme induction) while others decrease their activity (enzyme inhibition).

With the majority of anticonvulsant drugs in common use the rate at which the microsomal enzymes work is proportional to the serum concentration of the drug. Where biotransformation varies directly with the concentration of the drug in this way, metabolism is said to be governed by 'first-order kinetics' (*Figures 23.1a*). In this situation there will be a linear relationship between dosage and serum levels. When biotransformation is independent of the concentration (or quantity administered) of the drug it is said to be governed by 'zero-order kinetics', and in this situation the relationship between dosage and serum concentration will not be linear (*Figure 23.1b*).

These differences in the kinetics of drug metabolism are of paramount importance in the use of phenytoin. This drug is metabolized by first-order kinetics at a very low serum concentration, but as the serum level reaches the therapeutic range the enzyme system becomes saturated, reaches its maximum rate of action and is then governed by the laws of zero-order kinetics. The rate of action of the enzyme system, when saturated, cannot be exceeded and consequently small increments in dosage will produce a disproportionate steep rise in the serum phenytoin level. The clinical implication of this is that it is much easier to produce toxicity with this compound than with other anticonvulsants, and therefore monitoring of serum levels of phenytoin is particularly important because of the saturable nature of its metabolism (Aird and Woodbury, 1974; Richens, 1976).

Optimal dosage schedule

When an anticonvulsant drug is given orally in a single dose, the concentration in the plasma will rise to a peak and thereafter decline at a rate dependent upon the speed of its elimination, i.e. metabolism and excretion. Absorption and distribution on the one hand and elimination on the other produce an exponential curve when drug concentration is studied in relation to time. The *plasma half-life of a drug* is the time taken for the plasma concentration to fall by one-half once the elimination phase has been reached. Generally, the optimal dosage schedule for any drug involves administration at intervals equal to its biological half-life if a sustained drug effect is to occur. A steady rate of plasma plateau level is usually attained after four to five half-lives.

Although there is considerable variation between the half-lives of the various anticonvulsants, it does not usually lead to practical difficulties in administration. In general, it seems more convenient for the majority of patients to take their daily dosage in two equally divided doses (morning and evening). The patients or their parents are more likely to remember to administer the drug on such a schedule. Thrice daily dosage seems unnecessary except perhaps in very small children where biotransformation of the drug is rapid and in the case of a drug such as sodium valproate which has a short half-life. Although phenobarbitone has a very long half-life (36—72 hours in children), the usual twice daily dosage does not usually cause problems, although a once daily schedule should be adequate. The pharmacological principles discussed above are essential knowledge for anyone wishing to use anticonvulsant drugs wisely and in accordance with the tenets of scientific medicine.

DRUG INTERACTIONS

It is important to consider the interactions which may take place between antiepileptic drugs themselves and between these drugs and other therapeutic agents or endogenous substances. These interactions may occur during the absorption phase of a drug; for example when antacids are administered concurrently with phenytoin they interfere with its absorption. Drugs such as phenytoin which are highly bound to plasma proteins may be displaced from their binding sites by other drugs which are bound in the same way, but this is probably of little clinical significance. The most important interaction between drugs takes place at the cellular level in the liver. The activity of hepatic drug metabolizing enzymes can be enhanced or inhibited by other drugs. Enhancement occurs as a result of stimulation of enzyme production. Enzyme induction of this kind leads to increased degradation of the primary drug and increased excretion is a consequence. A decline in the level of the primary drug in the plasma ensues. Inhibition may occur because another drug competes with the primary drug for the same enzyme or because the second drug inactivates some of the enzymes involved in the metabolism of the primary drug. The result will be an increase in the level of the primary drug in the plasma.

Clinically important interactions

Although drug-drug interactions involving antiepileptic drugs are not infrequent, clinically significant interactions occur in only a minority of patients receiving the potentially interacting drugs. The most notable exception to this generalization is the combination of sulthiame and phenytoin and, to a lesser extent, with other anticonvulsants. Sulthiame is a potent inhibitor of microsomal enzyme activity. Indeed, it has been suggested that sulthiame has no intrinsic anticonvulsant properties and acts solely by raising the blood levels of other drugs when combined therapy is given (Richens, 1976). This inhibiting property of sulthiame is particularly important when the drug is used in combination with phenytoin. Marked increases in plasma phenytoin concentrations occur as a result of enzyme inhibition and toxic levels of the drug may occur with what is considered to be an average oral dosage. Other anticonvulsants which have a partial enzyme inhibiting effect are pheneturide and perhaps the benzodiazepines, although it seems more likely that the latter are enzyme inducers. Phenobarbitone has a complex action: initially it causes enzyme inhibition by competing with other drugs for the same enzyme pathway, and later it cancels out this effect by its powerful enzyme inducing action. Usually no clinically significant changes occur in plasma levels. Isoniazid and chloramphenicol can also inhibit phenytoin metabolism.

Drug-drug interaction between the enzyme-inducing anticonvulsants is not of great clinical significance. Possibly the only noteworthy one is that between carbamazepine and phenytoin. Carbamazepine reduces the half-life of phenytoin as a result of more rapid metabolism, consequent on enzyme induction, and a fall in plasma level occurs, but this only happens in some patients. It should be noted that some patients seem more susceptible to the effects of drug interaction than others, probably for genetic reasons.

The most important clinical effects of the potent enzyme inducers phenobarbitone, phenytoin, primidone and carbamazepine are felt by certain naturally occurring endogenous substances, and this aspect of the problem will be discussed later when the problems of chronic toxicity associated with the use of antiepileptic agents are described (*see* Chapter 24).

DRUG MONITORING IN EPILEPSY

It is appropriate to look at the methods of and indications for drug monitoring in epilepsy in the light of the relatively new knowledge about how the body deals with anticonvulsants. Spectrophotometric methods have been available since the late 1940s but have not been particularly reliable. Gas-liquid chromatography is widely used, is accurate and specific for a wide range of drugs and is extensively employed in research. However, it does require the services of a biochemist who is experienced in its use if reliable and reproducible results are to be obtained. Radioimmunoassay methods are employed for some drugs such as the benzodiazepines. The broader application of this method has been limited by its use of hazardous, expensive, unstable and radioactive chemicals and its use of complex expensive instrumentation. Enzyme immunoassay (EMIT) uses the selective affinity of antibodies for specific molecules to measure small amounts of chemical compounds in biological fluids, just as radioimmunoassay does, but replaces radioactive labels with enzyme labels. Although it was only recently introduced, it is already gaining widespread acceptance in the USA. It is quick, easily learnt, uses very small quantities of serum and the results are accurate and seem to correlate well with those obtained by gas-liquid chromatography. However, the reagents used are expensive and the method is confined to a limited but increasing range of anticonvulsants. Whatever method is employed, it is essential that the particular laboratory involved should belong to a quality control scheme such as that operated from St Bartholemew's Hospital, London, by Dr Alan Richens and serving monitoring centres throughout Europe.

Indications for monitoring

Richens (1976) has listed the following indications for drug monitoring in epilepsy:

1. When there is inter-individual variation in the rate of metabolism of drugs, as in the case in childhood
2. Where the phenomenon of 'saturation kinetics' occurs, as it does with phenytoin
3. Where the therapeutic ratio is low, i.e. when therapeutic doses are close to toxic doses
4. Where signs of toxicity are difficult to recognize clinically, as may occur in children or in the mentally handicapped
5. Where patients are on multiple drug therapy with the associated problem of drug interaction
6. Where other diseases of the gastrointestinal tract, the liver or the kidneys are present which may interfere with drug absorption or elimination
7. Where the patient's reliability in taking his medication is in doubt (so-called patient compliance)
8. Where the patient's seizures are refractory to treatment
9. Where therapeutic trials of a drug are being conducted.

The monitoring of drug levels in serum is most useful in the case of phenytoin for reasons related to the drug's metabolism and also because the drug's therapeutic range and toxic level are close. Phenytoin intoxication usually occurs at a serum concentration of 100–120 μmol/ℓ

(25–30 μg/ml). The therapeutic range and toxic level are less well defined for phenobarbitone. It is usually recommended that the serum level should exceed 43 μmol/ℓ (10 μg/ml) for a therapeutic effect to be obtained and toxic symptoms occur at levels of 108–215 μmol/ℓ (25–50 μg/ml). Primidone is metabolized into phenobarbitone and phenylethylmalonamide (PEMA) and all three substances possibly have anticonvulsant action. There is still confusion as to whether primidone or derived phenobarbitone has the major anticonvulsant effect and therefore both must be measured. Monitoring of carbamazepine is also done and it is suggested that serum levels should be 25 μmol/ℓ (6 μg/ml) or greater for therapeutic efficacy. Ethosuximide and sodium valproate levels may also be measured.

TABLE 23.1

Effective Therapeutic Levels of Anticonvulsant Drugs in Children (Pippenger, Penry and Kutt, 1978)

Phenobarbitone	64–172 μmol/ℓ (15–40 μg/ml)
Phenytoin	20–80 μmol/ℓ (5–20 μg/ml)
Primidone	37–55 μmol/ℓ (8–12 μg/ml)
Ethosuximide	283–708 μmol/ℓ (40–100 μg/ml)
Carbamazepine	25–42 μmol/ℓ (6–10 μg/ml)
Clonazepam	0.095–0.190 μmol/ℓ (0.03–0.06 μg/ml)
Sodium valproate	300–600 μmol/ℓ (50–100 μg/ml)

Phenytoin apart, the therapeutic ranges of the other commonly used anticonvulsants are still poorly defined (*Table 23.1*). Furthermore, it is a common experience of all who treat epilepsy that, particularly when the condition is mild, it may be controlled fully by relatively small doses of drugs (including phenytoin), and that the serum levels achieved in these patients may be well below the so-called therapeutic ranges. In a recent critical review of drug level monitoring in epilepsy, Brett (1977) emphasized the importance of reliability of the method used and was concerned about the necessity for repeated venepunctures in children attending out-patient clinics. He suggested that reliable micromethods for use with blood or saliva were urgently required for children. However, Gamstorp (1977), felt strongly that the availability and use of drug levels in clinics had led to better patient compliance because parents considered that their children were getting more individual attention and treatment. Nevertheless, it should always be remembered that it is the clinical response of the individual patient which is of paramount importance rather than an arbitrarily decided therapeutic level. It is important to continue to treat the patient and not a laboratory value.

DRUGS NOW COMMONLY USED

Despite new knowledge about drug levels, there is no doubt that in recent years clinicians have been using a much smaller range of drugs, using them more precisely and effectively and with as little polypharmacy

TABLE 23.2

Drugs in Common Use in the Treatment of Epilepsy in Childhood and Recommended Therapeutic Dosages

Phenobarbitone	4–5 mg/(kg . day) up to 20 kg only
Phenytoin	5–6 mg/(kg . day) up to 30 kg only
Primidone	20 mg/(kg . day)
Carbamazepine	20 mg/(kg . day)
Clonazepam	0.25 mg/(kg . day)
Sodium valproate	20–30 mg/(kg . day) up to 50 mg/(kg . day) in certain cases
Ethosuximide	20 mg/(kg . day)
Sulthiame	20–30 mg/(kg . day)
Acetazolamide	20–25 mg/(kg . day)

NB This table of dosages is meant as a guide. Some patients will not tolerate even the minimum doses recommended. Where a range of dosage is given, treatment should commence at the lower dosage. Drugs should be introduced slowly.

as possible in a condition as diverse and occasionally intractable as epilepsy (*Table 23.2*). The drugs in common use today are phenobarbitone, primidone, phenytoin, carbamazepine, the benzodiazepines (particularly clonazepam) and sodium valproate for the generalized major epilepsies, ethosuximide and sodium valproate for the generalized epilepsies of the petit mal type and carbamazepine, phenytoin and perhaps phenobarbitone or primidone for the partial epilepsies. Acetazolamide and sulthiame are also in occasional use.

The reader is referred to Livingston's (1972) textbook and to the excellent short monograph by Eadie and Tyrer (1974) on the pharmacological basis of anticonvulsant therapy for more detailed information

TABLE 23.3

Official Names of Antiepileptic Drugs

International nonproprietary name	Trade names
Phenobarbitone, phenobarbital	Luminal, Gardenal
Phenytoin	Epanutin, Dilantin
Primidone	Mysoline
Carbamazepine	Tegretol
Ethosuximide	Zarontin
Sodium valproate	Epilim, Depakine, Depakene
Diazepam	Valium
Nitrazepam	Mogadon
Clonazepam	Rivotril, Clonopin
Sulthiame	Ospolot
Trimethadione	Tridione
Acetazolamide	Diamox

Abstracted from: *Epilepsia* (1978), **19**, 430

about the various drugs. The monograph by Richens (1976) has already been referred to in the text and is indispensible reading for anyone interested in recent advances in this rapidly changing subject (*see Table 23.3*).

New drugs

Three important additions to the range of anticonvulsant drugs have been made in the past 15 years, namely carbamazepine the benzodiazepines and sodium valproate.

Carbamazepine

This is a tricyclic compound which is structurally related to imipramine. It has been in general use in Europe since 1962 and has been available in the USA in the past few years, although its use there in children has been restricted.

Carbamazepine is now established as a major antiepileptic drug and is not merely a supplemental medication. The best results with this drug have been achieved in patients with generalized seizures of the tonic-clonic type (grand mal) and in partial seizures of complex symptomatology (temporal lobe or psychomotor seizures). It also works well in other types of partial seizure such as those of benign focal epilepsy of childhood. It is very rarely effective in absences of the petit mal type and has little or no effect on the serious generalized epilepsies of early childhood which include infantile spasms and the myoclonic epilepsies.

Gamstorp (1976) summarized 10 years experience in the use of this drug in children. Approximately two-thirds of the children with focal seizures, including temporal lobe attacks, became seizure-free or were greatly improved on carbamazepine. Generalized major seizures also responded well. The main side-effects were an allergic skin rash, initial drowsiness, apathy and ataxia. Transient leucopenia frequently occurs at the time of initiation of carbamazepine therapy but earlier fears about possible bone marrow depression have not been borne out by prolonged experience. Gamstorp (1976) stated that she knew of no irreversible toxic or side-effects. Carbamazepine exerts a possible psychotropic effect with improvement in the patient's powers of attention and concentration, but this may be due in part to the fact that it does not have a depressant effect comparable with that produced by the older anticonvulsants such as phenobarbitone and phenytoin.

In the author's experience, carbamazepine has been the outstanding new anticonvulsant of the past 15 years and has stood up well to the test of time. It is extremely well tolerated by children of all ages and is a good drug for general use in paediatric practice, petit mal excepted (O'Donohoe, 1977). It is available in 100 mg and 200 mg tablets and as a syrup containing 100 mg/5 ml. The maximum dose is 20 mg/(kg·day) divided into morning and evening doses and it is strongly recommended that the drug should be introduced slowly to avoid side-effects. Experience is still accumulating about an appropriate therapeutic range in serum but probably $25-42\,\mu mol/\ell$ ($6-10\,\mu g/ml$) is close to the ideal.

Benzodiazepines

These drugs have been in use since the early 1960s and their use in epilepsy was extensively reviewed by Browne and Penry in 1973. Their most dramatic success has been in the treatment of status epilepticus where diazepam, given intravenously, is now the drug of choice. The treatment of status epilepticus has been discussed in an earlier chapter (*see* Chapter 6).

Clonazepam is undoubtedly the most important of the benzodiazepines for oral use in epilepsy and, in the author's view, it is a very valuable drug in childhood epilepsy. It has been criticized for producing side-effects in small children, notably tiredness, drowsiness and even somnolence and, sometimes, for causing irritability in a similar way to phenobarbitone. These side-effects can be reduced or even avoided by introducing the drug extremely slowly and gradually increasing the dose over a period of weeks. A rather troublesome side-effect in babies and small children is the occurrence of salivary or bronchial hypersecretion. This is more common in the relatively immobile developmentally retarded infant or child, and supervision of the airway may be necessary in hospital. However, this side-effect usually diminishes with time. Clonazepam, like the other benzodiazepines, has no serious toxic effects.

As has been discussed in earlier chapters, clonazepam is particularly valuable in the treatment of the most difficult varieties of epilepsy of early childhood, especially infantile spasms and the myoclonic epilepsies (*see* Chapters 4 and 5). It can also be very effective in generalized epilepsy of the petit mal type which is unresponsive to ethosuximide or sodium valproate.

When clonazepam was first introduced it was used in patients who were not satisfactorily controlled by existing medication. Experience since then has shown that clonazepam, in contrast to other anticonvulsants, is effective to some degree in controlling all types of seizure and that it should now be tried as initial therapy in place of conventional anticonvulsants in generalized seizures of the grand mal type and in partial seizures, both simple and complex; it does, however, seem to work better in the former.

It must be admitted that the sedative side-effect of clonazepam can sometimes necessitate stopping the drug and that this may occur even after a very slow introductory phase. The drug is available in tablet form in 0.5 mg and 2 mg sizes, and in some countries it is also available as a syrup containing 2.5 mg of clonazepam in 5 ml of syrup. The usual daily dosage is 0.5–1 mg in infants, 1–3 mg in young children and 3–6 mg in children of school age. In comparison with most drugs for epilepsy, the dosage of clonazepam should depend on the child's age, clinical response and tolerance, and it must be adapted to meet individual requirements. A certain amount of tolerance to the anticonvulsant properties of clonazepam may develop with the passage of time, but to a lesser degree than with other benzodiazepines. The drug may be given on a weight per day basis using 0.25 mg/(kg· day), but care should be taken that this does not lead to excessive doses in some children. Most important of all, initial doses should not exceed 0.25 mg at night in infants and small children and 0.5 mg at night only in older children. The determination of serum levels in man usually requires radio-immunoassay techniques and thus the therapeutic range is still poorly defined. Steady-state concentrations may not be reached until approximately six weeks of continuous therapy have elapsed (O'Donohoe and Paes, 1977).

Finally, the drug is also available for intravenous use and can be used as an alternative to diazepam commencing with an initial dose of 0.05 mg/kg which is given slowly. It has the same disadvantages as diazepam in respect of respiratory centre depression.

Sodium valproate

The third new drug which must be described in detail is *sodium valproate*. It is, in fact, a very old drug which was first synthesized almost a century ago. Serendipity led to the discovery of its anticonvulsant properties in 1963.

Sodium valproate, also known as dipropylacetate, differs markedly in structure from other anticonvulsant drugs and is thought to act by inhibiting GABA breakdown. GABA acts by providing an inhibitory effect on the propagation of seizure discharges in the brain.

This drug is rapidly absorbed after oral administration and is strongly bound to serum proteins. It is quickly eliminated: metabolism to a glucuronide conjugate in the liver being followed by excretion in the urine. The plasma half-life is only 7–9 hours, and as a consequence it may be necessary to give sodium valproate more often than twice daily, although this is still a controversial point. Levels in serum can be assayed by gas-liquid chromatography but there is still debate about an appropriate therapeutic range. It probably lies between 300–600 μmol/ℓ (50–100 μg/ml).

Sodium valproate is relatively lacking in sedative side-effects. Gastro-intestinal side-effects are more common but may be avoided by gradual introduction of the drug. It acts as a microsomal enzyme inhibitor, although probably only briefly, which may result in elevated plasma levels of phenytoin and/or phenobarbitone if these are used in combination with it. In high dosage, as mentioned in an earlier chapter (*see* Chapter 7), it may inhibit blood platelet aggregation with associated prolonged bleeding times and thrombocytopenia. Mild hair loss may occur in some patients. There have been reports of dysmorphogenic effects in animals but none in humans. It is still an expensive drug compared with its competitors.

The first report of the anticonvulsant properties of sodium valproate came from France in 1963 (Meunier *et al.* 1963), and it was widely used in Europe for several years before becoming available in the UK in 1975. Jeavons and Clark (1974) reported enthusiastically on its clinical efficacy in generalized epilepsies. It is now licensed for use in the USA. The best results in the generalized epilepsies have been reported in those patients whose EEGs showed spike and wave discharges and where attacks consisted of absences with or without automatisms. It is certainly a very useful drug in petit mal but the author does not think that it has necessarily superseded the well tried and cheaper drug, ethosuximide, in this condition. Jeavons, Clarke and Maheshwari (1977) considered it to be the drug of first choice in the myoclonic epilepsies of childhood and regarded it as being superior to clonazepam. The author would not agree with this view and considers that both drugs are valuable and not necessarily interchangeable in the therapy of these difficult epilepsies.

Sodium valproate seems to be most effective in those children with myoclonic epilepsy who have normal neurological and mental status although so-called symptomatic cases may also respond. It should also be considered for use in children with generalized major tonic-clonic seizures, particularly those of the primary type. It has the advantage, unlike phenobarbitone and phenytoin, of not being sedative. Patients who have been on the older drugs are often more lively and alert when sodium valproate is substituted as alternative medication and this is an important factor in children where school performance is concerned. Its lack of side-effects may also make it suitable for prophylactic use in febrile convulsions and trials are currently in progress to assess its value in this problem. Sodium valproate does not seem to be particularly effective in the control of partial seizures, either simple or complex (temporal lobe). However, it is undoubtedly the drug of choice for photosensitive epilepsy and for myoclonic epilepsy of adolescence (Jeavons, Clark and Maheshwari, 1977; Harding, Herrick and Jeavons, 1978).

This drug is available in 200 mg tablets and as a syrup containing 200 mg sodium valproate in 5 ml of syrup. Initial dosage in children over 20 kg should be 400 mg daily irrespective of weight with spaced increases until control is obtained. This is usually achieved with a dosage of 25 mg/(kg· day), but in intractable cases up to 50 mg/(kg· day) may be needed. This higher dosage should not be exceeded without monitoring plasma levels of the drug, and the possible effects on blood platelet function should be remembered. Those who have monitored levels of the drug in plasma have reported wide variations in the results obtained, and the individual response of the patient to this new anticonvulsant is probably of first importance, as indeed it is with many of the older drugs also.

INTRACTABLE EPILEPSY

With such a wealth of new drugs available and with greatly increased knowledge about how the older drugs work, it may seem surprising that epilepsy still proves intractable in some patients. There are many reasons for this and the majority of them have little to do with actual failure of the medication.

First, the patient may not see a doctor with an interest in the problem of epilepsy. The doctor may select the wrong drug for a particular type of epilepsy or give the right drug in the wrong amounts, i.e. too little or too much. He may show lack of patience with the problem or resign from it prematurely.

Secondly, the patient (or his parents) may arbitrarily change the anticonvulsant or change from doctor to doctor without showing patience with the problem or even optimism about it. Many parents will only accept full seizure control and are plunged into despair by even an occasional attack. This attitude also produces a feeling of anxiety and pessimism in the patient. It is difficult to convince some patients that a child is better off living an essentially normal life between occasional nonincapacitating seizures than being seizure free and in a perpetual state of drug-induced drowsiness and confusion. In adolescence, a disorderly or disorganized way of life may lead to poor seizure control, for example lack of adequate sleep, excess of alcohol, overwork and exhaustion and emotional difficulties.

Thirdly, treatment may fail because there is a serious associated brain disease. Many of the progressive degenerative disorders of the central nervous system involving changes in the neuronal grey matter may present with intractable epilepsy. The frequent association between frontal lobe lesions and status epilepticus has been emphasized by Rowan and Scott (1970), and this situation also obtains in childhood even though, of course, the majority of cerebral tumours in children are subtentorial. Actual structural disease of the brain in any highly epileptogenic area is likely to lead to difficulties with seizure control and this is seen, for example, with mesial temporal sclerosis causing temporal lobe epilepsy. Diffuse brain disease, such as occurs in some moderately and many severely mentally handicapped children, is frequently the cause of intractable seizures and these children are often victims of polypharmacy in attempts to control their fits. The lack of facilities for the investigation and treatment of epilepsy may lead to poor results being obtained and this has produced a demand for the establishment of special centres and clinics for the condition.

Finally, 'just keep taking the tablets' is far from being a joke where epilepsy is concerned. It has been estimated (Grass, 1974) that simply getting patients to take their medication regularly and in the right doses will improve epilepsy control by 15–20 per cent overall. The importance of regular medication cannot be over-stressed since haphazard treatment or the sudden withdrawal of treatment (as may happen with the misguided practice of stopping treatment before an EEG) can lead to the occurrence of status epilepticus. However, it must be admitted, as Gordon (1974) has written, that the child who continues to suffer from seizures, in spite of treatment given in appropriate dosage over a reasonable period of time, is still seen too often to allow any complacency about our ability to treat epilepsy. He stressed that a great deal of work obviously still needed to be done on discovering the cause of epilepsy because only this could lead to more rational methods of treatment for all affected children.

REFERENCES

Aird, R. B. and Woodbury, D. M. (1974). *The Management of Epilepsy.* Springfield, Illinois: Charles C. Thomas

Brett, E. M. (1977). 'Implications of measuring anticonvulsant blood levels in epilepsy.' *Devl Med. child Neurol.* 19, 245–251

Browne, T. R. and Penry, J. K. (1973). 'Benzodiazepines in the treatment of epilepsy: A review.' *Epilepsia,* 14, 277–310

Eadie, M. J. and Tyrer, J. H. (1974). *Anticonvulsant Therapy: Pharmacological Basis and Practice.* Edinburgh, London, New York: Churchill Livingstone

Gamstorp, I. (1976). 'Carbamazepine in the treatment of epileptic disorders in infancy and childhood.' In *Epileptic Seizures – Behaviour – Pain,* pp. 98–103. Ed. W. Birkmayer. Bern, Stuttgart, Vienna: Hans Huber

Gamstorp, I. (1977). 'A review of children with temporal lobe epilepsy.' In *Tegretol in Epilepsy. Proceedings of an International Meeting,* pp. 1–3. Macclesfield, Cheshire, England: Geigy Pharmaceuticals

Gordon, N. S. (1974). 'Why does medical treatment of epilepsy sometimes fail ?' In *Epilepsy. Proceedings of the Hans Berger Centenary Symposium,* pp. 187–191. Eds P. Harris and C. Mawdsley. Edinburgh, London, New York: Churchill Livingstone

Gordon, N. S. (1976). 'The control of anti-epileptic drug treatment.' *Devl Med. child Neurol.* 18, 535–537

Grass, E. R. (1974). Personal communication

Harding, G. F. A., Herrick, C. E. and Jeavons, P. M. (1978). 'A controlled study of the effect of sodium valproate on photosensitive epilepsy and its prognosis.' *Epilepsia,* 19, 555–565

Jeavons, P. M. and Clark, J. E. (1974). 'Sodium valproate in the treatment of epilepsy.' *Br. med. J.* 2, 584–586

Jeavons, P. M., Clark, J. E. and Maheshwari, M. C. (1977). 'Treatment of generalised epilepsies of childhood and adolescence with sodium valproate (Epilim).' *Devl Med. child Neurol.* 19, 9–25

Livingston, S. (1972). *Comprehensive Management of Epilepsy in Infancy, Childhood and Adolescence.* Springfield, Illinois: Charles C. Thomas

Meunier, G., Carraz, G., Meunier, Y., Eymard, P. and Aymard, M. (1963). 'Proprietes pharmacodynamiques de l'acide n-dipropylacetique.' *Thérapie,* 18, 435–438

O'Donohoe, N. V. (1977). 'Tegretol in everyday paediatric practice.' In *Tegretol in Epilepsy. Proceedings of an International Meeting*, pp. 10–12. Macclesfield, Cheshire, England: Geigy Pharmaceuticals

O'Donohoe, N. V. and Paes, B. A. (1977). 'A trial of clonazepam in the treatment of severe epilepsy in infancy and childhood.' In *Epilepsy: The Eighth International Symposium*, pp. 159–162. Ed. J. K. Penry. New York: Raven Press

Pippenger, C. E., Penry, J. K. and Kutt, H. (1978). *Antiepileptic Drugs: Quantitative Analysis and Interpretation*, pp. 321–333. New York: Raven Press

Richens, A. (1976). *Drug Treatment of Epilepsy*. London: Henry Kimpton

Rowan, A. J. and Scott, D. F. (1970). 'Major status epilepticus: A series of 42 patients.' *Acta neurol. Scand.* **46**, 573–584

CHAPTER 24

The Adverse Effects of Drug Therapy in Epilepsy

Drug effects may be classified as desired or therapeutic and undesired or adverse. Adverse reactions may be acute or chronic or occasionally idiosyncratic.

Phenytoin

The acute toxic effects of phenytoin are well known, particularly nystagmus, ataxia and tremor. These effects in association are sometimes called 'Dilantin inebriety' in the USA. Severe toxic effects, including tonic brain stem seizures, have been described in adults taking excessive doses of the drug and acute psychotic reactions may take place. An acute toxic encephalopathy of this nature may occasionally occur abruptly in patients on average doses of the drug who unexpectedly develop high blood levels. Apart from the tonic seizures and behavioural changes, dystonic reactions and choreoathetosis may also be seen.

Patel and Crichton (1968) pointed out that the acute toxic effects of phenytoin may easily pass unnoticed in children (particularly young children), that nystagmus may not occur and that ataxia may not be detected or may even be mistaken for an epileptic manifestation in the young. Precise diagnosis may be made more difficult by the presence of drowsiness and behavioural disturbances and because excessive amounts of the drug may make the epilepsy worse. Various studies have shown that there is a correlation between the concentration of the drug in plasma and the signs of acute toxicity: the higher the concentration

(100–120 μmol/ℓ (25–30 μg/ml)) the more severe the toxic signs. The occurrence of acute toxicity following the introduction of sulthiame with phenytoin has already been mentioned (*see* Chapter 23). All of these acute toxic effects are readily reversible although there are reservations about the cerebellar signs which will be discussed later.

Phenobarbitone

The most well known acute toxic effect of phenobarbitone is, of course, drowsiness. However, tolerance usually develops to this effect over a period of weeks and it gradually disappears.

The stimulatory effect of phenobarbitone in young children has already been described in the chapter on febrile convulsions, and the resulting irritability, aggressiveness and overactivity may be persistent and intolerable and necessitate withdrawal of the drug. Phenobarbitone may also have a dulling effect on attention and perception which can result in an individual being unable to maintain vigilance over long periods of time and being capable of only short periods of attentiveness. The implications for learning and school performance are obvious.

Primidone and the benzodiazepines

These drugs have rather similar effects to phenobarbitone, although the benzodiazepines only rarely cause aggressiveness and irritability in small children. Drowsiness can be a problem, however, but slow introduction of the drugs and the passage of time usually lead to tolerance developing. Primidone can sometimes produce alarming personality changes (Mysoline madness) and the EEG can be useful in distinguishing this from a consequence of a deterioration in the patient's epileptic state.

Carbamazepine

Acute toxicity from carbamazepine is unusual and is dose related. Dizziness, diplopia and gastrointestinal symptoms occur with high doses. There is a curious toxic effect which has been reported in adults and which is due to the fact that carbamazepine has a potentiating effect on the action of the antidiuretic hormone 8-arginine vasopressin (AVP) on the renal tubules. In toxic doses carbamazepine may occasionally lead to water retention and even water intoxication (Ashton *et al*. 1977). Very rarely carbamazepine causes an acute psychosis (O'Donohoe, 1973).

IDIOSYNCRATIC REACTIONS

Before dealing with chronic toxicity a word should be said about idio-syncratic reactions. Idiosyncrasy can be defined as a peculiar or unique characteristic distinguishing an individual, and Booker (1975) has written an excellent review of this aspect of anticonvulsant therapy. Idiosyncratic reactions are very unusual and some, at least, are probably genetically determined. Booker (1972) described a group of individuals

TABLE 24.1

Serious Individual Reactions to Anticonvulsant Drugs (after Booker, 1975)

Area affected or condition produced	Drug
Skin (exfoliative dermatitis, Stevens–Johnson syndrome)	Potentially all drugs
Liver	Trimethadione, phenytoin, carbamazepine, acetazolamide, sulthiame, succinimides
Renal	Trimethadione, succinimides, acetazolamide
Bone marrow	Trimethadione, succinimides, carbamazepine
Lupus erythematosus	Phenytoin, trimethadione, primidone, succinimides
Thyroiditis	Phenytoin, trimethadione
Initiation of a myasthenia gravis state	Phenytoin, trimethadione
Lymphoma	Phenytoin, trimethadione, primidone
Haemorrhage in the newborn	Phenytoin, primidone, phenobarbitone
Precipitation of porphyria	Phenobarbitone, phenytoin, succinimides
Hyperglycaemia	Phenytoin

who seem unable to metabolize primidone to phenobarbitone and who develop lethargy and drowsiness on small doses of the drug. Kutt *et al.* (1964) described an individual with an inability to metabolize phenytoin and there are other people who metabolize phenytoin at an increased rate. Serious individual reactions may involve the skin (e.g. rashes, ex-foliative dermatitis and the Stevens–Johnson syndrome), the bone marrow (e.g. aplastic anaemia), the liver (e.g. cholestasis and hepato-cellular damage), and the immunological system (e.g. a lupus erythematosus syndrome), and any one of several drugs may be responsible (*Table 24.1*).

CHRONIC TOXICITY

Chronic toxicity due to anticonvulsants has been brilliantly reviewed by Reynolds (1975) and his article is essential reading for anyone interested in the problem. What follows is largely derived from that source.

The fact that anticonvulsant drugs are usually administered for prolonged periods of time, often for a major portion of the patient's life, allows for the appearance of chronic toxic effects which are not seen with other drugs given for limited periods of time. Furthermore, epilepsy is a symptom which begins before the age of 20 years in over three-quarters of affected individuals and it often begins in early childhood and tends to recur despite therapy. This may lead to therapy being life-long in some instances. The early onset of epilepsy may also mean that growing tissues are exposed to the effects of drugs during vulnerable stages of development.

Reynolds (1975) considered that there was a general lack of awareness in the profession with regard to the problems of chronic drug toxicity and that the ill-effects of overdosage and polypharmacy may be attributed to other causes, including psychological factors. Many clinicians will have seen small children on multiple drugs (for example numbering 10 in one case seen by the author) and leading a twilight zombie-like existence as a result.

Gordon (1967) drew attention to a fact which is familiar to most people dealing with epilepsy, namely that when treatment is stopped, for some reason or other, the fits may subsequently occur less frequently. He suggested that it was possible that anticonvulsant treatment in these patients passes over the top of the therapeutic curve and starts to have a deleterious effect on the patient. It is well known, for instance, that in temporal lobe epilepsy the epileptic discharges are most likely to be recorded in the EEG during drowsiness and sleep. Therefore, if the patient is made excessively drowsy by treatment an increasing frequency of seizures may result. Furthermore, certain drugs, such as phenytoin, act as convulsants in toxic doses.

Central nervous system effects

The chronic toxic effects on the central nervous system have received particular attention, especially the possible damage inflicted on the cerebellum by phenytoin. The acute cerebellar syndrome produced by phenytoin has already been described (*see* page 258). The question of whether chronic phenytoin toxicity can permanently damage the cerebellum by causing Purkinje cell loss is still *sub judice*. Reynolds (1975) thought that it did whereas Dam (1970) thought that the Purkinje cell loss was due to frequent and severe seizures causing anoxic damage. The author sides with Reynolds in this argument and is influenced by a case seen personally. It may be that both theories are partially true and that repeated severe seizures and consequent brain damage may make the cerebellum more vulnerable to the chronic toxic effects of phenytoin (Iivanainen, Viukari and Helle, 1977).

The production of an acute toxic encephalopathy with certain anticonvulsants such as phenytoin, phenobarbitone, primidone and carbamazepine has already been mentioned. It has also been suggested that a *chronic encephalopathy*, with an insidious deterioration in intellectual functioning and in behaviour as its main characteristics, can also occur where high doses of anticonvulsants are used for prolonged periods. Such a syndrome may be mistaken for degenerative disease of the central nervous system, particularly in patients who are already mentally handicapped. The role of folate deficiency in the causation of such a deterioration will be discussed later, and it is important to remember that in this context there are many factors contributing to the development of mental illness in epilepsy including underlying brain damage, uncontrolled seizures and psychological, social and genetic influences. A chronic encephalopathic illness due to chronic drug toxicity should usually be reversible when the drugs are reduced or discontinued (Vallarta, Bell and Reichert, 1974).

Haemopoietic effects

Effects on the haemopoietic system have been recognized for many years. Aplastic anaemia has occurred rarely with the hydantoins and more frequently with the oxazolidine-diones such as trimethadione and paramethadione. Megaloblastic anaemia was first described in patients on phenytoin by Mannheimer *et al.* (1952) but the incidence is extremely low. Macrocytosis is more common, however, in those on phenytoin therapy. Both megaloblastic anaemia and macrocytosis are consequences of folate deficiency and respond to folic acid therapy. *Folate deficiency* has mainly been reported in patients on the three drugs commonly used in major generalized seizures, namely phenytoin, phenobarbitone and primidone, and it has been variously recorded as occurring in between 27 per cent and 91 per cent of these (Reynolds *et al.*, 1972). Subnormal folate levels have also been reported in the cerebrospinal fluid of epileptic patients on these drugs. Vitamin B_{12} levels are usually normal in the blood and the cerebrospinal fluid. The aetiology of folate deficiency is not certain. Malabsorbtion of the vitamin has been suggested but it seems more likely that the metabolism of folic acid in the liver is interfered with or enhanced by a process of enzyme induction engendered by the anticonvulsant drugs. The more rapid turnover leads to lower serum folate levels and a lower cerebrospinal fluid level is a consequence.

The clinical importance of folate deficiency is uncertain, apart from being responsible for megaloblastic anaemia and macrocytosis. Normally the level of folate in cerebrospinal fluid is about three times that in serum and Reynolds (1975) has suggested that this implies an important role for the vitamin in neuronal function. It has also been suggested that the antiepileptic action of drugs may be mediated, at least in part, by their antifolate activity. If this is the case then replacement therapy with folic acid in depleted patients should aggravate their seizures. However, the evidence for such an effect is still unconvincing (Grant and Stores, 1970). Perhaps a more important effect of folic acid replacement therapy is the improvement in mental state which has been reported to occur in some patients on replacement therapy (Reynolds, 1967). He reported increased alertness, drive, interest and energy in these patients, but others have not confirmed his results and controversy continues on this question. The role of folate deficiency in causing the chronic intellectual deterioration or encephalopathy in those on long-term therapy is a part of this controversy. One hard piece of evidence in favour of the theory is that there is a very high incidence of neuro-psychiatric illness in those adult patients who develop the rare megaloblastic anaemia while on anticonvulsant medication. Folic acid replacement therapy should be cautious (5 mg/day) in view of the possibility of aggravating seizures, at least in some patients.

One other important haemopoietic effect in paediatric practice is the production of *coagulation defects* with bleeding which has been reported in some neonates whose mothers were taking phenytoin and/or phenobarbitone (Mountain, Hirsch and Gallus, 1970). Clinically, the condition is slightly different from the usual haemorrhagic diseases of the newborn in that the bleeding tends to occur earlier, usually in the first 24 hours. The drugs cross the placenta and interfere with the immature liver enzyme mechanisms responsible for the production or release of vitamin K dependent clotting factors. The neonate has little transplacental and no intestinal source of vitamin K. Prevention can be achieved by giving mothers on anticonvulsants small doses of the vitamin before delivery or the neonate may be given vitamin K 1 mg at birth.

Metabolic bone disease

Metabolic bone disease associated with anticonvulsants was first reported in 1967 when Schmid reported rickets associated with epilepsy in children. Since then there have been many reports of osteomalacia in adults and rickets and bone fractures in children. The former may be easily overlooked and, particularly in mentally subnormal children on long-term anticonvulsant therapy, aching bone pain may also escape the notice of parents or attendants. The occurrence of metabolic bone disease is related to multiple drug therapy, to relatively high doses of drugs and to the duration of therapy. Phenobarbitone, primidone and phenytoin have been the main drugs implicated. Apart from radiological changes, investigations usually show a reduced serum calcium level, an elevated alkaline phsophatase reading and a normal serum phosphate concentration.

The bone changes are due to vitamin D deficiency brought about by drug induction of liver enzymes involved in the metabolism, especially hydroxylation, of vitamin D in the liver (Dent *et al.*, 1970). The metabolism of the vitamin is both enhanced and diverted along pathways which result in more inactive metabolites. Treatment consists of giving vitamin D and usually the dose required is significantly higher than that needed to correct simple dietary deficiency. It has been suggested that children with epilepsy should receive supplemental vitamin D while on anticonvulsant therapy, especially if they live in areas where exposure to sunlight is limited. It is interesting that the enzyme-inducing anticonvulsants have a similar enhancing effect on the metabolism of the contraceptive pill so that increased doses may be required for the desired prophylactic effect. The same effect on steroid metabolism may occur with cortisol.

Connective tissue disease

Long-term anticonvulsant medication, particularly with phenytoin, can affect connective tissue in various ways. This may occur as a result of an effect on collagen metabolism, or on fibroblast proliferation or may, perhaps, be related indirectly to the effects on liver metabolism as already described. The fact that phenytoin therapy is associated with a deficiency of circulating immunoglobulin A may also be important in the production of these toxic effects, but the exact mechanisms are unknown. The best known effect is the production of *gum hypertrophy* in children who are taking phenytoin (*Figure 24.1*). Livingston and Livingston (1969) estimated that this occurred in 40 per cent of patients on the drug and that it was more prevalent in children. It occurs with normal serum levels and is unrelated to dosage. It usually begins 2–3 months after commencing treatment with the drug, reaches its maximum in 9–12 months and usually regresses over 3–6 months after treatment is discontinued. Maximum hypertrophy occurs in areas of salivary contact. Phenytoin is excreted in saliva and this may be significant in causation, and the immunoglobulin A content of saliva is also reduced in such patients. Poor oral hygiene aggravates the condition so that it may also have a chronic infective basis. Reducing the dosage of the drug is not usually successful: it must be stopped if regression is to be achieved.

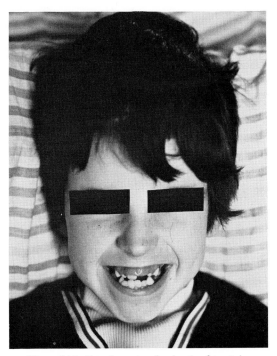

Figure 24.1. Gum hypertrophy due to phenytoin

Long-term anticonvulsant therapy can also cause *coarsening of the facial tissues,* including enlargement of the lips and nose. This appears to be due to a generalized thickening of the subcutaneous tissues of the face and scalp, and may be a particularly unsightly effect in adolescent girls. Those with marked changes have usually been on multiple drugs for severe seizures and this situation is especially likely to be found among the mentally handicapped. Phenytoin is the main culprit and gum hypertrophy is usually an associated finding. Falconer and Davidson (1973) reported two sets of twins in whom one of each pair developed facial coarsening while on anticonvulsant drugs whereas the non-epileptic twin was unaffected in each case.

Hirsuties

This is another unsightly effect of phenytoin therapy and Livingston, Peterson and Boks (1955) reported it in 5 per cent of their patients on this drug (*Figure 24.2*). Hirsuties is also a particularly embarrassing side-

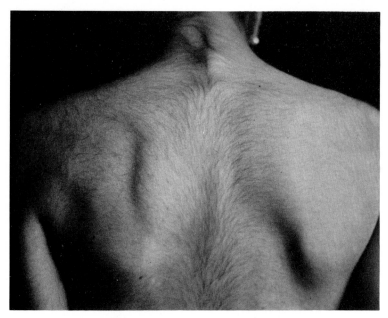

Figure 24.2. Hirsuties due to phenytoin

effect in girls and alternative treatment should be considered. In the author's experience this condition usually regresses when phenytoin is stopped, although others, including Livingston (1972), disagree on this point. Some pigmentation of the skin may also be seen with phenytoin occasionally.

Hyperglycaemia

A hyperglycaemic effect has also been reported in some patients on phenytoin or phenobarbitone, more commonly with the former drug. This appears to be due to interference by the drugs with the normal insulin response to glucose stimulation. Phenytoin should be used with caution in diabetic patients.

TERATOGENICITY

Before concluding the subject of drug toxicity in epilepsy, the terato-genic risk of anticonvulsants given in pregnancy needs to be mentioned. Meadow (1968) first drew attention to the association between con-genital abnormalities and maternal epilepsy. Janz (1975) reviewed the subject in detail and concluded that the risk of having a child with congenital abnormalities was 2–3 times higher than in the general population. Congenital heart disease, hare-lip with or without cleft palate and microcephaly have been the most common malformations reported. Debate has centred around whether the epilepsy itself is responsible for the increased tendency to produce a malformed infant or whether the drugs are responsible. Various studies of the problem strongly suggest that the drugs are responsible and that the fit fre-quency in the mothers of malformed babies is not significantly different from that in mothers of normal babies (Richens, 1976). However, Janz considered that if anticonvulsant drugs do act as teratogens, then their effect is weak and the degree of risk involved is not enough to justify discouraging a woman on such medication from having a child.

Nearly all the commonly used anticonvulsants, given during preg-nancy, have been incriminated as teratogens. In many instances, however, a combination of drugs was used and it was difficult to identify a causal relationship between a particular drug and the occurrence of an abnormality. As a result of animal experiments the hydantoins have been most frequently suspected of having a teratogenic effect in humans. Loughnan, Gold and Vance (1973) reported minor but clinically characteristic skeletal malformations occurring in seven infants of epileptic mothers taking phenytoin. These were hypoplasia of the nails and distal phalanges and, in five of the seven cases, there were associated major anomalies. They suggested that these visible abnormalities might serve as clinical 'markers' for more serious hidden defects in an affected infant.

The avoidance of phenytoin as an anticonvulsant during pregnancy has been recommended by some. Janz advised against the use of com-binations of anticonvulsants in pregnancy and suggested that if possible a single drug might be used with careful monitoring to avoid toxic serum levels, particularly in early pregnancy. However, the danger of pre-cipitating severe fits or status epilepticus by over-cautious treatment should be remembered because either might present an even greater danger to the fetus than the low risk of drug teratogenicity. The possible teratogenic role of folate deficiency consequent on anticonvulsant medication has given rise to speculation, but there is no agreement about the value of folic acid supplements in preventing the development of malformations.

GENERAL REMARKS

It will be seen from the above that individuals with epilepsy have to contend not only with having fits and with the psychological problems created by epilepsy, but also quite frequently with the pharmacotoxic effects of the drugs used to control their seizures. There are obviously strong arguments for keeping antiepileptic drugs to a minimum because of the risks of side-effects and toxic effects. This is not necessarily meant as an argument against the drug therapy of epilepsy, but rather as a plea that anticonvulsant medication should be carefully planned and controlled and that the dosage should not be left to chance. Accurate diagnosis of the patient's particular epileptic problem, as far as that is possible in each individual case, is a necessary forerunner of wise and beneficial treatment.

Gordon (1976) has stressed that the same arguments used to limit the use of anticonvulsant drugs also apply to decisions on the *duration of therapy*. Many of the toxic effects described are more likely to occur with long-term therapy, and this is a problem of great importance in children where developing tissues may be exposed to the adverse effects of drugs. There are many factors which influence duration of therapy including the type of epilepsy being treated, the severity of the fits which have occurred, the evidence (or lack of it) of structural brain damage or abnormality, the association of a strong family history and the age of the patient.

Livingston (1972) recommended that effective and well-tolerated medication should be continued in all patients in full dosage for at least four years from the time of the last seizure and that the medication should be withdrawn gradually over a further one or two years. He recommended continuing treatment beyond the four year period if the end of that period coincided with the onset of puberty.

Holowach, Thurston and O'Leary (1972) also favoured continuing drug treatment for four asymptomatic years followed by a staged withdrawal over a period of months, depending on the type of epilepsy. Shorter periods of treatment were used in uncomplicated petit mal. They found an unquestionable correlation between seizure type and the success or failure of withdrawal of medication. The primary generalized epilepsies (grand mal, petit mal) did best while those with partial seizures, particularly of the temporal lobe type, and patients with multiple seizure types fared worst. Unlike Livingston (1972), they did not find that the onset of puberty had a significant effect on the incidence of relapse after withdrawal of medication.

Summing up on this problem, the author agrees with Gordon (1976) that hard and fast rules should not apply in making decisions about withdrawing treatment. Each case should be considered on its merits and all available clinical and EEG data should be carefully considered. In view of the known risks of prolonged anticonvulsant medication, it is probably better to err on the side of withdrawing treatment sooner rather than later, provided the withdrawal is done cautiously. It is better to risk the occasional recurrence than to treat a number of children unnecessarily.

CONCLUSIONS

The various considerations expressed concerning the toxic effects of anticonvulsant drugs emphasize the present unsatisfactory state of the drug treatment of epilepsy, despite the advances made. Reynolds (1976) referred to the large number of patients with epilepsy and to the early age of onset in many and considered that there was no other group of patients who consumed so many drugs for so long. He thought that existing knowledge concerning these drugs was often not applied to the treatment of patients, resulting in the administration of excessive numbers of drugs in excessive amounts. There is, as he says, an urgent need for the development of new and more effective drugs and this constitutes a major challenge in clinical medicine today. Hopefully, the increasing world-wide interest in epilepsy and its treament by basic scientists, clinicians, the pharmaceutical industry and various supporting agencies will ensure that the challenge is met successfully.

REFERENCES

Ashton, M. G., Ball, S. G., Thomas, T. H. and Lee, M. R. (1977). 'Water intoxication associated with carbamazepine treatment.' *Br. med. J.* 1, 1134–1135
Booker, H. E. (1972). 'Primidone toxicity.' In *Antiepileptic Drugs*, pp. 377–384. Eds D. M. Woodbury, J. K. Penry and R. P. Schmidt. New York: Raven Press
Booker, H. E. (1975). 'Idiosyncratic reactions to the antiepileptic drugs.' *Epilepsia*, 16, 171–181
Dam, M. (1970). 'The number of Purkinje cells in patients with grand mal epilepsy treated with diphenylhydantoin.' *Epilepsia*, 11, 313–320
Dent, C. E., Richens, A., Rowe, D. J. F. and Stamp, T. C. B. (1970). 'Osteomalacja with long-term anticonvulsant therapy in epilepsy.' *Br. med. J.* 4, 69–72
Falconer, M. A. and Davidson, S. (1973). 'Coarse features in epilepsy as a consequence of anticonvulsant therapy.' *Lancet*, 2, 1112–1114
Gordon, N. S. (1967). *Communication to the British Epilepsy Association Symposium in Manchester, England.* Unpublished
Gordon, N. S. (1976). 'The control of anti-epileptic drug treatment.' *Devl Med. child Neurol.* 18, 535–537
Grant, R. H. E. and Stores, O. P. R. (1970). 'Folic acid in folate-deficient patients with epilepsy.' *Br. med. J.* 4, 644–648

Holowach, J., Thurston, D. L. and O'Leary, J. (1972). 'Prognosis in childhood epilepsy.' *New Engl. J. Med.* **286**, 169–174

Iivanainen, M., Viukari, M. and Helle, E. P. (1977). 'Cerebellar atrophy in phenytoin-treated mentally retarded epileptics.' *Epilepsia,* **18**, 375–386

Janz, D. (1975). 'The teratogenic risk of antiepileptic drugs.' *Epilepsia,* **16**, 159–169

Kutt, H., Wolk, M., Scheman, R. and McDowell, F. (1964). 'Insufficient parahydroxylation as a cause of diphenylhydantoin toxicity.' *Neurology, Minneap.* **1**, 542–548

Livingston, S. (1972). *Comprehensive Management of Epilepsy in Infancy, Childhood and Adolescence,* pp. 341–342. Springfield, Illinois: Charles C. Thomas

Livingston, S. and Livingston, H. L. (1969). 'Diphenylhydantoin gingival hyperplasia.' *Amer. J. Dis. Child.* **117**, 265–270

Livingston, S., Peterson, D. and Boks, L. L. (1955). 'Hypertrichosis occurring in association with Dilantin therapy.' *J. Pediat.* **47**, 351–352

Loughnan, P. M., Gold, H. and Vance, J. C. (1973). 'Phenytoin teratogenicity in man.' *Lancet,* **1**, 70–72

Mannheimer, E., Pakesch, F., Reimer, E. E. and Vetter, H. (1952). 'Die hamatologischen Komplikationen der Epilepsiebehandlung mit Hydantoinkorpem.' *Medsche. Klin.* **47**, 1397–1401

Meadow, S. R. (1968). 'Anticonvulsant drugs and congenital abnormalities.' *Lancet,* **2**, 1296

Mountain, K. R., Hirsch, J. and Gallus, A. S. (1970). 'Neonatal coagulation defect due to anticonvulsant drug treatment in pregnancy.' *Lancet,* **1**, 265–268

O'Donohoe, N. V. (1973). 'A series of epileptic children treated with Tegretol.' In *Tegretol in Epilepsy. Report of an International Clinical Symposium,* pp. 25–29. Ed. C. A. S. Wink. Manchester: C. Nichols and Co. Ltd. and Macclesfield, Cheshire, England: Geigy Pharmaceuticals

Patel, H. and Crichton, J. U. (1968). 'The neurologic hazards of diphenylhydantoin in childhood.' *J. Pediat.* **73**, 676–684

Reynolds, E. H. (1967). 'Effects of folic acid on the mental state and fit frequency of drug treated epileptic patients.' *Lancet,* **1**, 1086–1088

Reynolds, E. H. (1972). 'Diphenylhydantoin: Hematologic aspects of toxicity.' In *Antiepileptic Drugs,* pp. 247–262. Eds D. M. Woodbury, J. K. Penry and R. P. Schmidt. New York: Raven Press

Reynolds, E. H. (1975). 'Chronic antiepileptic toxicity: A review.' *Epilepsia,* **16**, 319–352

Reynolds, E. H. (1976). 'Unsatisfactory aspects of the drug treatment of epilepsy.' *Epilepsia,* **17**, xiii–xv

Richens, A. (1976). *Drug Treatment of Epilepsy.* p. 129. London: Henry Kimpton

Schmid, F. (1967). 'Osteopathien bei antiepileptischer Dauerbehandlung.' *Fortschr. Med.* **9**, 381–382

Vallarta, J. M., Bell, D. B. and Reichert, A. (1974). 'Progressive encephalopathy due to chronic hydantoin intoxication.' *Am. J. Dis. Child.* **128**, 27–34

CHAPTER 25

Surgical Treatment of Epilepsy

It is not proposed to deal in any detail with the surgical treatment of epilepsy in childhood. The reader is referred to the comprehensive reviews by Earl Walker in Livingston's textbook (1972) and by Dodson *et al.* (1976). The primary treatment of epilepsy in childhood should consist of the control of seizures be medical means, if possible, and of close attention to psychological and social considerations connected with the epilepsy. It is likely that modern anticonvulsant drugs will provide complete or partial control of seizures in up to 75 per cent of patients suffering from different varieties of epilepsy, with varying degrees of success and failure depending on the type of epilepsy from which the patient suffers. Of the remaining 25 per cent of patients who prove intractable to medication, only a small fraction will be suitable for or amenable to surgical treatment, but recent reviews, particularly those of Dodson *et al.* (1976), suggest that improved methods of investigation and more sophisticated surgical techniques are likely to lead to increasing interest in the surgical treatment of epilepsy in the future.

SELECTION OF CASES

For a child with intractable epilepsy to be considered for surgery the seizures should be focal in origin and arise from a circumscribed area of one side of the brain, preferably not an area concerned with important functions such as speech or motor control. There has always been a natural reluctance to submit a child to a surgical procedure which is necessarily destructive to some extent, mainly because of the possibility that the attacks will disappear or diminish considerably in frequency and severity with advancing age. Furthermore, the last 25 years have seen the development of several effective new anticonvulsant drugs and there is always the possibility that one of these may control the patient's epilepsy or that research in the future may provide an answer. However, it should be remembered that intractable epilepsy over a period of years may have a permanent adverse effect on the child's learning and development and also lead to a very poor quality of life. Frequent convulsions, particularly episodes of major status epilepticus, may lead to a permanent lowering of intellectual capacity and the long-term use of anticonvulsant drugs may have a similar effect, as described in detail elsewhere (*see* Chapter 24).

Wilder Penfield pioneered the surgical treatment of epilepsy with a focal origin during the years from the late 1920s onwards. His experiences are described in his classic book (Penfield and Jasper, 1954), and the results were later reviewed by Rasmussen (1969), who reported a success rate in controlling the patient's epilepsy of between 30 per cent and 45 per cent.

The Montreal school of neurosurgeons have always emphasized that, because the seizure activity does not arise from the lesion itself but from the adjacent epileptogenic cortex, this marginal tissue must also be excised. It seems paradoxical that surgical excision, which of itself produces focal brain damage and glial scarring, should act to prevent the continuation of clinical epilepsy. However, this is the case and, although the weak epileptogenicity of surgical scars *vis-à-vis* other scars is not fully understood, it is probably related to the histological components of scars produced by acquired brain damage and the proportions of gliotic and cellular tissue present. There is some evidence that when astrocytes are functioning normally they act by taking up potassium released during seizure discharges and that the clearance is much slower in gliotic tissue. Although local removal of small areas of cortex for the treatment of intractable partial epilepsy has been little used in childhood so far, it seems possible that, with the aid of technological and surgical advances, it will be increasingly employed in the future. This aspect of neurosurgery in childhood is fully discussed in the outstanding review by Dodson *et al.* (1976).

TEMPORAL LOBE EPILEPSY

The surgical treatment of intractable partial seizures of complex symptomatology originating in the temporal lobes has already been referred to in the chapter on temporal lobe epilepsy (*see* Chapter 10). There is now fairly universal agreement on the conditions suggested by Falconer (1965) and Rasmussen (1969) which need to be fulfilled before operation is undertaken. These include the following:

1. Failure to respond to a really adequate trial of drug treatment, which should include monitoring of serum levels
2. Evidence of a predominantly or wholly unilateral disorder, as shown by inferior or anterior temporal spikes in the EEG — if these are bilateral, they must be at least four times more frequent on the side to be operated upon
3. A period of observation long enough for there to be reasonable certainty that all potentially epileptogenic areas have manifested themselves and that spontaneous regression is unlikely
4. The patient should have an IQ of 60 or more.

Jensen (1975) reviewed the world experience of temporal lobe surgery between 1928 and 1973 and found that of 885 patients in whom the criteria just mentioned were fulfilled, 43.6 per cent were entirely free of seizures after operation, 18 per cent had their seizures reduced by three-quarters or more and in a further 16.5 per cent the seizures were reduced by a half or more. Further analysis of the results showed that surgery which was limited to a superficial or partial removal of the temporal lobe had fewer successful results than those in which the deeper structures were removed, including parts of the amygdala, uncus and hippocampus. Patients with bilateral abnormalities also did less well following surgery. The mortality from the operation was less than 1 per cent. Persistent hemiparesis occurred in 2.4 per cent, transient hemiparesis in 4.2 per cent and complete homonymous hemianopia in 8.3 per cent. Temporary dysphasia also took place but did not persist.

The value of surgery for intractable temporal lobe epilepsy is definitely established, and up to two-thirds of the patients will derive significant benefit from this type of treatment. Falconer pioneered temporal lobe resection for intractable temporal lobe epilepsy and advocated the earlier use of the operation in children who fulfilled the usual criteria. In 40 children, aged 15 years and younger who were operated on and follow-up for 1–24 years, 22 were seizure free, seven had only an occasional seizure, five had their seizures reduced by half and only six subjects failed to benefit from surgery. The best results were obtained in those patients with mesial temporal sclerosis (Davidson and Falconer, 1975).

HEMISPHERECTOMY

In 1950 Krynauw reported excellent results following total removal of the affected hemisphere (hemispherectomy) for patients with the triad of infantile hemiplegia, intractable epilepsy and uncontrollable behavioural disturbance. Enthusiasm for the operation has waxed and waned since then. Wilson (1970) reviewed the subject, basing the survey on personal experience of the operation in 50 patients. He reported that the operative mortality was low, that the abolition of seizures could be expected in about 70 per cent of patients and that there was a reduction in the frequency of seizures in a further 15 per cent. Improvement in behavioural disorders could be expected in over 90 per cent of the cases. No amelioration of spasticity or improvement in power occurred in the hemiplegic limb and sensory deficits could become worse, but overall physical capacity was often improved. Marginal enhancement of intellectual function could occur, further deterioration was usually prevented and, socially, the patient was more acceptable.

Wilson (1970) emphasized that case selection must be strict; i.e. the following criteria should appertain:

1. The basic personality should be good
2. The IQ should not be too low
3. Institutionalization should not have been prolonged
4. Parental collaboration should be good
5. Cerebral involvement should be essentially or predominantly uni-lateral.

Detailed investigation to establish the last point should precede surgery. The main complication of the operation is the occurrence, in up to 40 per cent of cases, of a delayed persistent chronic subdural haemorrhage into the operative cavity resulting in granular ependymitis and obstructive hydrocephalus of the remaining hemisphere. This process may present clinically with a variety of symptoms including headache, drowsiness, irritability, return of epilepsy, stupor and coma, and may be fatal ultimately. Treatment of the complication is by removal of the products of haemorrhage, correction of the secondary hydrocephalus by a shunt and inhibition of the meningeal reaction to the breakdown products of blood by the use of glucocorticoids. Wilson recommends some modifications of the original operative techniques which help to prevent this complication occurring.

Other techniques

At present, other surgical techniques such as lobotomy, division of the corpus callosum and the production of subcortical destructive lesions

stereotactically have not been used in the treatment of childhood epilepsy.
Recently, there has been increasing interest in the use of electrical
stimulation of the cerebellar cortex by implanted electrodes in cases
of intractable major generalized seizures of the grand mal type. The
procedure attempts to harness the natural inhibitory function of the
cerebellum, is still very experimental, and it has only been employed
in adults. For a discussion of both this and the surgical techniques just
mentioned, the reader is referred to the excellent review by Richardson
(1976). The neurosurgical management of the epilepsies in all age
groups is dealt with in the book by Purpura, Penry and Walter (1975),
and Cooper (1978) has edited a review of cerebellar stimulation in man.

REFERENCES

Cooper, I. S. (1978). Ed. *Cerebellar Stimulation in Man.* New York: Raven Press
Davidson, S. and Falconer, M. A. (1975). 'Outcome of surgery in 40 children with
temporal lobe epilepsy.' *Lancet,* 1, 1260–1263
Dodson, W. E., Prensky, A. L., De Vivo, D. C., Goldring, S. and Dodge, P. R.
(1976). 'Management of seizure disorders: selected aspects. Part II.' *J. Pediat.*
89, 695–703
Falconer, M. A. (1965). 'The surgical treatment of temporal lobe epilepsy.'
Neurochirurgia. 8, 161–172
Jensen, I. (1975). 'Temporal lobe surgery around the world. Results, complications,
and mortality.' *Acta neurol. Scand.* 52, 354–373
Krynauw, R. A. (1950). 'Infantile hemiplegia treated by removing one cerebral
hemisphere.' *J. neurol. Neurosurg. Psychiat.* 13, 243
Penfield, W. and Jasper, H. (1954). *Epilepsy and the Functional Anatomy of the
Human Brain* London: J. and A. Churchill and Boston: Little Brown and
Company
Purpura, D. P., Penry, J. K. and Walter, R. D. (1975). *Advances in Neurology,
Vol. 8: Neurosurgical Management of the Epilepsies.* New York: Raven Press
Rasmussen, T. (1969). 'The role of surgery in the treatment of focal epilepsy.'
Clin. Neurosurg. 16, 288–314
Richardson, A. E. (1976). 'Neurosurgery.' In *A Testbook of Epilepsy,* pp. 296–
313. Eds J. Laidlaw and A. Richens. Edinburgh, London, New York: Churchill
Livingstone
Walker, A. Earl (1972). 'Surgical treatment of epilepsy.' In *Comprehensive Manage-
ment of Epilepsy in Infancy, Childhood and Adolescence,* pp. 406–436. Ed.
S. Livingston. Springfield, Illinois: Charles C. Thomas
Wilson, P. J. E. (1970). 'More second thoughts on hemispherectomy in infantile
hemiplegia.' *Devl Med. child Neurol.* 12, 799–800

CHAPTER 26

The Prognosis of Epilepsy–
General Aspects of the Problem

The problems of prognosis for children with epilepsy are controversial. They are difficult to write about because of arguments about classification and terminology, and often because of uncertainty about the long-term outcome. Throughout this book the prognoses for different types of epilepsy under the rubric of the *International Classification* (Gastaut, 1970) have been considered. This is probably a better way to look at the problem than to consider all types of epilepsy together, although the latter method also has certain advantages.

Varieties of epilepsy

As a rule, authors have found that children with primary generalized epilepsy of the grand mal type or the petit mal type respond best to medication while those with complex partial seizures of the temporal lobe variety do relatively badly (Rodin, 1968). Holowach, Thurston and O'Leary (1972) followed-up a large group of children for up to 12 years after withdrawal of medication in an attempt to determine relapse rates. They were found to be at their lowest in major generalized epilepsy (grand mal), after febrile seizures and in petit mal epilepsy and at their highest in those with temporal lobe epilepsy and with multiple seizure types. Relapse rates were also high in cases with neurological and psychological deficits.

The question of prognosis in petit mal has always been controversial, and this is largely because few terms are so loosely applied, although few clinical disorders are so clearly defined. The name is constantly being given to different kinds of epileptic attack which have one feature only in common – they are not full-scale grand mal convulsions – but the distinction between true petit mal and minor attacks of other kinds is vitally important because the treatment and prognosis are different. Rodin (1968), after reviewing the literature on petit mal, found that the condition was relatively rare and that when stricter criteria were employed it was found more infrequently. He also found that the seizures tended to decrease in number and intensity as the child got older. He commented that approximately a third to a half of patients with petit mal tended to develop grand mal seizures later in life and that this was more likely to happen where the condition began after the age of 8–10 years (see Chapter 7).

Prognosis and age of onset

Prognosis may also be looked at from the point of view of the age of the child. Some of the most serious seizure disorders occur in infancy and early childhood, for example neonatal convulsions, infantile spasms and the secondary generalized epilepsies of the myoclonic type. Equally true, however, is the fact that febrile convulsions, the most common seizure disorder in this early epoch of life, has a very good prognosis. In those young children in whom prompt remission of epilepsy is obtained with or without treatment, the prognosis is good. Holowach, Thurston and O'Leary (1972) stressed that the possibility of stopping treament before the age of eight years usually implied a good long-term prognosis for a seizure disorder. The resistance to therapy, the chronicity of epilepsy, the occurrence of different seizure types and the association with mental defect and neurological and psychological disorders are all poor prognostic indicators in the young child. The chances for a patient to achieve complete freedom from his seizures depends particularly on the intensity of his seizure disorder and its duration, and both of these aspects are usually prominent when the epilepsy is symptomatic of a serious underlying brain disorder.

Primary and secondary causation

In general, the prognosis for childhood epilepsy tends to be better when the patient's epilepsy appears to be due to constitutional and/or hereditary factors, what Rodin (1968) called a 'specific seizure propensity', than when it is secondary to known cerebral damage or structural abnormality. Those varieties of childhood epilepsy in whose aetiology genetic factors are important are usually associated with a favourable long-term prognosis, for example true petit mal, febrile convulsions, benign focal epilepsy and photosensitive epilepsy. A study group reporting to the World Health Organization on juvenile epilepsy in 1957 expressed the opinion that: 'the prognosis of the type of epilepsy in which genetic factors predominate is better than for the other types as regards the number of fits, their responsiveness to treatment and the infrequency of undesirable psychological changes.' But, since that time we have realized that a seizure disorder which is primarily genetic in origin, for example a febrile convulsion, may damage an area of the brain, such as one temporal lobe, thereby leading to a later chronic epilepsy (Ounsted, Lindsay and Norman, 1966).

LONG-TERM STUDIES OF PROGNOSIS

Rodin (1968), following his exhaustive study of prognosis in epilepsy generally, was dismayed to find that there had been no substantial improvement in *long-term remission* rates of epileptic patients in the past 60 years. In 1972 he noted that it was a general opinion that 60–80 per cent of all patients could be satisfactorily controlled by current medication, but if one established as one's criterion complete cessation of seizures for a two-year period and looked at the world's literature from that point of view, only a third of all patients reached such a standard. He further stated that this state of affairs was virtually the same for all studies regardless of what drugs or combinations of drugs were used. He recommended that we ought not to be satisfied with treatment that leads to improvement, i.e. reduction in frequency and severity of seizures, and that we should only be content with their complete cessation. The person with continuing epilepsy faces many disadvantages of a social, educational and vocational nature, quite apart from the medical difficulties consequent on his seizures and the need for long-term (sometimes life-long) drug therapy. We must agree with Rodin (1968) when he says that the search must continue for better treatment, both by drugs and by other methods, which will lead to complete cessation of attacks and thereby to a better quality of life for those with epilepsy.

The fact that this *quality of life* is still far from satisfactory is shown by the revealing survey of Harrison and Taylor (1976). They followed-up a group of children who were part of a sample originally studied by Dr Christopher Ounsted in Oxford between 1948 and 1953. These children were originally identified only on the basis that they had come for treatment through having had at least one seizure in early childhood. Over 200 patients were successfully followed-up after 25 years and particular attention was given to the long-term prognosis in relation to medical, social and educational problems. Although nearly two-thirds of the sample suffered minimal ill-effects, the problems of the remainder were considerable: 10.1 per cent of the patients had died, and of the survivors 11.2 per cent were confined to institutions while 6.6 per cent were invalids at home. Overall the educational achievement of the sample was good but there were also a considerable number of educational problems. Continuing epilepsy was associated with greatly reduced educational and occupational achievement in contrast to the group in remission. The authors found themselves in disagreement with the statement that the great majority of people with epilepsy are able to live useful and normal lives, and they pointed out that the consequences of epilepsy for a third of their patients were very serious indeed. They also pointed out that this finding correlated with the public image of epilepsy as a serious and chronic disorder, and it revealed why the public was frightened by it and prejudiced against its sufferers. Yannet (1949) had come to very similar conclusions when he wrote: 'While there has been much written on the subject of prognosis in epilepsy, it is difficult to evaluate adequately. The primary reason for this is that surveys, as a rule, were concerned almost exclusively with the effect of treatment on the incidence of seizures alone. Unfortunately, this fails to take into account the many other factors that determine whether an epileptic child is living a relatively normal life in his community. It is conceivable that an emotionally well adjusted child having three to five spells a year is infinitely better off than a child having one spell a year but seriously handicapped by personality deviations resulting from untreated tensions in the home directly related to the epileptic state.' These problems of the epileptic child have been considered in the chapters on emotional and psychological aspects of epilepsy and on learning disorders (see Chapters 18 and 19). Reference to the EEG examination in relation to prognosis will also be found in Chapter 21. In general, where the EEG is normal or becomes so during treatment, a favourable outcome may be expected in children.

SUMMARY

In summary, one may say that patients who are normal in other respects, except for their epilepsy, tend to have a good prognosis, especially if they have certain types of seizures such as primary generalized epilepsy of the grand mal type or true petit mal. The prognosis worsens with long duration of illness, resistance to medication, association with neurological and intellectual deficits, the occurrence of different seizure types in the same individual and following the onset of one of the serious varieties of epilepsy early in infancy and childhood.

However, to sound a more modern and hopeful note Livingston (1972), in a review of approximately 20 000 patients followed-up at his clinic over 35 years, found that there was complete control of seizures in 60 per cent, that the seizures were reduced in frequency and/or severity in another 25 per cent so that the patients were able to live essentially normal lives, and that the seizures were refractory to all therapeutic measures in the remaining 15 per cent. Goodman (1969) put the situation pithily for all age groups when he wrote that 60–70 per cent of all patients can be seizure free and that 15–20 per cent have considerably reduced seizure frequency.

One of the problems in the past has been that controlled trials of anticonvulsant drugs have been few and far between in the voluminous literature on the subject and the true clinical efficacy of these drugs is often difficult to assess accurately. Perhaps the most hopeful feature is that we are only just beginning to experience the effects of prevention in epilepsy, the effects, for example, of better neonatal care, of better management of status epilepticus in early childhood and of attempts to prevent post-traumatic epilepsy by prophylactic treatment with conventional anticonvulsant medication. We are also seeing the advent of new and effective drugs to replace some of the old ones which may influence the long-term prognosis in the future. A better realization and understanding of the social, psychological and educational problems which beset children with epilepsy should forestall the development of secondary handicaps in affected individuals and thereby contribute in no small measure to an improved prognosis generally.

REFERENCES

Gastaut, H. (1970). 'Clinical and electroencephalographical classification of epileptic seizures.' *Epilepsia*, **11**, 102–113

Goodman, L. (1969). 'General summary of symposium on laboratory evaluation of antiepileptic drugs.' *Epilepsia*, **10**, 329–335

Harrison, R. M. and Taylor, D. C. (1976). 'Childhood seizures: a 25-year follow-up. Social and medical prognosis.' *Lancet*, **1**, 948–951

Holowach, J., Thurston, D. L. and O'Leary, J. (1972). 'Prognosis in childhood epilepsy.' *New Engl. J. Med.* **286**, 169–174

Livingston, S. (1972). *Comprehensive Management of Epilepsy in Infancy, Childhood and Adolescence*, p. 584. Springfield, Illinois: Charles C. Thomas

Ounsted, C., Lindsay, J. and Norman, R. (1966). *Clinics in Developmental Medicine, No. 22: Biological Factors in Temporal Lobe Epilepsy*. London. Spastics Society and Heinemann

Rodin, E. A. (1968). *The Prognosis of Patients with Epilepsy*. Springfield, Illinois: Charles C. Thomas

Rodin E. A. (1972). 'Medical and social prognosis in epilepsy.' *Epilepsia*, **13**, 121–131

World Health Organization (1957). 'Juvenile Epilepsy. Report of a Study Group.' *WHO Report Series, No. 130*, Geneva, Switzerland: WHO

Yannet, H., Dreamer, W. C. and Barba, P. S. (1949). 'Convulsive Disorders in Children.' *Pediatrics*, **4**, 677

CHAPTER 27

The Prevention of Epilepsy

Lennox (1960) referred briefly to this problem and commented: 'The preventive aspects of epilepsy have not received the attention their importance deserves. In comparison with many chronic diseases, the onset of seizures is predominantly in childhood; contributing causes are many and widely various; and the prevention of sequelae may be as important as prevention of the disease itself. Finally, and here the contrast is sharpened, the sequelae may be as much social as physical.' Apart from these comments, there was little in the literature about prevention until the excellent short review of the problem by Taylor and Bower (1971) and the publication of the Proceedings of the Fifth International Symposium on Epilepsy, held in London in 1972, in which the main theme had been prevention (Parsonage, 1973).

However, prevention of any condition presupposes a knowledge of its origins, and it is necessary to consider these again in the case of epilepsy. Aicardi (1976), in his review of the problems of prevention, noted that seizures in children fell into two broad aetiological categories, first, those resulting from organic brain anomalies, whether due to abnormal development or to brain insults occurring during fetal life, at birth, or postnatally, and secondly, those resulting from functional disturbances in the brain and body generally, about whose nature we understand relatively little and which are, at least in part, genetically determined. These two categories partially overlap, since some genetic factors induce seizures through causing organic brain abnormalities, e.g. tuberose sclerosis.

Genetic aspects

Our attack on the aetiological roots of epilepsy should probably begin with attempts to modify the genetic origins of epilepsy. Genetic factors play an important role in the primary generalized epilepsies such as primary grand mal, petit mal, benign focal or centrotemporal epilepsy, in some of the primary or cryptogenic myoclonic epilepsies and also in febrile convulsions. However, our knowledge of how genetic mechanisms work in the transmission of epilepsy is limited except in certain specific conditions such as tuberose sclerosis and phenylketonuria, where precise Mendelian laws operate.

The genetics of the epilepsies were reviewed by Refsum (1973). Examples of conditions in which epilepsy may be a symptom of a recessively inherited metabolic disorder include maple-syrup urine disease, phenylketonuria and galactosaemia, unless these conditions are treated by appropriate dietetic regimens. Degenerative conditions with a recessive inheritance which result in the storage of abnormal metabolites in neurones include Tay–Sachs disease (G_{M2} gangliosidosis), metachromatic leucodystrophy and neuronal ceroid lipofuscinosis (Batten–Vogt disease), and in all of these intractable seizures may occur.

Tuberose sclerosis, which frequently has epilepsy as a feature, appears to be inherited as an incomplete dominant trait with considerable variability with regard to penetrance and expressivity. Where one or other parent has tuberose sclerosis, the parents should be advised that 50 per cent of their offspring may be affected and that the risk may range from severe mental handicap with epilepsy to trivial cutaneous stigmas. They will then have to make up their own minds about the risks of procreation. In another condition with dominant inheritance, Huntington's chorea, it is probably sensible to assume that all children born to a marriage where one partner is affected by the disease are likely to be affected. There are also certain chromosomal aberrations which may be associated with epilepsy. Hereditary myoclonus epilepsy or Unverricht–Lundborg disease is a familial progressive disorder with a recessive inheritance in which epilepsy and mental deterioration are the main features (*see* page 97).

Epilepsy due to one of these rare disorders probably constitutes less than 1 per cent of the total incidence of epilepsy. In the majority of children with epilepsy in which inherited factors appear to be playing a significant role, the method of inheritance is far from clear. There are, however, certain situations in which the seizures seem to be the only manifestation of the genetic trait. Metrakos and Metrakos (1969), in a study based on clinical material, proposed the hypothesis that an EEG showing a relatively good background pattern but with interspersed paroxysmal bilaterally synchronous bursts of regular spike-wave complexes may be inherited as an autosomal dominant trait, and that environmental and genetic factors interact to precipitate the clinical seizures. Bray and Wiser (1965) described a familial variety of temporal lobe epilepsy with a good prognosis. Siblings of those affected by febrile convulsions have an increased risk of developing the same complaint.

Apart from these fairly well-defined situations, it is generally believed, from the results of studies in monozygotic and dizygotic twins suffering from 'idiopathic' and 'symptomatic' epilepsy, that the genetic hypothesis which best fits the facts is one of the polygenic influence. Refsum (1973) writes as follows: 'The hypothesis of a polygenic influence in interplay with environmental specific and unspecific factors would imply the concept of continuously varying, and approximately normally distributed tendency in the population towards having displayed a manifest epileptic attack, provided the individual has lived a number of years sufficient for the tendency to come to expression.' He concludes by saying that we know nothing definite about what the mode of reaction, which we call predisposition to epilepsy, depends on, but he considers that in the future we will achieve a deeper understanding of the neurophysiological and biochemical mechanisms involved.

Despite the considerable interest in the genetic aspects of epilepsy, relatively little can be expected from a genetic approach to prevention at present. Doose and his colleagues in West Germany have written extensively on selection of siblings of epileptic children for prevention on the basis of EEG abnormalities and summarized his results in 1973 (Doose and Gerken, 1973). He believes that siblings of patients whose EEGs exhibit spike-wave patterns at rest and following intermittent photic stimulation and which may also show what he terms 'abnormal theta rhythms' are at considerable risk of developing epilepsy and should perhaps have drug prophylaxis.

BRAIN DAMAGE

Epilepsies resulting from acquired brain damage offer greater opportunities for prevention. Prenatal infections such as rubella can now be prevented by the immunization of girls before puberty, and a vaccine against cytomegalovirus infection may be generally available in the future. Congenital syphilis is rarely seen today and toxoplasmosis can be recognized and treated in pregnancy. Perinatal brain damage, particularly that caused by anoxia, is an important cause of later epilepsy and improved obstetric management and better paediatric care of the neonate should contribute significantly to prevention. The development of neonatology has been marked, especially in recent years, by spectacular improvements in mortality and morbidity which are associated with important advances in the understanding of physiological disturbances in the newborn and with innovations in their management. The benefits and real and possible hazards of these methods and treatments are excellently reviewed by Baum, MacFarlane and Tizard (1977). The incidence of mental defect, visual and hearing disability and major and minor neurological handicaps in children who might have died as neonates without the availability of mechanical ventilation is described by Marriage and Davies (1977), and presumably many of these children will develop symptomatic epilepsy consequent on brain damage. A marked decline in the incidence of low-birth-weight spastic diplegia has been reported from both Great Britain and Sweden (Davies and Tizard, 1975; Hagberg, Hagberg and Olow, 1977), and has been ascribed to better neonatal care. However, a similar decline has not occurred in other types of cerebral palsy such as spastic hemiplegia. It is perhaps reasonable to hope that there may be a corresponding decline in epileptogenic brain damage. The early detection and treatment of hypoglycaemia in the newborn, for example, has been a very significant advance in preventing such damage. The practice of late feeding of low-birth-weight infants, which was fashionable in the 1950s, led to hypoglycaemia and hyperbilirubinaemia and continued until Smallpiece and Davies (1964) pointed out its inherent dangers.

Malnutrition in infancy

The evidence is now convincing that malnutrition in infancy permanently affects the minds of children who have been so afflicted by interfering with brain growth at a critical period (Winick, 1969). The time element is critical: both animal and human data demonstrate that the earlier the malnutrition the more severe and permanent are the effects. It appears that after infancy the brain is much more resistant to the effects of malnutrition. It also seems possible that the infant whose mother was malnourished is more at risk than the infant born to a well-nourished mother. Therefore, it would seem that the first priority should be the elimination of malnutrition in infancy and perhaps even prenatally. The problem of malnutrition is world-wide, affecting perhaps half of the world's population and is linked to the problems of intellectual impairment in general and consequently indirectly to epilepsy.

Infectious diseases of the CNS

The young developing brain is highly susceptible to any kind of insult. Infections are very common during the first few years of life and are one of the possible causes of brain damage and convulsions. As with so many of the advances in this subject in the last 25 years, Ounsted (1951) was the first to emphasize the important significance of convulsions occurring in children with purulent meningitis. He demonstrated a close association between failure of treatment and the occurrence and intensity of convulsive seizures. Age was the important determinant and purulent meningitis is commonest in infancy. Ounsted showed that status epilepticus in this age group was a relatively common complication of meningitis and was often fatal. He recommended routine prophylaxis with phenobarbitone in all cases of meningitis and rapid and intensive treatment of established convulsions. In recent years the early diagnosis and effective treatment of neonatal meningitis has lead to improved results, although many infants still die or are left permanently brain damaged. Aicardi (1973), writing about the role of infections in the aetiology of childhood epilepsy in his large series showed that infection was involved in causing one chronic epilepsy out of five and two occasional convulsions out of three. He included prolonged febrile convulsions as an important aetiological cause of chronic epilepsy later. Prompt recognition of infection, effective treatment, particularly where infections are complicated by seizures, and prophylactic anticonvulsant treatment to prevent further febrile convulsions are all helpful in the prevention of chronic epilepsy.

Other preventible causes

Diseases of infancy such as gastroenteritis, a world-wide problem especially in those who do not enjoy the benefits of breast-feeding, may result in brain damage through the production of hyperosmolar hypernatraemic dehydration. Mental retardation, epilepsy and cerebral palsy are sequelae in up to 11 per cent of the survivors from this metabolic disorder (Macauley and Watson, 1967). The best means of rehydrating hypernatraemic infants remains controversial but, although there is still debate about the proper concentration of saline solution to use, all are agreed about the importance of slow reduction of hyperosmolarity if death, convulsions and irreversible brain damage are to be avoided (Chambers, 1975). Hogan (1976) pointed out that the exact nature of the rehydrating solution is not of major significance, but the volume administered and the rate of rehydration are of vital importance. If too great a volume of saline solution is given too rapidly the child becomes oedematous and develops raised intracranial pressure, and stupor and convulsions may follow.

There are many other situations in paediatrics where the prevention of epilepsy may be achieved by an attack on its aetiological roots. The problems of post-traumatic epilepsy are dealt with in a separate chapter (*see* Chapter 13). In early infancy and childhood vaccination and immunization may confer protection against serious diseases, although, unfortunately, pertussis immunization is under a cloud at present. Febrile convulsions have already been dealt with at length (*see* Chapter 6), and one of the major problems is that the initial seizure is often the longest and most damaging. Stopping such seizures quickly and trying to find those at risk of developing such a seizure are likely to contribute significantly to the prevention of later chronic epilepsy.

Health education, in the broad sense, is also important in the prevention of epilepsy. There is increasing awareness, for example, of the special risks in adolescence in this respect when one considers the cultivation of regular and temperate habits, particularly with regard to alcohol: overhydration, especially when combined with alcoholic excess, provokes seizures. The risks of head injury and the dangers of drug abuse are also greater at this period of life. Drugs such as barbiturates, if abused, may, on withdrawal, lead to convulsions in persons who would otherwise not have suffered from them.

Three levels of prevention

Thomas (1973) suggested three levels of prevention of epilepsy and its consequences as follows:

1. Prevention of the onset of epilepsy
2. Prevention of recurrence of manifestations
3. Prevention of consequences of epilepsy — psychological, social and economic.

Aicardi (1976) thought that the prevention of epilepsy could be approached through an attack on its aetiological roots, by limitation of the complications of fits and by avoidance of the psychosocial consequences of seizure disorders. Taylor and Bower (1971) wrote about what they called the 'secondary handicaps' of epilepsy and felt that good seizure management should be the basis of their prevention. The clinician should use drugs as intelligently and effectively as possible, employing as few drugs as are necessary and avoiding overdosage and toxicity. Tower (1978), in a keynote address to the Ninth International Symposium on Epilepsy in Amsterdam in September, 1977, chose the problem of world-wide prevention as his theme and emphasized that the achievement of therapeutic levels of anticonvulsants in the blood had improved control enormously in the preceding quinquennium and that fewer drugs were required for seizure management. He speculated about the possibility of a dip-stick saliva test to measure drug levels more easily in the future.

SUMMARY

In summary, therefore, it can be seen that prevention of epilepsy implies attempts to avert its onset by better understanding of the genetic problems involved; by better prenatal, perinatal and neonatal care; and by more effective therapy of potentially brain-damaging illnesses in infancy and early childhood. It involves the prevention of recurrence of the manifestations of epilepsy by better case finding, by earlier and more accurate diagnosis and by better management. It implies the prevention of complications of epilepsy (the 'secondary handicaps') which may be psychological, social or economic. It requires a determined effort by all concerned with the condition to combat the public attitudes to epilepsy which are still influenced so strongly by fear and prejudice. The prevention of epilepsy and the succour of its victims should be special concerns of all physicians and others concerned with the care of children.

REFERENCES

Aicardi, J. (1973). 'Epileptic attacks accompanying or following acute infantile infections acquired during the first three years of life.' In *Prevention of Epilepsy and its Consequences*, pp. 28–31. Ed. M. J. Parsonage. London: International Bureau for Epilepsy
Aicardi, J. (1976). 'Prevention of epilepsy in children.' *Devl Med. child Neurol.* 18, 381–383
Baum, D., MacFarlane, A. and Tizard, J. P. M. (1977). 'The benefits and hazards of neonatology.' In *Clinics in Developmental Medicine, No. 64: Benefits and Hazards of the New Obstetrics*, pp. 126–138. Eds T. Chard and M. Richards. London: Spastics International and Heinemann
Bray, P. F. and Wiser, W. C. (1965). 'Hereditery characteristics of familial temporal-central focal epilepsy.' *Pediatrics*, 36, 207–211
Chambers, T. L. (1975). 'Hypernatraemia: a preventable cause of acquired brain damage ?' *Devl Med. child Neurol.* 17, 91–94
Davies, P. A. and Tizard, J. P. M. (1975). 'Very low birthweight and subsequent neurological defect (with special reference to spastic diplegia).' *Devl Med. child Neurol.* 17, 3–17
Doose, H. and Gerken, H. (1973). 'Possibilities and limitations of epilepsy prevention in siblings of epileptic children.' In *Prevention of Epilepsy and its Consequences*, pp. 32–35. Ed. M. J. Parsonage. London: International Bureau for Epilepsy
Hagberg, B., Hagberg, G. and Olow, I. (1977). 'The panorama of cerebral palsy in Swedish children born 1954–74.' *Neuropädiatrie*, 8, 516–521
Hogan, G. R. (1976). 'Hypernatraemia – problems in management.' *Pediat. Clins N. Am.* 23, 569–574
Lennox, W. G. (1960). *Epilepsy and Related Disorders*, p. 1000. London: J. and A. Churchill and Boston: Little Brown and Company
Macauley, D. and Watson, M. (1967). 'Hypernatraemia in infants as a cause of brain damage.' *Archs Dis. Childh.* 42, 485–491

Marriage, K. J. and Davies, P. A. (1977). 'Neurological sequelae in children surviving mechanical ventilation in the neonatal period.' *Archs Dis. Childh.* **52**, 176–182

Metrakos, J. D. and Metrakos, K. (1969). 'Genetic studies in clinical epilepsy.' In *Basic Mechanisms of the Epilepsies*, pp. 700–708. Eds H. H. Jasper, A. A. Ward and A. Pope. Boston: Little, Brown and Company and London: J. and A. Churchill

Ounsted, C. (1951). 'Significance of convulsions in children with purulent meningitis.' *Lancet*, **1**, 1245–1248

Parsonage, M. J. (1973). Ed. *Prevention of Epilepsy and its Consequences.* London: International Bureau for Epilepsy

Refsum, S. (1973). 'Genetics of epilepsies.' In *Prevention of Epilepsy and its Consequences*, pp. 11–14. Ed. M. J. Parsonage. London: International Bureau for Epilepsy

Smallpiece, V. and Davies, P. A. (1964). 'Immediate feeding of premature infants with undiluted breast milk.' *Lancet*, **2**, 1349–1352

Taylor, D. C. and Bower, B. D. (1971). 'Prevention of epileptic disorders.' *Lancet*, **2**, 1136–1138

Thomas, M. H. (1973). 'The ultimate challenge of epilepsy prevention.' In *Prevention of Epilepsy and its Consequences*, pp. 5–9. Ed. M. J. Parsonage. London: International Bureau for Epilepsy

Tower, D. B. (1978). 'Epilepsy: A World Problem.' In *Advances in Epileptology, 1977*, pp. 2–26. Eds H. Meinardi and A. J. Rowan. Amsterdam and Lisse: Swets and B. V. Zeitlinger

Winick, M. (1969). 'Malnutrition and brain development.' *J. Pediat.* **74**, 667–679

CHAPTER 28

Prospects for the Future

Epilepsy has always been a world-wide problem and one for all age groups, but particularly so for children and adolescents. Tower (1978), in his introductory address to the International Symposium on Epilepsy in 1977, took 'Epilepsy: A World Problem' as his theme and pointed out that the world population could be expected to increase by more than 50 per cent during the next two decades and that 75 per cent of that increase would occur outside Western Europe and North America. He reminded his audience that increasing populations inevitably mean more epilepsy unless preventative steps are taken.

Prevention is really of the essence if epilepsy is to be a diminishing problem in the future. In the developed countries there is clear evidence that brain injury can be prevented by improved antenatal and perinatal care. Hagberg, Hagberg and Olow (1975a, 1975b, 1976) have reported that the incidence of cerebral palsy has fallen successively and significantly, in an unselected series of cases of cerebral palsy in Sweden, from 2.2/1000 live births in the period 1954–1958 to 1.3/1000 live births in the period 1967–1970. Similar falls in incidence have been reported from other countries. There has been a dramatic decline in the occurrence of spastic diplegia consequent on low birth weight in Sweden, even though the percentage of low-birth-weight infants born remained constant through the years. Hagberg and his colleagues have ascribed these improvements to the fact that from the middle of the 1950s onwards each county in Sweden, with populations of 200 000 to 400 000, centralized obstetrical and neonatal care to large central hospitals with well-developed services and adequate staffing. Since 1970 there has been no further decrease in the incidence of cerebral palsied children, but further gains have been achieved with a successive decrease in the perinatal and postneonatal mortality rates (Hagberg, Hagberg and Olow, 1977). Hagberg has not been impressed with the value of very active perinatal measures, such as respirator treatment, but he believes that the outcome for children treated in his intensive therapy unit has been good, mainly due to systematic efforts to compensate for hypoxia, acidosis, hypothermia, hypocaloric states and hypoglycaemia in the routine of neonatal care.

With improving care of this nature becoming more widely available, prenatal negative factors are now beginning to influence the series of events which may lead to the later development of the cerebral palsy syndrome or other brain damage syndromes such as epilepsy. Fetal growth retardation is particularly important in this respect and may be considered to be present when the birth weight is below the mean for gestational age and where toxaemia or bleeding or other adverse circumstances have occurred in pregnancy and have caused 'fetal deprivation of supply' (Hagberg, Hagberg and Olow, 1976). The common combination of fetal deprivation of supply and asphyxia and/or cerebral haemorrhage suggest that the brain is more susceptible to perinatal complications after negative intrauterine influences have operated. Additive interactions of many prenatal and perinatal factors may constitute the main predisposing cause of brain damage at birth today. For this reason systematic screening procedures to detect fetuses at risk are essential, and when a threatening situation is discovered expert care will be needed to avoid further deterioration in the situation and to bring the fetus to extrauterine life at the optimal time, in best possible condition and with the minimum of perinatal trauma (Hagberg, 1978).

While this type of sophisticated prevention is engaging the attention of paediatricians and obstetricians in the developed countries, it is pertinent to remember that in countries like India childhood infections are still a major cause of epilepsy and that in Nigeria cerebral malaria with associated seizures presents considerable problems. Cysticercosis with cerebral complications is an especially prevalent cause of seizures in Mexico and in Papua New Guinea (Tower, 1978). Malnutrition is especially severe in many of the developing countries and the consequences predispose to many epileptogenic factors, mitigate against effective resistance to infection and may even interfere with the metabolic responses to drugs such as anticonvulsants. It is clear that established public health measures and better nutrition have major roles to play in the prevention of epilepsy, and bodies such as the World Health Organization are of paramount importance in this area.

Theoretical advances in the field of epilepsy concern concept and terminology. The concept of the epilepsies, rather than epilepsy, is gaining widespread recognition. Seizures must be seen as a behavioural manifestation of an enormously diverse group of underlying states of brain dysfunction rather than having a single cause. Such a viewpoint gives proportion to one's expectations about the epilepsies. If there is no single epilepsy then there cannot be a single cause or cure. With reference to terminology, the growing use of the *International Classification* of the Epilepsies (Gastaut, 1970) has promoted clarity of thinking and communication among those working with patients with epilepsy and in research.

NEW CONCEPTS IN THE PATHOPHYSIOLOGY OF THE EPILEPSIES

Probably the most fundamental recent advance in the understanding of *the pathophysiology of the epilepsies* has been the discovery of the kindling effect. This phenomenon is described in detail elsewhere (*see* Chapter 13). A question of fundamental importance in the causation of epilepsy is what causes a particular group of cells or a region of the brain to become epileptogenic. It is likely that the answer will ultimately be a complex one and will depend on the coexistence of a number of interrelating factors, including the kindling effect. Research into the causes of epilepsy in infancy and early childhood is likely to be particularly fruitful because of the known vulnerability of the immature brain to traumatic and metabolic insults, especially hypoxia, ischaemia and fetal deprivation of supply (Hagberg, Hagberg and Olow, 1976). When damage occurs at this stage of the brain's development neuronal dropout, alterations in dendritic arborization and spine formation and the distortion of cell bodies and axons seen in chronic foci in animals and man (together with the accompanying change in afferent inputs) may all play a role in making a group of neurons epileptogenic (Pedley, 1978). The remarkable work of Purpura (1975) on normal patterns of neuronal growth and differentiation and on the functional consequences of aberrant neuronal development may be fundamental to our understanding of these matters. For example, Huttenlocher (1974) has demonstrated deficient dendritic development in the brains of children with mental retardation and infantile spasms.

It is obvious, however, that not all glial scars are epileptogenic and that only a rough correlation exists between the extent and type of tissue damage and the occurrence of clinical seizures. Other mechanisms must be important in the generation of epileptic activity and these must involve the cellular properties of neurones in an epileptic focus and also the ionic microenvironment of the cell. There has been argument as to whether the 'epileptogenic tendency' resides in the collective behaviour of a pool of nerve cells or in the altered state of single 'epileptic' neurones. This distinction is probably artificial since, while a group of neurones is necessary to generate epileptic events, there must be some fundamental abnormality affecting the cells comprising the group. No evidence yet exists with regard to the critical size of the neuronal aggregate necessary to produce epileptic potentials.

Disorders of spike generation in neurones have been described. Neurones normally fire orthodromically, that is, from the cell body outwards via the axon. In epileptic foci, Gutnick and Prince (1972) described a phenomenon termed 'backfiring' in which the neurones fire antidromically, that is, the action potential is initiated ectopically in the axon and then propagates into the cell body. 'Backfiring' or ectopic spike generation, appears to be a feature unique to the epileptic process and it has been postulated that it provides a kind of built-in powerful recurrent excitatory mechanism in the neurone. It has been speculated that the conversion from orthodromic to antidromic firing may provide a general cellular mechanism for the profound increases in excitability and synchronization of cortical neurones which are characteristic of focal seizure development.

Based on a number of observations showing that the extracellular potassium ion concentration increased during seizure activity, it was proposed that potassium accummulation in the brain's extracellular spaces would lead to increasing levels of excitability, ultimately resulting in epileptic discharges. While it is now considered that changes in extracellular ionic potassium are not directly related to epileptogenesis (Pedley, 1978), it is known that the amount of potassium released during interictal and ictal discharges varies at different cortical depths, thereby creating a gradient across the cortex which will have differential effects on the excitability of vertically disposed neurones. Furthermore, ionized potassium may also play a part in, or even initiate, the abnormal excitability of nerve terminals that results in the type of ectopic spike generation already described.

The role of the astrocytes in dealing with extracellular potassium has already been mentioned in another chapter (*see* Chapter 25). Reactive changes in astrocytes, commonly termed gliosis, are not invariably associated with epilepsy, but epileptic foci are invariably associated with gliosis. One of the principal reactions of astrocytes is the swelling which they exhibit in response to the presence of excess ionized potassium in the extracellular fluid. This swelling reflects their property of 'buffering' or taking up excess ionized potassium released from neurones during hyperactivity of the type occurring during ictal or interictal discharge (Tower, 1978). If the astrocytes function normally, much if not all of the released potassium should be 'buffered' or removed by them to maintain a normal perineuronal extracellular milieu. However, it has been demonstrated experimentally that the clearance rate of released potassium ions in epileptic foci may be less than one-half of normal, presumably reflecting disordered astrocytic function.

There has also been considerable interest in the part played by ionized calcium in epileptogenesis. Ionized calcium is critically related to the association between a neurone's membrane potential and the conductance mechanisms for sodium and potassium. In general, increases in ionized calcium stabilize the cell membrane by increasing the amount of depolarization necessary to reach the threshold for spike generation. Conversely, decreasing ionized calcium enhances neuronal excitability. Ionized calcium is essential for neurotransmitter release at presynaptic terminals and it is suggested that phenytoin may exert its anticonvulsant action at this point by influencing calcium influx into axons and synapses.

One of the most active areas of research into epileptogenesis concerns the transmission of the nerve impulse from one nerve cell to another. Direct local cell-to-cell communication in the nervous system is mediated by specific excitatory or inhibitory chemical transmitter agents. There is storage of the neurotransmitters in the cell of origin, a mechanism for release is available, specific receptor sites on the target cell are present and there are specific responses to such reception within the target cell. In the normal situation there exists a balance between excitatory and inhibitory neurotransmitters, and any imbalance may be significant in determining epileptogenicity. For example, it has been demonstrated experimentally that certain convulsants, such as penicillin and pentylenetetrazole, act as specific antagonists of the inhibitory transmitter GABA, presumably by interfering or combining with the GABA receptors. In contrast, the barbiturate pentobarbitone prolongs or enhances GABA-mediated inhibition (Ransom and Barker, 1976; MacDonald and Barker, 1977). Research into excitation and inhibition at the synaptic level has been paralleled by neurophysiological work at the level of groups of cells forming an epileptic aggregate. It is now believed that epileptic activity may disrupt normal brain function in animals and man not just by incorporation of neurones into an epileptic focus but also by widespread inhibition evoked in areas of brain remote from the actual focus, particularly at a subcortical level (Pedley, 1978). The phenomena which lead to the failure of these intrinsic control mechanisms and permit seizures to occur are unknown.

NEW TECHNIQUES IN INVESTIGATION

Reference has already been made elsewhere in this book to the impact of newer methods of investigation on the understanding of the epilepsies in the future (*see* Chapter 21). The most important of these new techniques is probably CT scanning. *Regional cerebral blood flow studies* and *metabolic mapping* with radioactive desoxyglucose are two new related experimental techniques. In the first technique, a radioactive substance is injected into the patient's or animal's blood. Regions of the brain which are active for whatever reason have increased blood flow. Regional changes in blood flow are reflected in focal accentuations in radioactivity as detected by multiple sensors arranged over the hemispheres. This technique has been said to detect epileptic foci not evident in the EEG. A structurally altered sugar molecule is used in the second technique which is taken up by active cells as if it were glucose but is not further metabolized, and it accumulates in areas of high metabolic activity. Radioactive labelling of the molecule allows the spread of activity to be mapped as a seizure focus begins to involve other brain areas (Lewis, 1976).

Apart from CT scanning, there have been *technological advances* permitting intensive monitoring of the patient with epilepsy and these have already been described elsewhere. This technique may be particularly important in the differential diagnosis of attacks of various kinds and also in the investigation of intractable or refractory epilepsy. The two main techniques in use are the telemetered EEG combined with simultaneous recording on video-tape of the clinical features of the seizure and its electrical correlate, and the use of the 24-hour cassette recorder for long-term monitoring of ambulant patients or patients pursuing their normal daily activities at home or at work (*see* Chapter 21). *Seizure warning devices* which monitor the individual's brainwave patterns have also been developed experimentally. The device picks up warning signs of an attack and alerts the individual by producing a low-pitched noise. The person carrying the device may then have time to move away from any physical hazard or even retire to a more private place. Parents worry exceedingly about the risks which their children may run in busy thoroughfares or while bicycling and clearly a device of this nature, if it becomes a practical proposition, will have a significant place in paediatric epileptology.

Perhaps the most significant advance in treatment in recent years has been the widespread use of accurate techniques for measuring levels of anticonvulsant drugs in the blood. The results of this development in the management of anticonvulsant therapy in North America and in Western Europe have been dramatic. Sherwin's (1978) results in Montreal show that less than one-half of their patients with epilepsy were controlled and nearly 40 per cent had frequent seizures before utilizing blood level determinations of drugs to improve seizure management. Within five years, just by adjusting drug dosage on the basis of optimal blood levels, some 75 per cent of their patients were well controlled, and less than 10 per cent still had frequent attacks. However, if blood level estimations of anticonvulsant drugs are to be part of the medical armamentarium in developing countries, it will be necessary to develop simpler methods of testing for these levels. It is easier to perform EMIT from the technician's standpoint than is gas-liquid chromatography and the results are reliable. 'Dip-stick' methods, using saliva or a drop of blood from a finger prick, might provide an answer in the future. The future will also see the development of new anticonvulsant drugs, perhaps deriving from the great increase in knowledge about neuro-transmitter agents. However, Tower (1978) has estimated that the research and development processes involved in producing a new drug in the USA may cost between 16 and 40 million dollars. Something which is certainly needed in the future, where new anticonvulsant drugs are concerned, is the use of carefully *controlled clinical trials in epilepsy* which have been sadly lacking up to now, as Richens (1976) has emphasized. As an example, he gave the case of ACTH therapy for infantile spasms. Although used for this serious epilepsy since 1958 there is still no objective evidence that it does any more than produce an immediate reduction in the number of seizures. The dilemma about its use and efficacy in the syndrome of infantile spasms is a good illustration, according to Richens, of how the lack of early controlled studies can impede medical progress since many clinicians would now argue that, in the absence of better treatment, it would be unethical to withhold ACTH therapy in such a serious condition. As a consequence, it is impossible to create the opportunity of initiating a trial in which an untreated group is compared with a group treated with ACTH.

Meanwhile, the search continues for *new methods of treatment* other than with anticonvulsant drugs. The use of surgery may increase as CT scanning reveals hitherto hidden structural lesions in patients with epilepsy. Cerebellar stimulation is an experimental technique which seeks to control seizures by electronic stimulation of part of the brain. The long-range effects of such stimulation on brain tissue are unknown and, for that and other reasons, it is not likely to find a significant application in paediatrics. However, other related techniques may be developed in the future which may find a place in the treatment of children.

TREATMENT BY CONDITIONING TECHNIQUES

On several occasions in this book, attention has been drawn to the fact that environmental conditions external to the epileptogenic tissue may be a major cause of potentiating or attenuating the seizure disorder. Alterations in the internal milieu of the body or in homeostasis or in the external environment may all operate in this way. The increasing knowledge of such relationships has given rise to attempts to modify the frequency and severity of seizures by behavioural intervention and treatment. The various procedures may be classified into three main categories as follows:

1. Reward and punishment programmes
2. Self-control and psychotherapy
3. Psychobiological techniques.

These various aspects are fully reviewed by Mostofsky and Balaschak (1977). Treatment of this nature has been applied in patients who experience many and severely disrupting seizures and for whom pharmacological management has failed and/or for whom surgery is not possible. Seizure disorders are notorious for their cyclic exacerbations and remissions which are quite often without any logical explanation. The protagonists of behavioural therapy would say that such biorhythmic effects are the results of psychosomatic mechanisms influencing central nervous system functioning.

Biofeedback

Perhaps the psychobiological method which has excited most interest has been *biofeedback*, a therapy based on the concept that individuals can develop a degree of control over involuntary physical processes through conditioning. The brain, as we have seen, does not function independently of what happens in its surroundings. The various senses take information from these surroundings to the brain. This information influences the activity of the brain and the brain in turn influences other parts of the organism. For example, if the incoming information is of a threatening character, feelings of fear and stress arise and these emotions are accompanied by increased muscular tension and by changes in breathing and heart rate. The individual may not be conscious of these changes but if the effects are visualized by means of electronic devices they can then be fed back to the subject. He then becomes aware, through light or sound signals, of the stress effects which are present in the biological sphere. This process is called biofeedback. It has been used to teach people to relax in threatening or stressful situations.

In 1963, Brazier described a 13—14 Hz EEG rhythm recorded from the sensorimotor cortex in cats. It has been called the sensorimotor rhythm or SMR. Subsequently it was demonstrated that the presence of this rhythm in cats was accompanied by immobility and with increased resistance to drug-induced epileptic seizures. Observations of SMR in cats is relatively easy because it is a dominant rhythm whereas detection of 12—14 Hz activity in humans is complicated by the presence of other activity such as the alpha rhythm. However, it is claimed that patients can be trained to change their EEG patterns by biofeedback techniques. These consist of detecting the SMR patterns by recording over the central or Rolandic fissures and, when the specific pattern is present, a feedback signal is presented to the patients telling them that they are producing it. The signal may be visual or auditory. Additional feedback cues may be fed to the patient when he produces epileptic discharges in his EEG. By means of regular training sessions the patient may be trained to increase the amount of SMR present and so inhibit seizure activity in his EEG and reduce the frequency of clinical epilepsy (Sterman, MacDonald and Stone, 1974). Research in this remarkable technique may eventually make it possible to give patients the ability to modulate their own brain waves and hence learn to reduce their seizures through voluntary control, initially through the use of biofeedback equipment and later by themselves. It is only fair to point out, however, that there are many who question the validity of these techniques in controlling epilepsy, not least because of their placebo effects (Gastaut, 1975).

EDUCATION

Ignorance, prejudice and superstition still surround epilepsy in all parts of the world, although the emphasis may differ from country to country. Even in those countries where most people smile about superstitions and old wives' tales, there remains a widespread and deep-rooted feeling about epilepsy which bars the acceptance of people with epilepsy as ordinary fellow citizens. Too often, even today, the sufferer from epilepsy may feel with John Clare (Quiller—Couch, 1939):

I am ! Yet what I am who cares, or knows ?
My friends forsake me like a memory lost.
I am the self-consumer of my woes;
They rise and vanish, an oblivious host,
Shadows of life, whose very soul is lost.
And yet I am — I live — though I am toss'd
Into the nothingness of scorn and noise,
Into the living sea of waking dream,
Where there is neither sense of life, nor joys,
But the huge shipwreck of my own esteem
And all that's dear. Even those I loved the best
Are strange — nay, they are stranger than the rest.

Medical care which reduces or stops the patient's seizures, and social care which helps him to adjust to society and the problems presented by his complaint, cannot have their full effect unless society changes its attitudes about epilepsy and those who suffer from it. *Education* must be the key to changing public attitudes and in this respect most has been accomplished in many countries by those people with epilepsy who have formed associations in order to take an active part in fighting their own battles. The primary aims of these associations are to combat prejudice against the disorder and to help all people with epilepsy to lead normal lives. The medical profession should be equally diligent in ensuring that medical students are adequately informed about this common and world-wide problem and that the teaching of epileptology takes its proper place in specialist training and in the continuing education of family doctors (Stores, 1975).

Lennox (1960) wrote: 'A convulsion is a beacon light in medical symptomatology. The path lighted by its rays reaches to the far limits of recorded medical history.' Never before has there been such intense international interest in epilepsy as there is today – in fundamental research, in the aetiology and clinical presentation of the disorder, in treatment, and, above all, in the possibility of prevention.

The physician who deals with children in whatever capacity is in the forefront of the battle against epilepsy since the majority of the potentially brain-damaging conditions occur in the paediatric age group and because 90 per cent of patients with epilepsy develop their initial symptoms before 20 years of age. An attempt, inevitably incomplete because of the scope and complexity of the subject, has been made in this book to provide the essential information to enable him to help the child with epilepsy.

REFERENCES

Brazier, M. A. B. (1963). 'The problem of periodicity in the electroencephalogram: studies in the cat.' *Electroenceph. clin. Neurophysiol.* **15**, 287–298

Gastaut, H. (1975). 'Comments on "Biofeedback" in epileptics.' *Epilepsia,* **16**, 487–490

Gutnick, M. J. and Prince, D. A. (1972). 'Thalamocortical relay neurones: Antidromic invasion of spikes from a cortical epileptogenic focus.' *Science,* **176**, 424–426

Hagberg, B. (1978). 'The epidemiologic panorama or major neuropaediatric handicaps in Sweden.' In *Clinics in Developmental Medicine, No. 67: Care of the Handicapped Child*, pp. 111–124. Ed. J. Apley. London: Spastics International and Heinemann

Hagberg, B., Hagberg, G. and Olow, I. (1975a). 'The changing panorama of cerebral palsy in Sweden 1954–1970. I. Analysis of the general changes.' *Acta paediat. Scand.* **64**, 187–192

Hagberg, B., Hagberg, G. and Olow, I. (1975b). 'The changing panorama of cerebral palsy in Sweden 1954–1970, II. Analysis of the various syndromes.' *Acta paediat. Scand.* **64**, 193–200

Hagberg, B., Hagberg, G. and Olow, I. (1976). 'The changing panorama of cerebral palsy in Sweden 1954–1970, III. The importance of foetal deprivation of supply.' *Acta paediat. Scand.* **65**, 403–408

Hagberg, B., Hagberg, G. and Olow, I. (1977). 'The panorama of cerebral palsy in Swedish children born 1954–1974.' *Neuropädiatrie*, **8**, Suppl. pp. 516–521

Huttenlocher, P. R. (1974). 'Dendritic development in neocortex of children with mental defect and infantile spasms.' *Neurology, Minneap.* **24**, 203–210

Lennox, W. G. (1960). *Epilepsy and Related Disorders*, p. 1065. London: J. and A. Churchill

Lewis, J. A. (1976). 'Recent advances in epilepsy.' *J. electrophysiol. Technol.* **2**, 322–323

MacDonald, R. L., and Barker, J. L. (1977). 'Pentylenetetrazol and penicillin are selective antagonists of GABA-mediated post-synaptic inhibition in cultured mammalian neurons.' *Nature*, **267**, 720–721

Mostofsky, D. I. and Balaschak, B. A. (1977). 'Psychobiological control of seizures.' *Psychol. Bull.* **84**, 723–750

Pedley, T. A. (1978). 'The pathophysiology of focal epilepsy: neurophysiological considerations.' *Ann. Neurol.* **3**, 2–9

Purpura, D. P. (1975). 'Dendritic differentiation in human cerebral cortex. Normal and aberrant developmental patterns.' In *Advances in Neurology, Vol. 12: Physiology and Pathology of Dendrites*, pp. 91–116. Ed. G. W. Kreutzberg. New York: Raven Press

Quiller–Couch, A. Sir (1939). Editor. 'Written in Northampton County Asylum; John Clare 1793–1864.' In *The Oxford Book of English Verse, 1250–1918*, New edn, p. 735. Oxford: Clarendon Press

Ransom, B. R. and Barker, J. L. (1976). 'Pentobarbital selectively enhances GABA-mediated post-synaptic inhibition in tissue cultured mouse spinal neurons.' *Brain Res.* **114**, 530–535

Richens, A. (1976). 'The controlled clinical trial in epilepsy.' In *Drug Treatment of Epilepsy*, pp. 82, 154–169. London: Henry Kimpton

Sherwin, A. L. (1978). 'Clinical pharmacology of ethosuximide.' In *Antiepileptic Drugs: Quantitative Analysis and Interpretation*, pp. 283–295. Eds C. E. Pippenger, J. K. Penry and H. Kutt. New York: Raven Press

Sterman, M. B., MacDonald, L. R. and Stone, R. K. (1974). 'Biofeedback training of the sensorimotor electroencephalogram rhythm in man: Effects on epilepsy.' *Epilepsia*, **15**, 395–416

Stores, G. (1975). 'Teaching medical students about epilepsy.' *Devl Med. child Neurol.* **17**, 518–519

Tower, D. B. (1978). 'Epilepsy: A World Problem.' In *Advances in Epileptology, 1977*, pp. 2–26. Eds H. Meinardi and A. J. Rowan. Amsterdam, Lisse: Swets and B. V. Zeitlinger

The MCT-Based Ketogenic Diet

(with the assistance of Caitriona Murphy, SRD, formerly Senior Dietitian, Our Lady's Hospital for Sick Children, Dublin.)

The ketogenic diet is used in cases of epilepsy which have not responded to conventional medication (*see* Chapter 5). The effects of the diet correspond to the degree of ketosis achieved. Rises in serum lipids and other metabolic changes such as disturbed water and salt balance are also thought to be significant in producing a therapeutic effect (Gordon, 1977).

The use of medium-chain triglycerides (MCT) in recent years has meant that carbohydrates need not be rigidly restricted, resulting in a more palatable and more easily prepared diet (Huttenlocher, Wilbourn and Signore, 1971). However, Livingston, Pauli and Pruce (1977) maintain that the modified diet is not as effective in controlling seizures as is the standard diet in which the amount of fat (in grams) is four times the amount (in grams) of carbohydrate and protein combined. Readers who are interested in the details of the standard ketogenic diet should consult Livingston (1972). In the standard diet, normal dietary fats are used to supply approximately 88 per cent of the total calorie intake in order to produce the desired effect. Because MCT oil is more ketogenic, only 50–70 per cent of the total calories need to be supplied by this preparation. This results in greater palatability and allows a more generous allowance of protein and carbohydrate in the diet.

As has been emphasized in Chapter 5, the diet is more likely to succeed when the parents are interested, cooperative and able to gain a detailed understanding of the regimen. Initially, the children should be admitted to hospital for stabilization on the diet.

The diet is initiated by fasting the patient while allowing 50 per cent of the normal fluid intake or a maximum of 1000 ml/24 hours, given as water or as low calorie drinks (nor more than 50 calories/24 hours). Any drugs being administered should be free of carbohydrates. Nothing else is given until the patient is strongly ketotic and this is usually achieved after approximately 36 hours. Ketosis should be confirmed by blood and urine tests.

TABLE 1

Basic Recipe for MCT-based Ketogenic Diet

	Protein (g)	Fat (g)	Carbohydrate (g)	Calories	Fluid (ml)
8 ml 50 per cent MCT emulsion	–	4.0	–	33.2	8
5 g skimmed milk powder	1.8	0.1	2.6	16.7	–
Water to 100 ml	–	–	–	–	About 90
Total	1.8	4.1	2.6 g	49.9	100

The 50 per cent MCT emulsion is prepared by liquidizing equal quantities of MCT oil and cold boiled water with 25 g of gum acacia per 1000 ml of fluid

The next step is to introduce the MCT-based ketogenic diet while still maintaining a restriction of fluids. The basic recipe for the diet is given in *Table 1*. It has a concentration of 4 per cent MCT and provides 65 per cent of total calories as MCT. The mixture is offered in small frequent drinks and the patient is advised to sip it slowly. Possible side-effects (vomiting, diarrhoea and abdominal pain) are usually avoided in this way, but if they should occur further water is added while still maintaining the overall restriction of fluids.

If, after 24 hours, the diet is being well tolerated, the concentration of MCT is increased to 5 per cent, providing 70 per cent of the total calories (i.e. 10 ml of 50 per cent MCT emulsion per 100 ml of mixture instead of 8 ml). When it is clear that this concentration of MCT is being tolerated and if ketosis is being maintained, solid food may be introduced gradually.

The basic recipe with 5 per cent MCT oil is continued as a milk substitute, flavoured if necessary with low-calorie syrups or coffee essence and the like, and the patient is encouraged to drink up to 800 ml daily, preferably before solid food is taken. The 50 per cent MCT emulsion, flavoured if desired, is used in measured quantities before food to achieve ketosis and provide calories.

Solids are introduced slowly, and they are gradually increased in amount over approximately five days. Preference is given at this early stage to foods requiring small amounts of MCT emulsion in order to maintain ketosis. Fluid restriction is continued only if ketosis is not being maintained. The patient is considered to be stabilized on the diet when ketones are regularly present and when the diet is fully accepted and tolerated.

A normal calorie intake and minimum recommended dietary allowance of protein are given, both based on the child's dietary history, age and weight. Approximately 60 per cent of the total calories need to be provided by MCT oil, 1 ml of which produces 8.3 calories. Approximately 30 per cent of the remaining calories will be provided by protein and carbohydrate and the intake of fat other than MCT oil need not be limited unless the child is overweight. Foods are weighed and calorie content and amounts of MCT oil required to balance their antiketogenic effects are worked out by parents from lists and specimen diets provided by the dietitian. Exchange lists are used to vary the diet. Dietitians calculate the antiketogenic effects of the various foods from the knowledge that 10 per cent of fat is antiketogenic, 58 per cent of protein is antiketogenic and carbohydrates are entirely antiketogenic.

The MCT-based diet is nutritionally inadequate and sugar-free 'Ketovite' tablets (one three times a day) and 'Ketovite' liquid (5 ml once daily) are given. Calcium supplements may be unnecessary if sufficient of the basic MCT skimmed milk mixture is drunk daily. Otherwise, additional calcium is required. Sufficient iron should be provided by first-class protein foods, vegetables and cereal foods. The family doctor should be warned against prescribing additional medications with a syrup (i.e. carbohydrate) base but, if these have to be administered, then additional MCT oil to compensate for their antiketogenic effect will be required. Regular support and supervision by a dietitian are essential, particularly during the introductory stages of the diet and in the early weeks of treatment, if successful dietetic management is to be achieved.

Acceptance of the MCT is usually not a problem once the patient realizes that food will not be given until the MCT drink has been consumed. Sometimes, ketosis may be difficult to maintain in the morning and this may require an increase in the daily intake of oil. As a rule side-effects are few, even when the concentration of fat is 50 per cent, and are discussed below.

Problems with the diet

Urine testing for ketones is performed with 'Ketostix'. If the test is only weakly positive and especially if seizures recur coincidentally, the diet should be readjusted as follows:

1. Give 20–30 ml of MCT emulsion without any food and repeat two-hourly if necessary until ketosis is re-established
2. Increase the MCT allowance by 20–25 per cent above the recommended dose for specific foods
3. Reduce the fluid intake to 50 per cent of the recommended fluid intake or to 1000 ml/24 hours, whichever is the lesser
4. Reduce the food intake to three small meals a day and preferably use foods of protein origin.

If vomiting, abdominal pain or diarrhoea occur, solid food should be discontinued. The MCT basic recipe only is given to the limits of the patient's tolerance with instructions that it should be sipped slowly. The aim should be to maintain ketosis. Other fluids of minimal calorie value may be administered to sustain hydration while, if possible, avoiding a reduction in ketosis. Gradual re-introduction of solids should take place as the patient's symptoms diminish.

Should the patient 'cheat' on the diet by taking extra foods, the antiketogenic effect may be counteracted by giving a suitable extra amount of MCT emulsion.

The ketogenic diet, as described above, is very flexible for situations such as a change in meal pattern, holidays, school lunches and so on. All that is required is to calculate the amount of MCT emulsion needed for use with a particular food. The diet also encourages the full consumption of MCT thereby enhancing the ketogenic effect. Patients need not feel that their diet is particularly restricting apart from the stipulation that MCT emulsion must be drunk in measured quantities before solid food is consumed.

REFERENCES

Gordon, N. S. (1977). 'Medium-chain triglycerides in a ketogenic diet.' *Devl Med. child Neurol.* **19**, 535–538
Huttenlocher, P. R., Wilbourn, A. J. and Signore, J. M. (1971). 'Medium-chain triglycerides as therapy for intractable childhood epilepsy.' *Neurology,* **21**, 1097–1103
Livingston, S. (1972). *Comprehensive Management of Epilepsy in Infancy, Childhood and Adolescence,* pp. 380–405. Springfield, Illinois: Charles C. Thomas,
Livingston, S, Pauli, L. L., and Pruce, I. (1977). 'Ketogenic diet in the treatment of childhood epilepsy.' *Devl Med. child Neurol.* **19**, 833–834

Glossary

Approved name	USA Trade name	UK Trade names
Acetazolamide	Diamox	Diamox
Benztropine mesylate	Benztrophine mesylate	Congentin
Carbamazepine	Tegretol	Tegretol
Chloramphenicol	Amphicol	Chloromycetin
Chlormethiazole edisylate		Heminevrin
Clonazepam	Clonopin	Rivotril
Dexamethasone	Decadron, Hexadrol	Decadron, Oradexon
Dextroamphetamine, dexamphetamine sulphate	Dexedrine	Dexedrine
Diazepam	Valium	Valium
Diazoxide	Hyperstat	Eudemine
Diphenhydrochloride	Benadryl	Bendryl
Ethosuximide	Zarontin	Zarontin
Frusemide, Furosemide	Lasix	Lasix
Imipramine	Imavate, Presamine	Tofranil
Isoniazid	Niconyl, Nydrazid	Rimifon
Lignocaine	Anestacon	Xylocard
Mannitol	Mannitol	Osmitol
Methylphenidate hydrochloride	Ritalin	Ritalin
Metaclopramide	Reglan	Moxolon
Nitrazepam	no available in USA	Mogadon
Paraldehyde	Paral	
Paramethadione	Paradione	Paradione
Penicillin	Hyasorb, Pfizerpen G	Crystamycin
Pentylenetetrazole, leptazol	Metrazol	Cardiazol
Pheneturide	not available in USA	Benuride

Phenobarbitone, phenobarbital	Eskabarb, Stental	Luminal, Gardenal
Phenytoin	Dilantin, Dilabid	Epanutin
Primidone	Mysoline	Mysoline
Reserpine	Raurine, Serpate	Serpasil
Sodium valproate	Depakene	Epilim
Sulthiame	not available in USA	Ospolot
Thiopentone	Pentothal	Intraval, Pentothal
Troxidone	Pentothal, Tridione	Tridione

Index